Epidemiology for Canadian Students

Epidemiology for Canadian Students

Principles, Methods & Critical Appraisal

Third edition

Scott B. Patten MD, PhD

www.brusheducation.ca

21 22 23 24 25 5 4 3 2 1

Printed and manufactured in Canada

Brush Education Inc.
www.brusheducation.ca
contact@brusheducation.ca

Cover and interior design: Carol Dragich, Dragich Design.
Cover images: iStock.com/csheezio—dandelion image; iStock.com/urbancow—crowd.
Permission for Dobrow et al's consolidated principles of screening (p. 271) provided by the author (M. J. Dobrow).

Library and Archives Canada Cataloguing in Publication

Title: Epidemiology for Canadian students : principles, methods & critical appraisal /
    Scott B. Patten MD, PhD.
Names: Patten, Scott B., 1962- author.
Description: Third edition. | Includes bibliographical references and index.
Identifiers: Canadiana (print) 20210157240 | Canadiana (ebook) 20210157267 |
    ISBN 9781550598964 (softcover) | ISBN 9781550598971 (PDF) | ISBN 9781550598988 (EPUB)
Subjects: LCSH: Epidemiology—Textbooks. | LCSH: Epidemiology—Canada—Textbooks. |
    LCGFT: Textbooks.

Classification: LCC RA651 .P38 2021 | DDC 614.4—dc23

We acknowledge the support of the Government of Canada
Nous reconnaissons l'appui du gouvernement du Canada | Canadä

Contents

List of Figures

First principles of epidemiology

1

What is epidemiology?

OBJECTIVES

- Define key epidemiological terms.
- Identify the historical roots of epidemiological reasoning.
- Describe the importance of epidemiology to health professionals.

Definition and terms

Epidemiology is the study of the distribution and determinants of disease in populations.

Let's break this down.

Distribution and determinants

The definition of epidemiology uses the terms *distribution* and *determinants*, which describe an important division in the field.

Distribution is the focus of descriptive epidemiology. The ability to describe the distribution of diseases is essential for developing hypotheses about their etiology, and for planning and evaluating health services.

Determinants are the focus of analytical epidemiology. A determinant is something that causes a disease (an etiological factor), or that influences the distribution of a disease in a population. For example, a risk factor is a determinant—one that increases the risk of disease. Factors that determine the chances of recovering or dying from a disease are also determinants, because they shape disease patterns in populations.

Descriptive and analytical epidemiology are different, but it's important not to make too much of this distinction. Many epidemiological studies have both descriptive and analytical goals.

Key point: Epidemiology has 2 major branches: descriptive epidemiology and analytical epidemiology.

Population

Epidemiology is a population-based science. Although epidemiology can be concerned with many different kinds of populations, it is always concerned with a population. It focuses on groups of people rather than individuals.

Studies that focus on individual people (case studies or case series) do not usually provide any epidemiological data. Epidemiological studies have the goal of advancing knowledge about populations.

The focus on studying populations does not mean that epidemiology is not relevant for individual people. Much of what we know about the health of individual people derives from epidemiological studies. What makes people sick? What keeps them healthy? What treatments are most likely to return sick people to health? Individual people have a multitude of individual differences. Studies of large groups of people make the effects of such differences cancel out—they bring into focus the health outcomes associated with various exposures in a way that is not possible at the individual level.

For example, defenders of smoking used to say that they knew somebody who smoked heavily and who did not develop any complications. They interpreted this observation as evidence that smoking was not harmful. But an individual case is a poor basis for determining whether smoking is harmful. It would be better to know what happens to large numbers of people who smoke, and to contrast this with the experience of large numbers of nonsmokers. This requires researching groups of people, but the knowledge gained is very relevant for individual decisions, such as whether to start or stop smoking. Studying large groups of people can teach us a lot (arguably most of what we know) about determinants of health and disease as they affect individual people.

In recent years, health sciences have begun to move in the direction of precision health, which means trying to understand and address origins of disease in individual people based on their personal characteristics. Many of the methods used in precision health research are modifications of methods that emerged from epidemiologic research. However, the foundation of epidemiology remains unchanged: understanding diseases and health outcomes in populations.

Key point: Epidemiology emphasizes groups of people rather than individuals, but it can teach us a lot about health risks that are important to individuals.

It is important to keep an open mind about what is meant by the term *population*. In epidemiology, a population can be almost any definable group. The most familiar type of population is defined geographically or politically—for example, the population of Nova Scotia. Epidemiologists are often interested in provincial populations because administration of health care is a provincial responsibility in Canada. Descriptive epidemiological information (e.g., the number of people in different regions of Canada with various types of cancer) is necessary for planning and administering services, and for formulating health policy. Some classic examples of descriptive epidemiology have recently been published by Darwich et al, who looked at the distribution of 2 important types of eye tumours in relation to personal characteristics, geographical location, and trends over time in Canada.[1,2] They reported that the incidence of invasive ocular surface squamous neoplasms was increasing over time and was higher in males. Such information is useful for planning services, and the male preponderance may help to generate hypotheses about causation. Descriptive epidemiology often describes the occurrence of disease in relation to time, place, and person in a defined population.

A population doesn't need to be a geographically defined group. The term *population* could also apply to, for example, recreational skiers, or women, or children with disabilities enrolled in a particular school system. Epidemiology is a way of answering questions about populations and the term *population* can be used to describe almost any group about which there is a question to be answered.

Key point: A population, in epidemiology, can be almost any identifiable group of people.

Disease

In epidemiology, *disease* is shorthand for almost any type of health outcome, including many that are not normally called a disease—for example, obesity, literacy, and hunger. This is partly because, in the literature, too many terms can lead to complex and cumbersome language.

Just to be clear: it would be perfectly correct to define epidemiology as the study of the distribution and determinants of health-related problems in populations.

Other key terms

Exposure refers to a determinant or potential determinant of health outcomes. For example, a person may be exposed to cigarette smoke, radiation, or psychosocial stress. Often, studies ask whether such factors are health determinants, so it makes sense to call these factors *exposures* until research confirms them as determinants. Investigations of a factor as a potential determinant of disease often reveal that some people have had exposure to the factor and others have not. When collecting data, the presence or absence of the factor can assume different values (in this case exposed or not exposed, yes or no)—in other words, exposure is a variable. The traditional distinction between an independent and dependent variable in experimental science roughly corresponds to exposure and disease, respectively, in epidemiology.

You may see definitions of epidemiology with the term *disease frequency* rather than just *disease* (e.g., "the study of the distribution and determinants of disease frequency in populations"). This wording emphasizes that epidemiological research tends to target groups of people rather than individuals. Other definitions specify "human populations" (e.g., "the study of the distribution and determinants of disease in human populations"). This wording aims to distinguish epidemiology from laboratory sciences, but it creates a problem by excluding veterinary epidemiology—human and animal epidemiologists use similar research methods and increasingly work together under a philosophy called "One Health."[3] With the emergence COVID-19 disease in 2019, the One Health philosophy has become even more prominent. The SARS-CoV-2 virus that causes COVID-19 is believed to have originated in bats.[4]

Inconsistent terminology is a difficult reality of epidemiology. It can be frustrating: people use terms differently, or use different labels for the same intended meaning. This book attempts to adhere to the most precise or most widely used terminology. However, since all health science students (and practitioners) need to access and understand the literature, it is necessary, to some extent, to embrace this diverse terminology, which means becoming familiar with its contradictions, variations, and nuances. In your own work and writing, though, you should aim to use the most specific and applicable terms available. This book will offer many suggestions about preferred terminology, but will also occasionally point out problems connected to the interpretation of specific terms.

History of epidemiology

The science of epidemiology originated in efforts to address epidemics of infectious disease in the nineteenth century.

John Snow is usually identified as a founder of epidemiology due to his work in public health in London, England. Snow was also an innovator in the field of anesthesiology, but he is now most famous for his investigation of cholera outbreaks. In the 1850s, Snow was able to link cholera deaths to sewage-contaminated drinking water. He also linked a point-source outbreak of cholera to a public water source, the Broad Street pump.[5] He accomplished this not by studying cholera patients in a hospital, morgue, or laboratory, and not by culturing cholera bacilli in a lab—instead, he examined the distribution of cholera deaths in relation to possible determinants. He identified a pattern of distribution consistent with water as the most likely source of infection. This contradicted a theory popular at the time that tainted air—a "miasma"—caused cholera outbreaks. Snow's approach was innovative and represented a major public-health milestone. The London School of Hygiene and Tropical Medicine commemorated his legacy in 2013, the bicentenary of his birth.[6]

The story of John Snow highlights 2 defining characteristics of epidemiology.

First, epidemiology uses probability and statistical reasoning. This broke with scientific conventions at the time, which were more directly aligned with logic and mathematics. During the cholera outbreaks Snow studied, not everyone exposed to sewage-contaminated water developed cholera, and not everyone with cholera was directly exposed to sewage-contaminated water. But people who were exposed had a higher probability of getting cholera—according to Steven Johnson, 6 in 10 drinkers of water from the Broad Street pump developed cholera, compared with only 1 in 10 of nondrinkers.[5] If you look at historical postulates for linking infectious agents to disease such Koch's postulates (see Table 1), Snow's approach might seem fuzzy and undisciplined, but it has come to dominate health science research—at least research involving human subjects. This is true even within the sphere of medical therapeutics. Today, for example, a drug is "efficacious" if it produces a desired outcome more often than placebo. If Koch's postulates were used assess the effectiveness of drugs (e.g., "everyone should improve when given the drug, no one should improve without the drug" etc.), it would be almost impossible for therapeutics to advance.

TABLE 1. KOCH'S POSTULATES[7]

---

1. The infectious agent must be found in abundance in all individuals with the disease, but should not be found at all in healthy individuals.

2. It must be isolated and cultured from a diseased individual.

3. The cultured infectious agent should cause disease in a healthy individual (creating a new case of the disease).

4. The infectious agent must be isolated from the new case and confirmed as identical to the original infectious agent.

Second, the John Snow story highlights the ability of epidemiology to deliver effective public health strategies before the biology of a disease is clear. The cholera bacillus was not isolated until decades after Snow's work,[8] but his work produced effective public health action. To this day, safe drinking water is the key strategy to controlling diarrheal diseases such as cholera—more effective and more important than treatments targeting the infectious agents themselves (e.g., antibiotics). Similarly, and more recently, several sub-Saharan African countries have reduced under-5 mortality, not through directly treating children, but through mosquito-control measures that in turn control malaria.[9]

Key point: Epidemiological methods originated in studies of infectious diseases, but are key to understanding health and disease in general.

Is epidemiology important to health professionals?

Epidemiology is a foundational health science. A great deal of contemporary health research and the majority of studies conducted with human subjects use epidemiological principles and methods.

The most notable exception is qualitative research, which typically does not draw on epidemiological methods (epidemiology is a decidedly quantitative field). Even qualitative researchers, though, need to read the quantitative literature, which requires knowledge of epidemiology. In addition, researchers often combine qualitative methods with epidemiological approaches in mixed-method studies. For example, Riley et al[10] applied mixed methods to study continuity of care between cardiac rehabilitation services and primary care practices in Ontario. They collected quantitative data from discharge summaries and responses provided in physician interviews. Qualitative data came from semistructured telephone interviews conducted with the same physicians that were transcribed and analyzed using a technique called *grounded analysis*. They identified major gaps in communication between cardiac rehabilitation programs and primary care physicians. In another example of mixed methods, Hong et al[11] used both qualitative and quantitative methods to identify reasons for inappropriate visits to emergency departments in patients with atrial fibrillation. They combined a statistical analysis of data collected using a telephone survey of 356 patients that had recently come to emergency departments in Ontario, Nova Scotia, Alberta, and British Columbia. They also recorded narrative statements that were analyzed using qualitative methods. The quantitative and qualitative results both pointed to disease-related anxiety as an important determinant of these visits.[11]

Key point: Epidemiology is a foundational health science. Understanding the basics of epidemiology enables better understanding of the contemporary health research literature.

The foundational role of epidemiology in health science research makes it an especially important field to study. A solid grasp of epidemiology is also essential for practising health care professionals. Interpretation of diagnostic signs and symptoms, as well as interpretation of test results, depends on concepts from epidemiology. Even the randomized controlled clinical trial—the most important study design for evaluating treatments—is built on epidemiologic foundations.

In a world dominated by technology, it is easy to imagine that a discipline such as epidemiology might become obsolete. After all, how can comparisons between groups of people possibly compete with advanced medical imaging or molecular biology? But consider: How can we gauge the risks and benefits of emerging technologies for health? The answer to this crucial question depends on the foundational concepts and strategies of epidemiology. For example, advances in pharmacology lead to the development of new drugs, but it will all come to nothing—all the investment of time, money, and technology in drug development—if the drugs cannot be shown effective and safe in the real world. This part hinges on epidemiologic data.

Key point: Technological advances create a need for epidemiological research. Epidemiology is a more essential and vibrant discipline now than ever before.

The COVID-19 pandemic has underscored even further the importance of epidemiologic thinking and epidemiologic data. In a paper published in the *Lancet* in January 2020, Chaolin Huang et al described 41 patients admitted to hospital in Wuhan with a new type of pneumonia,[12] and they reported that a novel coronavirus had been isolated from respiratory-tract secretions collected from these patients. In an observation reminiscent of Snow's, these authors reported that 27 of the 41 patients had direct exposure to the Huanan Seafood Market. The market was closed on January 1, 2020.[13] However, a new case in Thailand was reported on January 13, in Japan on January 16, and in Korea on January 19. On March 11, the World Health Organization officially declared COVID-19 a pandemic. Unlike the cholera epidemics investigated by Snow, person-to-person transmission of the SARS-CoV-2 virus (the virus that causes COVID-19 disease) led to its propagation around the world. However, in parallel to the historical example, fighting the disease meant reducing exposure to its main determinant (an infectious person) via public health strategies, which for the SARS-CoV-2 virus included physical distancing, self-isolation, mask wearing, and quarantine.

Modern health care systems are driven by data. In Canada, the publicly funded health system has a responsibility to respond to the needs of Canadians, and the administration of this health system means collecting massive quantities of data. Increasingly, these administrative data sets are used to drive health system decisions, to monitor the functioning of the health system, and to track the impact of diseases. Research designed to make the health system better—health services research—is also firmly planted on a foundation provided by epidemiology. In our information age, and with the advances of evidence-based medicine, epidemiology will become increasingly important.

Thinking deeper

Epidemiology in symbols

Epidemiology is the study of the distribution of disease in populations. This is a starting point for expressing epidemiological ideas in symbols, because it implies a division between members of a population that have a disease and members that don't. You can express this as A (for people with a disease) and B (for people without a disease). This expression is called *complementary* because each person either has, or does not have, the disease. The total number of people in the population, then, may be denoted N such that $A + B = N$.

Table 2 embodies the distinction between having a disease or not. This table has 1 row with population values and 2 columns that describe the distinction. It is therefore a 1×2 ("one by two") table.

TABLE 2. 1×2 TABLE FOR A POPULATION

Disease	No disease	Total
A	B	N

It is easy to see how a 1×2 table can be used to represent the amount of disease in a population. However, epidemiology is concerned with the distribution of disease in populations—so, it is useful to have a table that contains, or represents, a comparison of disease frequency in several groups. A good place to start is with consideration of an exposure. If we divide a population of size N into exposed and not-exposed categories, we can construct a table that depicts the number of people with and without disease in each group. In this case, the cross-tabulation of disease and exposure has something to say about the relationship between exposure and disease. Indeed, examination of this exact contingency (the exposure-disease contingency) is a central paradigm of epidemiologic research. This kind of table is called a 2×2 contingency table. A 2×2 contingency table has 4 cells based on 2 variables that can each assume 2 values (see Table 3).

TABLE 3. 2×2 CONTINGENCY TABLE

	Disease	No disease
Exposed	A	B
Not exposed	C	D

In Table 3, note that A and B have different meanings than in Table 2. In Table 2, A included all of the people with the disease. In Table 3, A includes only a portion of those with the disease (those also exposed). The remaining portion (C) includes those who have the disease but are not exposed. Similarly, B now represents only those without disease who are exposed, and D represents those without the disease who are not exposed.

A word of caution about 2×2 contingency tables: some books and papers present disease status in the table rows rather than the columns (the reverse of Table 3). This changes the meaning of the symbols A, B, C, and D (assuming that their row and column positions remain the same), and the meaning of row totals ($A + B$ and $C + D$) and column totals ($A + C$ and $B + D$). A subscript to denote exposure and disease status conveys these totals with clarity (see Table 4). Note that Table 4 includes the 2 × 2 contingencies, and also places noncontingent counts in the margins. For example, $N_{disease}$ is the number with the disease irrespective of exposure status. These row and column values are called *marginal sums* since they appear in the margins of the 2 × 2 table.

TABLE 4. 2 × 2 CONTINGENCY TABLE WITH ROW AND COLUMN TOTALS

	Disease	No disease	Row totals
Exposed	A	B	$N_{exposed}$
Not exposed	C	D	$N_{nonexposed}$
Column totals	$N_{disease}$	$N_{no\,disease}$	

The cells of a 2 × 2 contingency table allow important comparisons. For example, the frequency of disease in the nonexposed component of the population is $C/N_{nonexposed}$. Since diseases do not distribute randomly in populations (they instead distribute in relation to their determinants), it is very interesting to know how $A/N_{exposed}$ compares to $C/N_{nonexposed}$.

Questions

1. In 2006, Bernstein et al[14] applied a case-identification algorithm to administrative data for inflammatory bowel diseases to identify cases of these diseases in 5 Canadian provinces. The case definition allowed estimation of the number of cases in each province, one of the research objectives of the study.

   a. Administrative data derive partially from physician-billing invoices and hospital-discharge summaries. Do you think this is a good way to identify cases of disease?

   b. Would you classify this study as primarily descriptive or primarily analytical?

   c. Does it concern you that only 5 provinces were included? Why or why not?

   d. Is it important to know how many people have this disease? Why or why not?

2. Maxwell et al[15] studied 2779 clients receiving services from community care access centres in Ontario from 1999 to 2001. Nearly half of these clients had daily pain, but one-fifth of those in pain received no analgesic treatment. The investigators were concerned that the needs of these clients were not being met.

   a. Is this study "population based"?

   b. Do you think that this study qualifies as an epidemiological study?

   c. Why did the investigators need such a large sample?

   d. What is the descriptive value of their result?

   e. Can you think of a role for this finding in the planning or administration of health services?

3. Tyas et al[16] studied risk factors for Alzheimer disease in Manitoba. They used data from a longitudinal, population-based study of dementia conducted in that province. During 5 years of follow-up, subjects with fewer years of education were found to be at greater risk of Alzheimer disease.

a. Based on the information provided, would you regard this study as analytical or descriptive?

b. As you see it, what is the value of this kind of information?

4. Can you identify any similarities between the work of Bernstein, Maxwell, and Tyas, and the work of John Snow?

5. Imagine that you are John Snow and that you are advocating for safer disposal of sewage in nineteenth-century London.

a. You are accused of failing to appreciate the difference between correlation and causation, and thereby drawing a false conclusion about a causal link. How would you respond?

b. You are accused of knowing nothing of the etiology of cholera because you have no idea what the infectious agent is. How would you respond?

6. In a "case report," a clinician observes an interesting case and describes its characteristics.

a. Do you think that this qualifies as an epidemiological study?

b. A "case-series report" describes a group of cases of a disease. Do you think that a case-series report qualifies as an epidemiological study?

7. John Snow studied an infectious disease: cholera. Based on what you've learned from this chapter, do you think that epidemiology would be a useful approach for studying noncommunicable chronic diseases such as diabetes and high blood pressure?

8. Do you think that epidemiology will ever become obsolete? Why or why not?

9. "Precision health" is becoming increasingly popular. It seeks to avoid a one-size-fits-all way of thinking. For example, a molecular biological analysis of cancer cells from a specific person's tumour might lead to a particular treatment in preference to other possible treatments in that person. A risk factor may have different effects in people with 1 or more biological differences, such as different risk-factor profiles. By contrast, epidemiology focuses on groups of people. Do you think that precision medicine is a better approach than the approach taken by the science of epidemiology?

10. Some Canadian academic programs and research-funding organizations differentiate between health-services research and epidemiology. Health-services research examines and compares outcomes achieved by patients within the health system. Do you see health-services research as a completely different discipline from epidemiology, or do you see it as a subtype of epidemiological research?

2

Epidemiological reasoning

OBJECTIVES

- State the fundamental assumption of epidemiological research.
- Explain the key concepts of association, proportion, period prevalence, and point prevalence.
- Identify the 2 main sources of error in epidemiologic research: random error and systematic error (bias).
- Define critical appraisal.

The fundamental assumption

Epidemiology rests on this fundamental assumption: diseases do not distribute randomly in populations, but rather distribute in relation to their determinants.

Intuitively, this makes a lot of sense. If smokers, for example, are more likely to develop lung cancer, then a pattern of association (or, we could say "contingency") will emerge between smoking and lung cancer. Specifically, you would expect smokers to develop lung cancer more often than nonsmokers. You might also expect people with lung cancer to have been smokers more often than people without the disease. In the language of epidemiology, smoking and lung cancer are associated. If smoking and lung cancer were in fact distributed randomly in the population (if they were independent of each another and therefore not associated), the only value of studying their distribution would be descriptive: to determine how much smoking and lung cancer exists in the population.

Key point: Studying associations between exposures and disease is the "bread and butter" of analytical epidemiology.

Association and causation

Everyone has heard the truism that "correlation is not causation." In other words, an association between 2 variables does not mean that 1 is causing the other. Occasionally, a scientist challenges the value of epidemiological studies because of this—some laboratory scientists, for example, believe only a detailed understanding of the molecular underpinnings of a disease can substantiate causal association.

Certainly, many spurious correlations exist. Did you know, for example, that annual US spending on science, space, and technology correlates strongly (0.99) with the annual number of suicides by hanging, strangulation, and suffocation in the US?[17] This association is not causal—but does this sort of example mean that associations can never be considered causal? Not at all: the reason epidemiology can inform etiology is that, for epidemiologists, questions of cause are related to public health actions, not mechanistic conceptions of cause.

EPIDEMIOLOGY AND SMOKING

The question of whether smoking causes lung cancer is a good illustration. In 1950, Doll and Hill[18] published a study in the *British Medical Journal* called "Smoking and Carcinoma of the Lung: Preliminary Report." They began their study by carefully identifying cases of lung cancer (as well as certain other cancers) from a selection of hospitals in the UK. Doll and Hill interviewed the patients in each case to obtain a detailed record of the patients' smoking history. With this data, they classified the cases into smoking and nonsmoking groups, where exposure (smoking) was defined as anyone who had smoked at least 1 cigarette per day for at least 1 year. They applied the same interview and classification procedure to a comparison (control) group, whose subjects mirrored the lung-cancer group in terms of sex, 5-year age group, and where and when they were hospitalized. This allowed a comparison of the frequency of smoking in the lung-cancer and control groups (an approach that has come to be known as a case-control study). A large majority of the men in their sample were smokers, according to their definition. This included all but 2 (0.3%) of the male cancer patients and all but 27 (4.2%) of the controls. Doll and Hill used an exact statistical test to confirm that a difference this large, or larger, would be very unlikely to emerge by chance (the calculated probability was 0.00000064). They had confirmed an association between smoking and lung cancer.

The discovery of an association between smoking and lung cancer led to public health efforts to decrease the frequency of smoking. These efforts have been partially successful. In men, the frequency of daily or occasional smoking has diminished to 17.3% of males and 12.3% of females as of 2019.[19] This, in turn, has resulted in diminishing lung cancer incidence in recent decades,[20] although in recent years the incidence of cancers of the lung and bronchus have been fairly stable in Canada at about 57 per 100 000 population per year.

This progress happened even though no mechanism of causation between lung cancer and smoking had been identified. If the world of public health had waited for research to establish the mechanism, imagine the thousands of people who would have died. And waiting may have served no point: understanding the basic physiology may not have assisted in any way with the public health actions necessary for this progress. A strategy document published by Health Canada in 1999 listed the following strategic directions to reduce smoking: policy and legislation, public education, industry accountability and product control, research, and building capacity for action. None of this depends on molecular biology or even physiology.

Note the parallels between the epidemiology of smoking described in this chapter and the work of John Snow described in chapter 1. The power of epidemiological research to identify etiological connections in the absence of a thorough pathophysiological understanding is clear.

The "acid test" for an epidemiological assertion of cause involves public health action. Will a "cause" in the public health sense (diminishing the frequency of smoking) produce the desired public health effect (a lowering of the incidence of lung cancer)? Had the association between smoking and lung cancer not been causal, public health action would not have been justified and the incidence of lung cancer would not have changed as a result of efforts to discourage smoking. If epidemiological evidence confirms that a public health or clinical action will lead to improved health, then a causal effect has been identified.

Key point: Analytical epidemiologic studies are not often concerned with disease mechanisms (sometimes they are). However, they are often concerned with disease etiology.

EPIDEMIOLOGY AND THERAPEUTIC INTERVENTIONS

A corollary to this way of thinking can also be seen in the literature about the efficacy of treatment and the modern emphasis that is placed on evidence-based medicine. If health professionals are practising evidence-based medicine, they are taking actions that, according to evidence, will lead to the improved health of their patients. These choices do not usually hinge on detailed knowledge of pathophysiology and pharmacology. Health professionals need this knowledge, but this knowledge is not (according to evidence-based medicine) the key deciding factor when selecting among—for example—drug therapies. The key deciding factor comes from observations similar to those made by John Snow, and Doll and Hill—observations that derive ultimately from comparisons of frequencies in different groups of people. Note that, where drug therapies and other therapeutic interventions are concerned, randomized controlled trials are the most important way of delivering information about frequencies.

Key point: Epidemiological research can identify the causes of disease, but the concept of "cause" is often based on clinical or public health "effects."

Epidemiologic parameters

A parameter, in epidemiology, represents a characteristic of a population. Parameters usually need to be estimated (this is what epidemiologic research does!) and understanding such estimates involves understanding probability.

Proportion

Actions to reduce smoking, and choices about drug therapies, invoke the fundamental assumption of epidemiology and also the idea of comparison. There would be no value in comparing smokers to nonsmokers if the health outcomes at issue were purely random. Similarly, randomized controlled trials comparing different drug therapies would be of little value if treatment outcomes were random. If the results of a diagnostic test were not associated with the disease under evaluation, that test would be useless. The reality that health outcomes are not random makes exploration of those nonrandom elements (associations) valuable.

The fundamental assumption of epidemiology connects progress in health research to statistics—specifically to the link between frequencies (which can be observed in samples or populations) and probabilities, risks, and rates. Gaining the knowledge needed to improve health depends on estimating probabilities, risks, and rates (which must be known) from things like counts and frequencies (which can, at least, be observed).

Epidemiology has a precise term for the concept of frequency: *proportion.* A proportion is a type of ratio, so it consists of 2 numbers, 1 divided by the other. The top number in the ratio is the numerator and the bottom number is the denominator. The special characteristic of a proportion (as opposed to any other ratio) is that the contents of the numerator are contained in the denominator.

Imagine that you have flipped a coin 10 times, and the result is 5 heads and 5 tails. The proportion of the coin flips that are heads is 5/10. The numerator is 5 and the denominator is 10. The 5 heads are included with the 5 tails in the denominator of the ratio. This example, as artificial as it may be, illustrates an important point. If you flip a coin 10 times, you might observe exactly

5 heads. Indeed, this is the expected proportion based on the symmetry of the coin. However, it is also quite likely that you would only observe 3 or 4 heads rather than the expected 5. You would also fairly frequently observe 6 or 7 heads. Nothing about the coin changes, which means the observed proportion of heads in this small series is influenced by chance. Notice that if you had flipped the coin only twice, the vulnerability of this proportion (of heads) to chance is even greater. Based on the symmetry of the coin, we can surmise that 2-flip experiments repeated many times would produce the following proportions: 0/2, which would be observed one-quarter of the time; 1/2, which would be observed one-half of the time; and 2/2, which would be observed one-quarter of the time (in decimal form, the proportion of heads may be 0, 0.5, or 1). These proportions cover the whole range that a proportion can cover, from 0 to 1. Since the denominator of any proportion includes the contents of the numerator, a proportion can never be more than 1. In the case of our 2-flip example, the entire range of possible values is covered (0, 1, or 2 heads) and the probability of each of the various possible outcomes is quite high, suggesting that there is a lot of randomness in what happens when a coin is flipped twice.

THE LAW OF LARGE NUMBERS

There is something magical about proportions. The magic, however, only emerges when the coin is flipped many times, not just twice. If you have the time, try a little experiment: try flipping a coin 100 times, or 1000 times. Or play with an online simulated coin flipper. As the number of flips goes up, the proportion of heads that you observe gets closer and closer to one-half. This is the magic: when you flip a coin once, the proportion you observe will be either 0/1 or 1/1; when you flip it twice, the proportion you observe could be 0/2, 1/2, or 2/2; when you flip it 1000 times, the proportion you observe will predictably be very close to 1/2 (in the language of ratios it will be close to 500/1000, in the language of decimals it will be close to 0.50, and in the language of percentages it will be close to 50%).

The effect you observe as you increase the number of coin flips is an example of the law of large numbers. This law states that when an experiment with a random variable as an outcome is repeated many times, the result becomes closer and closer to an expected value.

To truly understand the power of the law of large numbers, you must reverse this line of reasoning. Imagine that you had a coin that might be a trick coin—let's say that it might have 2 heads or 2 tails—and that you had to flip the coin to figure this out.

If you flip the coin once, you won't be able to tell: you will observe either heads or tails, but because both outcomes are possible for a fair coin and a trick coin, you aren't going to learn very much about the coin.

If you flip the coin twice and observe heads each time, you might begin to think it's a trick coin: you know the probability of this happening is lower. The 2 flips are 2 independent events: if it's a fair coin, we can calculate the probability of seeing heads both times as the product of each event in isolation—0.5×0.5 or 0.5^2, which is 0.25 or 25% (this is the "one-quarter of the time" from a few paragraphs back).

What if you flip the coin 10 times and each time it's heads? The probability of this happening is 0.5^{10}, which is an extremely tiny number, approximately 0.001. Based on this very low probability, it would be safe to conclude that the coin is a trick coin. If the coin is flipped 5 times, the probability of observing 5 consecutive heads is less than 0.05 (it is 0.031), so you might say that you are more than 95% confident that it is not a fair coin.

The lesson here is that the law of large numbers goes both ways. It allows prediction of long-run probabilities when the expected value of an individual trial is known, but more importantly it allows knowledge to be gained about the probabilities that underlie observed proportions.

Flipping a coin results in heads or tails—a binary outcome. Binary outcomes are at the centre of many health-related questions. A person can have a disease or not, and can be exposed to a risk factor (drinking unsafe water, smoking) or not. A diagnostic test can be positive or negative, right or wrong, and so on.

Key point: A few observations of a binary outcome do not provide very much information about the probabilities associated with that outcome, but observing many independent observations provides a lot of information about those probabilities.

Prevalence

The law of large numbers and properties of coin flipping also apply to prevalence, another key concept in epidemiology.

Prevalence is the proportion of a population with a disease. Prevalence is an example of an epidemiologic parameter. Mathematically, it is a proportion and cannot therefore be less than 0 or more than 1. Epidemiologically, it represents a characteristic of a population: the amount of disease in that population. As with other proportions, prevalence has a numerator and a denominator. The numerator is the number of people with a disease and the denominator includes all members of the population. It should be noted that, occasionally, epidemiologists use the term *prevalence* to refer to the number of people in a population with a disease. However, most commonly, prevalence refers to a proportion as described here.

There are several types of prevalence: the most important is point prevalence, which is the proportion of a population with a disease at a particular point in time. How can knowledge about the prevalence of disease be obtained? Think about flipping a coin again: each flip of the coin is an event that produces either heads or tails. Now imagine this: instead of flipping a coin, you randomly select individual people from a population—say, the population of Canada—and determine whether they have a particular disease. Heads or tails? Disease or no disease? The probability that a member of this population has the disease will reflect the probability that Canadians in general have this disease. If it were possible to examine everybody in Canada and determine whether they had the disease, you could divide the number that have the disease by the total number of Canadians, leading to exact knowledge about the point prevalence of the disease. A sample of 1 person would not add very much to the state of knowledge on this question. As with a coin flip, that person will either have the disease or not, from which you can only conclude that the prevalence is either greater than 0 (if that person has the disease) or less than 100% (if the person does not). But a large sample, which consists of many independent observations, gives more information. The larger the sample—like the more flips of a coin—the stronger the expectation that the observed proportion reflects the underlying point prevalence.

Sources of error

The power of epidemiological research comes from the fundamental assumption of epidemiology and the law of large numbers: epidemiologists can understand disease distribution very clearly if their research studies have large samples. The value of epidemiology for planning services, generating causal hypotheses, identifying risk factors, identifying prognostic factors, and interpreting the results of tests follows logically from this. It would seem that the "sky is the limit," and that epidemiology can hardly fail to shed light on the distribution and determinants of any disease.

Unfortunately, it is not quite that simple. Things can go wrong in research.

Systematic error comes from flaws in study design that systematically bias study results. Imperfect measurement is an example of systematic error. In our discussion of coin flipping and random sampling, we assumed we had perfect measurement: that a head could be accurately discerned from a tail, and disease from no disease. Determining whether someone has a disease, however, isn't necessarily a simple matter. If measurement is imperfect, the law of large numbers does not work in the expected way.

Random error comes from chance. For example, it is not always possible to obtain the huge samples that can fully harness the law of large numbers. When sample sizes are too small, as with a small number of coin tosses, the observed disease proportions may fall far from the actual prevalence by chance alone. Random error always becomes smaller as sample size increases.

Extraneous factors can also lead to error—in ways that challenge the fundamental assumption itself. Diseases distribute in populations in relation to determinants, but what if a real determinant just happens to go together with some unimportant factor? It could fool a researcher into thinking that it—the unimportant, extraneous factor—was a cause of the disease. A researcher unaware of this possibility could mistake the extraneous factor for a determinant merely due to its tendency to distribute with a real determinant.

Key point: Epidemiology has a theoretical basis grounded solidly in the law of large numbers. However, in practice there are many potential pitfalls. Students and practitioners of the health sciences and health professionals need to be skilled in identifying vulnerabilities to bias in published epidemiological studies.

THE PURPOSE OF CRITICAL APPRAISAL

When epidemiologists design studies, they need to take deliberate steps to avoid sources of error. If you are training to be an epidemiologist, this will be a big part of your job: to design and conduct good studies.

When you read health research studies, you also need to think deliberately about sources of error. Faced with a study result, you need to ask yourself: What are all the ways that this study result could be wrong? This is called *critical appraisal*. It means that you don't read a study with the expectation that it is right. Instead, you try to attack it, looking for ways the study's methods make it vulnerable to error. Note that the skills required of an epidemiologist, and those required of a health professional critically appraising a study, are the same: both need to be able to understand all the ways in which this type of research can go wrong.

The principles of critical appraisal shape the health sciences literature. When a researcher submits a study to a journal for publication, the study goes through a process of peer review: experts in the field examine it critically, looking for vulnerability to error. Peer-reviewed journals consider studies for publication only if studies survive this kind of intellectual attack.

Thinking deeper

Expressing prevalence symbolically

The law of large numbers has a focusing effect on the parameter of prevalence. The vulnerability to random differences gets smaller and smaller when estimates of the parameter are based on larger and larger samples. What is going on here? And how can we express this idea symbolically?

In chapter 1, the disease status of a population was depicted using upper-case letters, *A* and *B*, in contingency tables. We can extend this symbolic approach to depict the prevalence of disease in a population and produce a formula for calculating this parameter:

$$\text{PREVALENCE} = \frac{A}{A+B}$$

Since *N* = *A* + *B*, the formula could also be written as:

$$\text{PREVALENCE} = \frac{A}{N}$$

Note that *prevalence* is uppercase (PREVALENCE): in this book's notation, this signifies that we are talking about the prevalence of the disease in an entire population. If a study examined every member of a population and determined, without error, the disease status for each person, the study, if repeated, would produce the same result every time. There is no chance involved. PREVALENCE is therefore not an estimate: it *is* the prevalence. PREVALENCE also functions as a probability: the probability that a randomly selected individual from this population has the disease.

Researchers do not usually have access to information about entire populations. In contingency tables, they may represent this symbolically with lowercase letters to depict disease status (see Table 5). The lowercase letters signal that the counts inside the table derive from a sample rather than from an entire population.

TABLE 5. 1 × 2 TABLE DEPICTING SAMPLE-BASED DATA

Disease	No disease	Total
a	b	n

If prevalence is calculated from Table 5, lowercase letters again signal the use of sample-based data:

$$\text{Prevalence} = \frac{a}{a+b}$$

Or, alternatively:

$$\text{Prevalence} = \frac{a}{n}$$

Here, *n* is the sample size. The probability of selecting any particular member of the population for the study sample is *n*/*N*.

RANDOM VARIABILITY, TRUE PREVALENCE, AND SAMPLE-BASED PREVALENCE

Recall that repeating a study to calculate PREVALENCE would result in exactly the same result every time, as long as there was perfect classification of A and B. Chance does not play any role here.

Chance, however, affects calculations of sample-based prevalence. For one thing, not just any a and b people will do for the calculation of sample-based prevalence. You have to assume that the probability of selecting any person from the population does not depend on their disease status. Remember the example of flipping a coin? It was understood that the long-run probability of heads would equal 0.5, because the symmetry of a coin means heads and tails should have equal probability. The same principle suggests that if sample-based prevalence is to tell us something about PREVALENCE, then each member of the population must have an equal probability of being selected. If people with disease (the A people) are more likely to be selected than people without disease, you would expect sample-based prevalence to be greater than PREVALENCE. If people with disease are less likely to be selected, sample-based prevalence will tend to underestimate PREVALENCE.

However, if each member of a population has an equal probability of selection and if measurement is perfect, the long-run probability that any person we select is an a is actually PREVALENCE. For the same reason that flipping a coin thousands of times will almost always result in a proportion of heads near 50%, a study involving thousands of subjects will almost always produce an estimated prevalence very close to PREVALENCE.

CALCULATING STANDARD ERROR

"Almost always" is a key consideration here. Estimated parameters, such as sample-based prevalence, are vulnerable to random variability. An important way to quantify the variability of a parameter is its standard error. The standard error of an estimated proportion (p)—such as prevalence—is provided by the following formula:

$$\text{Standard Error} = \sqrt{\frac{p \times (1-p)}{n}}$$

Actually, this is an approximation when it is calculated from a sample, but it is usually good enough. Note that n is present within the denominator of the fraction inside of the square root sign. This means that as n increases, this fraction will get smaller and smaller. The standard error, and therefore the variability associated with the estimate, will also get smaller and smaller. This formula helps to quantify the focusing effect of large samples.

A NOTE ABOUT FORMULA AND EQUATION FORMATS

This book uses the following formats to present and discuss formulas and equations.

- Formulas and equations that incorporate population-based data (data from an entire population) use uppercase letters for all variables. For example:

$$\text{PREVALENCE} = \frac{A}{A+B}$$

- Formulas and equations that incorporate sample-based data (data from a sample of a population) use lowercase letters, except for spelled-out variables. Spelled out variables use title case. For example:

$$\text{Prevalence} = \frac{a}{a+b}$$

Questions

1. According to data from Statistics Canada,[21] there were 2,273,800 people older than 17 with asthma in Canada in 2019. Assuming that this figure is correct and that the population of Canada older than 17 in that year was 30,378,269 at mid-2019,[22] what is the prevalence of asthma in Canada?

2. A study seeking to determine the frequency of delirium (a confusional state due to metabolic dysfunction in the brain) in psychiatric units identified a sample of $n = 401$. From this sample, 9 cases of delirium were identified.[23]
   a. What is the prevalence of delirium in psychiatric units?
   b. What is the estimated standard error of this proportion?

3. In your opinion, is point prevalence a more appropriate parameter for descriptive or analytical studies?

4. Some diseases do not affect entire populations. Prostate cancer, for example, does not occur in women, because women do not have a prostate gland. When calculating the prevalence of this disease, should the entire population be included in the denominator, or only the men?

5. There are various ways to quantify the impact of random variation on epidemiological estimates. Confidence intervals are 1 procedure. These will be described in more detail in a later chapter. In brief, a confidence interval provides a range of plausible values for a population parameter based on observations of a sample. When samples are small, there can be considerable random variation among estimates, and quantification of random error is essential. When samples are large, estimates are likely to be very close to the true value

and confidence intervals are less critical. Do you think there is any value in having confidence intervals for estimates that are based on an entire population?

6. Prevalence is sometimes reported as a number (e.g., "2500 people in this city have diabetes") and sometimes as a proportion (e.g., "7% of people in this city have diabetes"). List 1 advantage and 1 disadvantage of describing prevalence as a count rather than as a proportion.

7. A study is examining diabetes prevalence by assessing fasting blood glucose to identify cases of diabetes. On their way to the laboratory, the study participants randomly take different routes. Some of them pass doughnut shops and are unable resist purchasing and (secretly) eating doughnuts. The results of their blood tests are wrong: their blood sugar is higher than it would have been had they fasted, creating the false impression that they have diabetes. Since this occurred randomly, is this a form of random error?

8. A study assesses the prevalence of alcoholism by randomly visiting households and administering an interview that can detect this condition. Some of the participants don't understand some of the questions and just guess, providing random answers. Will this cause random or systematic error?

9. Does it seem unfair to you that scientists attempt to attack the results of their colleagues through criticism of their research methods? What is the justification for this critical stance?

10. Most epidemiological studies use samples because they do not have access to an entire population.

   a. Does this mean that they are always vulnerable to random error?

   b. The law of large numbers suggests that the proportion of independent outcomes observed in individual members of a study sample should begin to resemble the true underlying proportion as the number of independent observations gets larger and larger. However, the selection of individuals into a sample is not necessarily a set of independent observations. For example if one person selected has the disease, there is one less person in the population with the disease, so the next person selected will have a slightly different probability of having the disease. Does this mean that prevalence cannot be estimated accurately?

PART II

Fundamental descriptive parameters

Epidemiology has 2 basic parameter "families"— prevalence and incidence—that focus on the frequency or rate of single variables.

Prevalence and incidence are also the building blocks of more complex parameters that capture in more detail the effects of exposure on disease in populations.

The next 2 chapters look at, first, the basic parameters of prevalence and incidence, and then at more complex parameters.

Basic measures based on frequencies and rates

OBJECTIVES

- Distinguish the parameter families of prevalence and incidence.
- Define key parameters within each family.
- Describe the relationship between proportions and odds.
- Describe the relationship between prevalence and incidence.
- Define cumulative incidence and describe how to calculate it.

Parameter families

Epidemiology has 2 basic parameter "families"—prevalence and incidence—that focus on the frequency or rate of single variables. Later chapters describe parameters of more complexity, which compare disease distribution among, for example, exposure groups.

The formulas for calculating prevalence and incidence sometimes look the same—a confusing reality—but prevalence and incidence are entirely different concepts.

The prevalence family

POINT PREVALENCE, PERIOD PREVALENCE, AND LIFETIME PREVALENCE

Chapter 1 noted that epidemiological research has 2 main branches: descriptive epidemiology and analytical epidemiology. In descriptive epidemiology, prevalence is the basic parameter. Note that we are talking here about prevalence as a parameter, not as a sample-based estimate of prevalence, nor as the actual prevalence of a disease in an entire population (PREVALENCE). In most cases, the best, specific term for this parameter is *prevalence proportion*.

(Some people use the term *prevalence rate*, but a rate is different than a proportion, so this counts as sloppy terminology.)

As a parameter, prevalence includes point prevalence, period prevalence, and lifetime prevalence. In some unusual situations, this parameter can also be a count (simply a tally of diseased individuals) rather than a proportion—in these situations, you would call the parameter a *prevalence count*.

Point prevalence quantifies the amount of disease in a population at a point in time. Unless otherwise specified, the term *prevalence* refers to point prevalence.

The Canadian Multicentre Osteoporosis Study[24] produced a point prevalence estimate. This study used a random sample, based on household telephone listings, of 10 061 women and men aged 25 years and older, distributed approximately equally across areas served by 9 study centres. At the baseline time point, the data were used (among other things) to estimate the point prevalence of osteoporosis in women and men aged 50 years and older (the study used the criteria of the World Health Organization to define osteoporosis). The data showed the point prevalence of osteoporosis among Canadians in this age group was 15.8% for women and 6.6% for men.

The Canadian Study of Health and Aging[25] provides another example of estimating point prevalence. This study was based on a sample of 1835 subjects from a population of 283 510 Canadians who were age 85 and older at the time of the survey. The sampling procedures ensured that the sample represented both household residents in the community and people who were living in institutions. The study estimated the point prevalence of dementia in this age group as 28.5%.

Period prevalence is the proportion of a population that has, or has had, a disease at any time during a defined time interval, such as 1 year or 1 month. Statistics Canada employed period prevalence in the 2002 Canadian Community Health Survey: Mental Health and Well-being.[26] The survey used an interview to assess several conditions, including the 12-month period prevalence of depressive episodes. Investigators asked respondents whether they had experienced various symptoms during the preceding 12 months, and used an algorithm to determine whether respondents' symptoms fulfilled diagnostic criteria for 1 or more major depressive episodes. They estimated that 4.8% of the sample had experienced such an episode.[26] This is an example of a 12-month, or annual, prevalence estimate. The study was repeated in 2012 and showed that the annual prevalence estimate remained essentially unchanged at 4.7%.[27] The examples provided here come from the field of psychiatric epidemiology. Because mental disorders are often recurrent and can follow various patterns over time, period prevalence is often preferred over point prevalence in the mental health field.

For similar reasons, period prevalence has also been a popular estimate of migraine prevalence.[28]

Lifetime prevalence—an unusual type of prevalence—is the count or proportion of people in a population who have had a particular disease at some time in their life. Lifetime prevalence usually applies to diseases that transition in and out of active phases. In Canada, studies of mental illness use this parameter most. People who have had episodes of mental illness remain at risk for future episodes: it is reasonable to think their illness as a lifelong condition subject to recurrence and remission.

For some mental disorders, it is difficult to conceptualize prevalence in any other way than lifetime prevalence. For example, bipolar I disorder is characterized by a lifetime history of 1 or more manic episodes.[29] A manic episode is a discrete period in which a person has elevated mood and increased activity. Usually, people with bipolar I disorder have recurrent episodes of mania and also episodes of depression. However, many people who do not have bipolar disorder develop depression, so depressive episodes indicate a bipolar disorder only if preceded by an episode of mania. The national mental health survey conducted by Statistics Canada in 2002 provides an example of lifetime prevalence.[30] The survey administered a structured diagnostic interview to a sample of more than 35 000 Canadians.[31] It found that 12.2% of the population had had an episode of depression at some time in their life. When it excluded respondents reporting a past manic episode, it estimated the lifetime prevalence of depression as 10.8%.

Fiest et al[32] also used lifetime prevalence in estimating the prevalence of epilepsy. They used a systematic review methodology (systematic reviews are discussed in chapter 5) and found that the lifetime prevalence was 7.60 per 1000 persons. For comparison, the point prevalence was slightly lower at 6.38 per 1000 persons.

In another example, Stubbs et al[33] studied the lifetime prevalence of traumatic brain injury among homeless and marginally housed individuals. These authors also used a systematic review and found that more than half of their participants reported a lifetime history of traumatic brain injury.

A troubling characteristic of lifetime prevalence is that it is dependent on age. Whereas period prevalence has a specified interval of observation (e.g., 1 year), the interval of observation for lifetime prevalence depends on the age of the person being assessed. This means that lifetime prevalence does not quantify disease burden as clearly as point prevalence or period prevalence. Also, in practice, lifetime prevalence can be difficult to measure accurately, because it can require subjects to remember long-past signs and symptoms. Some experts argue that these problems make the parameter useless. In a 2010 paper, Dr. David Streiner of the University of Toronto and McMaster

University posed the question: "Has lifetime prevalence reached the end of its life?"[34]

Key point: Prevalence is the most common measure of disease burden. While the term encompasses several variants (types of period prevalence and lifetime prevalence), the most common meaning is the proportion of a population with a disease at a point in time (point prevalence).

EXPRESSING PREVALENCE PROPORTION

Except in unusual situations where prevalence is reported as a number (a count), prevalence is expressed as a proportion—for example, as a fraction, percent, or decimal. In a very small population, such as a group of students in an elementary school class, a fraction provides clear information.

For example, imagine that there are 25 students in a class. During influenza season, 5 of these students become ill with influenza. You could express the period prevalence as 5/25. You could also express it as a decimal (5/25 = 0.20), or as a percentage, which is the decimal form multiplied by 100 (0.20 × 100 = 20%). Many diseases have a much lower prevalence than our classroom example, which makes considering the clearest form of expression important. For example, a systematic review by Pringsheim et al[35] estimated that the prevalence of Huntington disease was 2.71 per 100 000—a form easier to digest than the decimal (0.0000271) or the percentage (0.00271%).

Proportions are intuitive and easy to understand because of their relationship to probabilities. If 5/25 students in a particular class became ill during an influenza outbreak, it is easy to understand that a student in that class had a 20% chance of becoming ill.

Another way to convey the same information uses odds. In our classroom example, this is the number of students who got the disease during the observation interval divided by the number who did not get the disease, or 5/20. The odds of having the disease, expressed as a decimal, are 0.25. As with proportions, you can think of odds as a probability—just like betting odds in horse racing, or when people say "the odds are stacked against you" meaning you have a low probability of success. Clearly, you could use odds rather than proportions to express prevalence, although in practice this is rare. When odds are used to express prevalence, it is especially important to use the most specific language possible: *prevalence odds.*

Key point: Prevalence can be expressed as a count, a proportion, or odds.

The incidence family

THE DIFFERENCE BETWEEN INCIDENCE AND PREVALENCE

The difference between incidence and prevalence is a key distinction in epidemiology. A firm idea of this distinction is the foundation for understanding more complex parameters.

Incidence refers to the new occurrence of a disease. The operative word here is *new*. To be a prevalent case, a person merely needs to have a disease. To be an incident case, a person needs to newly develop the disease. The Canadian Multicentre Osteoporosis Study and the Canadian Study of Health and Aging are examples of studies seeking to estimate both incidence and prevalence. Such studies are an important source of prevalence data because, to estimate incidence, they need to be able to exclude everyone who already has the disease (the prevalent cases).

INCIDENCE PROPORTION, INCIDENCE RATE, AND ATTACK RATE

As a parameter, incidence includes the incidence proportion, incidence rate, and attack rate.

An incidence proportion derives from observations over an interval of time. The interval of time—a risk interval—must be specified or the parameter is meaningless. Note the contrast here with point prevalence, which is like a snapshot at a specific point in time. An incidence proportion requires a risk interval: a 5% risk over 1 day is a completely different probability than a 5% risk over 1 hour or 1 year.

To measure an incidence proportion, it is necessary to first identify a population at risk. People who already have a disease at the beginning of a risk interval cannot newly develop the disease during the interval—so measurement involves assessing research subjects at a baseline time point, eliminating those who already have the disease, and assessing the (remaining) at-risk population over a risk interval to see how many develop the disease. The resulting proportion is an incidence proportion. Although it is also theoretically possible to measure incidence using odds rather than a proportion, this is rarely done.

Key point: Whereas prevalence in its various forms quantifies the amount of disease in a population, incidence proportions represent the risk of newly developing a disease during a specified time interval.

An incidence rate, like all rates, describes change in a quantity as a function of time. As an example of a rate, think about velocity. If you drive a car at a velocity (rate) of 60 kilometers per hour, you know you will travel 60 kilometres in 1 hour, 120 kilometres in 2 hours, and 30 kilometres in a half hour.

Note that *per hour* could also be written /*hour* (e.g., 60 km/hour) or—because the sign of an exponent changes depending on whether it is in the numerator or denominator of a ratio—*hour*$^{-1}$ (e.g., 60 km hour^{-1}). Incidence rates are like velocity: velocity describes the rate at which an object travels, and an incidence rate describes the rate at which people become ill. As with an incidence proportion, an incident rate presupposes that a person is not already ill: it applies to an at-risk population that excludes those who are already ill at the time that observation starts.

Unlike an incidence proportion, which has no time units, an incidence rate has person-time units. These are expressed as time^{-1} (the idea of "being a person" doesn't really need to be specified). The time units associated with incidence rates, while they are always in this form, are themselves arbitrary. Think back to the analogy with velocity: 60 km/hour is the same as 60 km/60 minutes or 1 km/minute—the rate does not change, only the units. Similarly, an incidence rate can use any time units—for example, days^{-1}, weeks^{-1}, months^{-1}, or years^{-1}. Epidemiologists aim to select time units that are easy to understand and maximally informative. For example, if the incidence rate for amyotrophic lateral sclerosis in Nova Scotia[36] is expressed as 2.24 per 100 000 person-years (2.24 per 100 000 year^{-1}), a planner can easily imagine the number of new cases likely to arise in at-risk populations in Nova Scotia in a given year. It wouldn't make much sense to report this incidence rate in person-seconds or person-days: this would produce correct, but tiny, numbers of little help to planners.

Key point: Incidence rates are not proportions and not odds: they are rates and expressed in person-time units.

An attack rate describes a special type of incidence proportion, where a particular disease corresponds with a particular risk interval.

For example, influenza produces seasonal epidemics in Canada, so the risk interval for influenza is sometimes defined as this seasonal period (November to April). Another example: in some "point source" outbreaks of infectious diseases, the behaviour of the infectious agent can define the risk interval. Say a group of wedding guests is exposed to food contaminated with toxins produced by *Staphylococcus aureus*: they are at risk for developing food poisoning within 6 hours. This 6-hour interval is an obvious choice as the risk interval for calculating the attack rate. During the COVID-19 pandemic people with exposures to known cases of the disease were asked to quarantine for 2 weeks, under the assumption that if they contracted the disease they would have symptoms within this interval. In other words, 2 weeks was taken as the relevant risk interval following an exposure to the virus.

If you are dismayed that anyone would call an incidence proportion a *rate*, you have reason—it is very misleading terminology (reminiscent of the unfortunate term *prevalence rate*). Nevertheless, it is a standard terminology.

Severe acute respiratory syndrome (SARS) was an important infectious disease outbreak in Canada[37] where attack rates were reported. The outbreak originated in Guangdong province in China in 2002 and was brought to Canada by travellers infected in Hong Kong in 2003, with the first known case arriving in Canada on February 23, 2003. The initial wave of the outbreak was followed by a second wave consisting of 74 cases reported between April 15 and June 9, 2003. Of these, 29 were health care workers and 28 were people exposed to the virus during hospitalization. Another 17 cases occurred among hospital visitors. Nursing staff at the hospital wards where most of the exposures occurred used a common nursing station, shared a washroom, and ate together in a lounge near the ward. The attack rate among nurses working in an orthopaedic section of the ward was approximately 40% and among those in a gynecology section was approximately 25%. Note that these attack rates are percentages, which are just a type of proportion. The risk interval associated with these estimates is the time period in which the outbreak occurred.

In the COVID-19 pandemic, a different version of the attack rate was important: the household secondary attack rate. This is defined as the proportion of residents of a household who develop the disease after another member of the household contracts it. An early estimate from China placed this at 17.1%,[38] whereas a Winnipeg estimate was 14.7%.[39]

Key point: Attack rates are a type of incidence proportion, and should properly not be called *rates* (but they are).

Basic mortality rates

Mortality rates are a kind of incidence rate. The population at risk for mortality consists of all those who are alive at a point in time. Every time somebody dies, the mortality event is their first (and only) occurrence.

There is a lot of information about mortality in Canada available from Statistics Canada through data tables that can be found on the Statistics Canada web page. The information system consists of numerous tables (more than 100 for mortality alone) that users can customize. These data tables are not limited to examination of mortality, nor even to health statistics, yet they contain a wealth of frequently updated health and mortality data.

Mortality rates are calculated by dividing the number of deaths in a year by the midyear population of that same year. On the surface, this sounds like a proportion, so it is tempting to call this a *mortality proportion*. However, there is a distinction. If you were calculating an annual incidence proportion, you would count the number of deaths that occurred during a year (January 1 to December 31), and divide this by the population at the start of the same year (January 1). A mortality rate uses the midyear population (the population on July 1), rather the population on January 1, because the midyear population reflects the occurrence of births and deaths (as well as immigration and emigration) during the year: assuming the population is in a steady state, it describes the person-time in the population. A person born on July 1 provides only half a person-year of time at risk of death, but a person who dies on July 1 also provides only half a person-year of time at risk. In a steady state population, births and deaths are equal and occur throughout the year. For this reason, this kind of mortality statistic can reasonably be called an *annual mortality rate* and is always reported with year^{-1} units.

The relationship between odds and proportions

Converting odds to proportions and vice versa
To report the basic parameters of prevalence and incidence, you can use proportions or odds—these are interchangeable. There is a formula for converting proportions to odds:

$$Odds = \frac{Proportion}{1 - Proportion}$$

And there is a formula for converting odds to proportions:

$$Proportion = \frac{Odds}{1 + Odds}$$

Odds and proportions have similar values for rare diseases
Here is another interesting characteristic of odds and proportions. When a disease is rare, the prevalence or incidence is quite similar whether expressed as odds or a proportion. Consider the formulas for a proportion and odds in sample-based data (so, using the a and b notation):

$$Proportion = \frac{a}{a + b}$$

$$Odds = \frac{a}{b}$$

When a is small, $a + b$ is very similar to b, and the 2 formulas produce a similar result. So, a disease with a prevalence of 1 in 10 000 (1 person of 10 000 has the disease), the proportion is 0.001 and the odds are almost identical at 0.001001. By contrast, if the proportion is 0.5 then the odds are 1.0, which is not very similar at all.

The relationship between prevalence and incidence

When prevalence and incidence are the same

Let's think about the classroom with 25 students again, where 5 students developed influenza during an outbreak. We could talk about the period prevalence proportion in this situation: the proportion of students with the disease (5/25) during a defined interval (in this case, the period of outbreak).

Could 5/25 also express an incidence proportion?

It could, if all 25 students were free of influenza at the start of the interval. In this case, the interval used to calculate the period prevalence proportion corresponds to the risk interval for calculating the incidence proportion. The 2 proportions are the same. It would also, of course, be correct to describe the incidence proportion as an attack rate in this case.

Prevalence, incidence, and endemic diseases

An endemic disease is defined as a disease whose prevalence has assumed fairly stable levels—a steady state—within a population. There is a very important relationship between prevalence and incidence in endemic disease.

Let's first clearly understand how endemic disease differs from outbreaks, epidemics, or pandemics of infectious disease. In outbreaks, epidemics, and pandemics, disease parameters are unstable. An epidemic occurs when disease exceeds normal, expected levels in a defined community, geographic area, or season. The terms *outbreak* and *epidemic* have similar meanings, but *outbreak* implies an infectious agent and a defined locale. Obesity, for example, currently exceeds expected, historical levels—we often talk about an epidemic of obesity,[40] but never an outbreak of obesity. Canada is also experiencing an epidemic of opiate overdose deaths.[41] A pandemic occurs when an infectious disease, such as influenza or SARS-CoV-2 (the virus that causes COVID-19 disease), sweeps across the globe and creates sequential epidemics in many different populations. In outbreaks, epidemics, and pandemics, the relationship between prevalence, incidence, and mortality is dynamic—there is no steady state. These situations are best understood as departures from a steady state.

The relationship between incidence and prevalence in endemic disease is key to understanding complex parameters in epidemiology. Think of the prevalence proportion as a pool made up of the members of a population with a disease. (Note that this concept of prevalence corresponds to point prevalence, not to period prevalence or lifetime prevalence.) There is an inflow to the prevalence pool (the incidence rate—the rate at which people without disease "flow" into the prevalence pool) and an outflow from the prevalence pool (because of mortality—people dying—or recovery from the disease). The size of the prevalence pool is determined by this inflow and outflow. If more people are getting the disease than are dying or recovering, the prevalence pool increases. If the opposite is true, the prevalence pool shrinks.

In a steady state situation (where inflow and outflow are equal), a simple formula describes the relationship between prevalence and incidence, and it is approximately true most of the time: prevalence is equal to the incidence rate multiplied by the mean duration of illness. More precisely, the prevalence odds are equal to the incidence rate multiplied by the mean duration of disease. The mean duration of illness is influenced by both recovery from the disease (if this is possible) and mortality. For an irreversible disease, the duration is determined only by the age of onset and mortality.

Since the mean duration of illness has time units and the incidence rate has $time^{-1}$ units, these units disappear in the calculation of the prevalence odds.

$$\text{Prevalence Odds} = \text{Incidence Rate}\left(t^{-1}\right) \times \text{Duration}\left(t\right)$$

A real-world example of this relationship is the global pattern of HIV infection. In highly developed countries with good access to antiretroviral treatment, which leads to greatly prolonged survival, HIV prevalence is higher relative to incidence than in countries with poor access to treatment. In some countries, longer survival means that diminishing or stable incidence has been associated with increasing prevalence over time.[42] If you look at the formula, you can see how this works. Imagine that the incidence does not change. Under this assumption, increasing duration—in this case due to longer survival as a result of antiretroviral treatment—will lead to increasing prevalence.

Key point: Point prevalence is approximately equal to the product of the incidence rate and the mean duration of illness.

This formula—which expresses the relationship between prevalence and incidence—helps epidemiologists estimate prevalence from information about incidence, and vice versa. For example, the Global Burden of Diseases study[43,44] aims to quantify and rank the burden of certain diseases in every country of the world. Burden can be due either to premature mortality or to living with a disease (due to the discomfort and dysfunction that diseases produce). To make these calculations, researchers need information about incidence, prevalence, and mortality, but sometimes do not have adequate data. So, they use mathematical models called DisMod models,[45] which flesh out the basic relationships among incidence, prevalence, and mortality. The current version of DisMod is DisMod-MR. When information is available for only 2 parameters, the models allow researchers to make an educated guess about the third.

The formula also leads to a qualitative understanding of the relationship between prevalence and incidence, which is particularly valuable. For example, it clarifies the motivations of clinical interventions for public health actions. The formula also shows that reducing incidence through prevention, even in the absence of improved treatment, will diminish the prevalence (and therefore burden) of a disease in a population. It also makes plain the role that the health system plays in population health. Better treatments abbreviate the duration of nonfatal diseases and reduce prevalence, even if incidence does not change. Better treatments may also improve survival (as opposed to curing a disease), which will increase the average duration of disease and, therefore, prevalence in the population.

Cumulative incidence

Cumulative incidence refers to the proportion of cases that accumulate over an interval of observation in an at-risk cohort—a concept very similar to incidence proportion. Indeed, the 2 terms are often used interchangeably. However, there is a subtle distinction: the incidence proportion usually uses the number of people in the at-risk cohort at a baseline time point in its denominator, but cumulative incidence is calculated in ways that take into account the fact that those who become ill during the observation interval are no longer at risk after their illness occurs.

Thinking deeper

Calculating cumulative incidence

Imagine a situation in which the 1-year incidence proportion for an irreversible disease is known to be 0.05. What would the cumulative incidence be after 2, 3, or 5 years?

It seems sensible to simply multiply the 1-year incidence proportion by the number of years—so, the 2-year cumulative incidence would be twice the 1-year proportion ($0.05 \times 2 = 0.1$). However, this wouldn't quite be correct. The reason lies in the basic definition of cumulative incidence.

Imagine that the at-risk population at baseline is $n = 100$. Since the incidence proportion is 0.05, it is reasonable to expect, on average, about 5 people will become ill during the first year. Let's assume that this is exactly what occurs. In the second year, there are no longer 100 people at risk of illness. Five of them have become ill, so now only 95 remain at risk. The number expected to become ill in the second year is now 0.05 of 95 people rather than 0.05 of 100.

The complement of a proportion is 1 minus that proportion. So if the risk of becoming ill during an interval is 0.05, the complement (the risk of not becoming ill) is 0.95. In the calculation of cumulative incidence, it is useful to think of the proportion of the population becoming ill as the complement of the number remaining well. Imagine that a 1-year cumulative incidence is equivalent to the annual incidence proportion. This equivalency could be written as:

$$\text{Cumulative Incidence}_{1\text{ year}} = 1 - (1 - \text{Annual Incidence Proportion})$$

At first glance, this seems like a silly formula. Why start with the proportion that does not have the disease at baseline and then subtract the complement of the proportion that gets the disease? The value of this expression becomes clear when there are a series of intervals, which is what cumulative incidence is all about. At this stage, the expression within the bracket can be used to represent the probability of staying well through the first year and also through the second year. Since these are independent probabilities, the joint probability is their product, such that for year 2:

$$\text{Cumulative Incidence}_{2\text{ years}} = 1 - (1 - \text{Annual Incidence Proportion}) \times (1 - \text{Annual Incidence Proportion})$$

Or, more simply:

$$\text{Cumulative Incidence}_{2\text{ years}} = 1 - (1 - \text{Annual Incidence Proportion})^2$$

And this leads to a more general way of anticipating cumulative incidence over a set of n risk intervals:

$$\text{Cumulative Incidence}_{n\text{ years}} = 1 - (1 - \text{Annual Incidence Proportion})^n$$

Returning to our hypothetical population in which the annual incidence proportion was 0.05 and the population size was 100, the last formula tells us the expected value of the 2-year cumulative incidence: $1 - (1 - 0.05)^2$ or 0.0975.

These formulas deal with only 1 factor that can arise from the relationship between a series of smaller risk intervals and a bigger risk interval comprising the smaller intervals: the shrinking of the population at risk as people become ill from the disease under investigation. These formulas are useful conceptually, but circumstances this simple do not occur often in the real world. For example, members of the monitored cohort may die, which would diminish the size of the at-risk population—the formulas do not address this. Similarly, they do not address reductions of the at-risk population due to other diseases or circumstances. A set of methods called *survival analysis* provides a solution to these problems.

EXPECTED CUMULATIVE INCIDENCE: THE EXPONENTIAL EQUATION

The following formula estimates the expected cumulative incidence after a period of observation measured in units of time (t) in a population with a specified incidence rate. This is called the *exponential equation*. Like the previous formulas, this formula only accounts for the diminishing population at risk as incident cases occur (it does not account for other characteristics that could compete with incidence in removing people from the at-risk population). Nevertheless, it is a useful formula.

$$\text{Cumulative Incidence}_t = 1 - e^{-\text{Incidence Rate} \times t}$$

Note that the e in the formula is the base of the natural logarithm, a constant (also an irrational number) that has an approximate value of 2.718. The term after the minus sign in the formula is the inverse logarithm, or exponentiation, of the negative value of the incidence rate multiplied by time.

This formula is not a good substitute for calculating incidence. If the research goal is to estimate a 10-year incidence proportion, then it's best to conduct a 10-year study (as opposed to conducting a 1-year study and using this formula to estimate 10-year cumulative incidence). However, the formula does allow helpful and convenient calculations. Watch out, though, for a common mistake in using this formula: don't forget that a negative sign precedes the incidence rate.

Questions

1. The following table describes the experience of 10 people susceptible to a very dangerous disease. A study of this small population begins on January 1 and observation ends on December 31. Each month, the subjects' health status is assessed and coded as follows: free of disease (grey), ill (black), or dead (white).

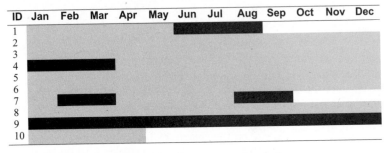

ID	Jan	Feb	Mar	Apr	May	Jun	Jul	Aug	Sep	Oct	Nov	Dec
1												
2												
3												
4												
5												
6												
7												
8												
9												
10												

   a. What is the annual period prevalence of this disease?

   b. What is the point prevalence in August?

   c. What is the 12-month incidence proportion of this disease?

   d. Calculate an annual mortality rate for this population.

   e. The experience of subject 7 indicates that this is a recurrent disease. Survivors reenter the population at risk. Under this assumption, calculate an incidence rate for this disease.

2. The following table describes the experience of 10 people susceptible to a rapidly fatal disease. A study of this small population begins on January 1 and observation ends on December 31. Each month, the subjects' health status is assessed and coded as follows: free of disease (grey), ill (black), or dead (white).

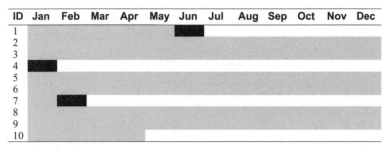

a. What is the annual period prevalence of this disease?
b. What is the point prevalence in August?
c. What is the 12-month incidence proportion of this disease?
d. Calculate an annual mortality rate for this population.
e. Calculate the incidence rate for this disease.

3. The following table describes the experience of 10 people with a highly recurrent condition. A study of this small population begins on January 1 and observation ends on December 31. Each month, the subjects' health status is assessed and coded as follows: free of disease (grey), ill (black), or dead (white). Assume that each of the episodes is a new, including the episode in month 1 in ID = 1.

a. What is the annual period prevalence of this disease?
b. What is the point prevalence?
c. This is a recurrent disease. Survivors reenter the population at risk. Under this assumption, calculate an incidence rate for this disease.
d. What are the prevalence odds? Explain whether you can also calculate the prevalence odds using the following formula: prevalence odds = incidence rate × mean duration.

4. Change the following proportions into odds:
a. 0.0009
b. 0.009
c. 0.09
d. 0.9

5. Dr. Frederick Banting of the University of Toronto received the Nobel Prize in 1923 for his discovery insulin to treat diabetes. Did this accomplishment make insulin-dependent diabetes mellitus more or less common?

6. What is the formula used to calculate period prevalence from an incidence rate and duration of time?

7. If the incidence rate for influenza is 0.25 month^{-1} during the winter months in a Canadian city, what is the annual incidence rate?

8. Assume that 1 in 5 people experience a mildly stressful life event each month. Suppose that a certain epidemiologist dislikes the use of months as time units in incidence-rate calculations. This epidemiologist calculates the annual incidence rate as follows:

Annual Incidence Rate = 0.02 month^{-1} × 12 months/year

Unfortunately, the result of this multiplication is greater than 1, which this (so-called) epidemiologist regards as being impossible, claiming that incidence cannot exceed 1. What, if anything, is wrong with this calculation?

9. Of the various members of the prevalence family (point, period, lifetime), which do you consider the best for quantifying disease burden?

10. Lifetime prevalence is sometimes erroneously described as the probability of developing a disease at some time during one's life. What is wrong with this interpretation?

4

Specialized mortality rates and composite measures of disease burden

OBJECTIVES

- Define and interpret key specialized measures of mortality: cause-specific mortality rate; age- and sex-specific mortality rate; perinatal mortality rate; infant mortality rate; postneonatal mortality rate; and case-fatality rate.
- Define and interpret key composite health indicators: QALYs and DALYs.
- Describe the role of these rates and indicators in monitoring population health.

Measures of mortality and disease burden

Chapter 3 introduced the 2 basic parameters of epidemiology—prevalence and incidence—and showed how to calculate these as true values and estimates.

There are situations, however, in which these parameters do not fully capture the burden of disease in a population.

This chapter describes parameters for these more complex situations. These parameters use mortality, prevalence, and incidence as building blocks.

Specialized mortality rates and parameters

Parameters that capture differences in the way diseases affect populations have considerable descriptive value. These include certain specialized parameters calculated from mortality data.

For example, some diseases have a large impact on mortality, such as cancer, cardiovascular disease, and cerebrovascular disease. Some diseases tend to kill young people, such as congenital anomalies, trauma, and suicide. Some, such as stroke, predominantly kill elderly people.

In addition, certain mortality rates, especially those for the very young, quantify more than just deaths. The number of children dying around the time of childbirth or in the first year of life is an important way of assessing the general level of social and health system development in a country.

Cause-specific mortality

A statement from the 1955 *United Nations Handbook of Vital Statistics Methods* highlights the importance of cause-specific mortality statistics: "It may truthfully be said that virtually every large-scale problem in preventive medicine has been brought to light—in part at least—by statistics of death, and further that the adequacy of remedial or curative action is, in the last analysis, reflected in these same statistics."[46] Cause-specific death statistics are among the oldest indicators of population health status. In England, "bills of mortality" (weekly mortality statistics) date to the seventeenth century.[47] Abstracts based on bills of mortality produced by William Farr were an important data source for John Snow's cholera investigations.[7]

Recall the calculation of a mortality rate (see page 32): the number of deaths in a particular year is counted in the numerator, and the midyear population is taken as an estimate of person-time for the denominator of the rate.

This calculation provides information about the rate at which people are dying, but not about the reasons for their death. Cause-specific mortality statistics address this deficiency. Here, the numerator represents the number of people dying of a specific cause, and the denominator is the midyear population at risk of dying from that cause.

When a cause of death affects only 1 sex (e.g., prostate cancer), the population at risk should only include that sex. For example, cause-of-death tables published by Statistics Canada[48] report a crude mortality rate for prostate cancer (22.4/100 000 in 2009) for men, but not for women. It would be misleading to report this rate for the entire population, since prostate cancer is not a health issue for women. Women are not members of the population at risk.

DATA SOURCES ABOUT CAUSE-SPECIFIC MORTALITY

Registration of death is required in all developed countries, making cause-specific mortality statistics among the most widely used health indicators internationally.

A registration of death requires completion of a certificate—usually by a physician, but also by specialized nurses in some provinces[49]—specifying the cause of death. In Canada, where responsibility for health care has been constitutionally assigned to the provinces, relevant vital-statistics legislation varies from province to province. The Vital Statistics Council for Canada works to coordinate and standardize documentation of causes of death (along with other issues, the council is also concerned with certification of births and changes of name). Medical certificates of death are entered into provincial mortality databases and, because of the shared standards, the databases can then be effectively aggregated into a national mortality database: the Canadian Mortality Registry.

Internationally, the World Health Organization (WHO) compiles international tables of cause-specific mortality for its member states. These international efforts have contributed to effective standardization of procedures for certification of causes of death. The WHO's system for classifying disease, the International Classification of Disease, or ICD, has become the standard classification. It is currently in its eleventh edition (ICD-11).[50] Another WHO classification is the International Classification of Functioning, Disability and Health, or ICF. Details of this classification are available on the WHO's website.[51]

A medical certification of death includes demographic information and information from the deceased person's medical history. It identifies an immediate cause of death (the direct cause of death—e.g., respiratory arrest), underlying causes of death (the disease or injury that initiated the sequence of morbid events leading directly or indirectly to death—e.g., carcinoma of the lung), and any antecedent causes of death that are judged to intervene in the sequence of events between the underlying and immediate causes of death. For example, a fall at home could be an underlying cause of death as follows: the fall caused a fracture, which led to surgery and immobility (an antecedent cause), which led to a terminal pneumonia. The last element in the sequence listed on a medical certificate of death is the immediate cause of death. Death certificates also provide an opportunity to list other associated conditions.

Cause-specific mortality data are made readily available in Canada through Statistics Canada data tables, which allow users to produce customized output from the national mortality database. The top 10 causes of death in Canada are:

1. malignant neoplasms (cancer)
2. heart disease
3. accidents
4. cerebrovascular diseases (e.g., stroke)
5. chronic lower respiratory diseases
6. diabetes
7. influenza and pneumonia
8. Alzheimer disease
9. intentional self-harm (suicide)
10. kidney disease

Some of them have sex-related differences: accidents rank third among leading causes of death in men, but rank fifth for women; suicide ranks eighth for men and fourteenth for women.[52]

When a death appears to be due to unnatural causes (e.g., suicide, accident), or when it is sudden or unexpected, it may trigger an investigation by a coroner's or medical examiner's office. (Note that the use of *coroner* or *medical examiner* depends on the province or territory.) The information collected by these offices can be used as a source of research data. Statistics Canada and the Public Health Agency of Canada have also developed a national database of mortality data from these offices, called the Canadian Coroner and Medical Examiner Database.

Key point: Information about mortality is readily available in most countries, including Canada, and is an important source of epidemiological data.

EPIDEMIOLOGICAL RESEARCH BASED ON CAUSE-SPECIFIC MORTALITY DATA

Many epidemiological studies in Canada have used mortality data.

In a well-known example, Ashmore et al[53] used exposure data from a registry of radiation exposure called the National Dose Registry of Canada to identify a cohort of 206 620 workers who were monitored for radiation exposure. They linked this exposure data to the national mortality database, which allowed them to identify a cohort of more than 5000. They used this cohort to investigate the possible role of radiation exposure in the incidence of cancer and other diseases.

A study by Hwang[54] identified a cohort of homeless men in Toronto in 1995. The Ontario Office of the Registrar General ascertained deaths in this population during 1995 to 1997 using provincial death certificates. Men aged 18 to 24 in this cohort were 8.3 times more likely to die than men in this age group in the general inner-city population. The causes of death were found to depend on age. In younger men, accidents, poisonings, AIDS, and suicide were more common causes of death; in older men, cancer and heart disease were most common, and accidental death was also common.

Aronson and Tough[55] investigated a series of 38 horse-related deaths in Alberta. Since these deaths were "unexpected," the medical examiner's office was a reasonable source of data, and the data were likely representative of accidental deaths related to horses. However, Aronson and Tough noted that only about half the deaths had undergone autopsy, so the exact cause of death may not have been known in all cases. The main finding of this study was that many of these deaths involved head injuries, suggesting that education about the value of helmets was an appropriate preventive strategy.

A study by Boyd et al[56] examined the role of trauma and asphyxia in deaths from avalanches. In collecting data for this study, the investigators reviewed avalanche fatalities that occurred between 1984 and 2005. They searched the database of the Canadian Avalanche Centre, where 220 deaths were recorded. Of those 220 deaths, 204 were also recorded in the databases of the British Columbia Coroners Service or the Chief Medical Examiner of Alberta. Again, about half the deaths ($n = 117$) underwent autopsy. They found asphyxia had caused 154 (or 75%) of the deaths and trauma had caused 48 (24%). Interestingly, they found that the frequency of death due to different causes depended on the nature of activities in which the victims were engaged. Trauma, for example, was the cause of death for 42% of ice climbers and only 9% of snowmobilers. Another study used coroners' data to describe all deaths classified as suicides between 1998 and 2012 in Toronto. Of 3319 suicides identified, 1.8% were homeless people and 6.9% were precariously housed people, indicating an over representation of these groups in this form of mortality.[57]

THE VALUE OF CAUSE-SPECIFIC MORTALITY DATA

For descriptive purposes, mortality data provide a lot of information about what people are dying from. This has obvious value for planning services and for generating hypotheses that analytical studies can evaluate.

However, each record of cause-specific mortality involves the judgement of the professional making the record. Some provinces have produced detailed manuals for completing certifications of death,[58] which may help standardize these judgements. Many Canadian physicians feel inadequately trained in death certification, though—a situation the quality of the data may reflect.

For example, it might make sense to record suicide as an immediate cause of death (e.g., using an International Classification of Disease code for self-inflicted injury)—but what should be viewed as a contributing cause? In some circumstances, mental disorders (such as depression) that are strongly associated with suicide might be coded as an underlying cause, but such disorders may sometimes be unknown or undocumented.

Other circumstances involve even more difficult, or arbitrary, judgements. A death whose immediate cause was cardiac arrest might have an underlying cause of drug overdose—which might, in turn, have occurred as a possible suicide attempt within the context of a substance use disorder.

Epidemiologists view the causal data contained in registration data with caution.

Key point: Mortality rates are a type of incidence rate. Everyone alive is at risk of death and death is always a new (incident) rather than an ongoing (prevalent) occurrence.

SURVEILLANCE

In addition to their value to research, mortality data are a classic source of surveillance data.

Unlike research, surveillance is an ongoing process that provides monitoring through the use of routinely available data sources. In addition, surveillance data must be analyzed, and the information communicated to people who plan and administer health services, or who mobilize public health responses to emerging threats.[59]

Key point: Surveillance differs from research in the sense that it is an ongoing process, and is inherently coupled with processes of data analysis and communication.

For these reasons, government ministries of health perform most surveillance activities. In Canada, all provincial governments participate in surveillance activities, and the federal government plays a role in the integration and analysis of surveillance data.

Examples of surveillance activities include:

Monitoring of infectious diseases by Canadian provinces: Provinces legislate certain infectious diseases as notifiable diseases. Labs, physicians, and other health professionals must then report cases of these diseases to public health authorities. This allows monitoring of the diseases and rapid response to outbreaks. In some cases, rapid response might mean targeting an individual (e.g., prompt treatment for someone with tuberculosis). In other cases, rapid response might mean targeting a population. This kind of surveillance is becoming increasingly important in Canada for certain infectious diseases. For example, falling vaccination rates for diseases such as pertussis (whooping cough) and measles have led to outbreaks requiring rapid implementation of supplementary vaccination programs. Another example: cases of food-borne illness—such as a 2008 listeriosis outbreak linked to a Maple Leaf Foods plant in Toronto, or the staphylococcal intoxication associated with "cronut burgers" at the 2013 Canadian National Exhibition, also in Toronto— have triggered closures of food-serving, -producing, and -processing facilities. The website of the Public Health Agency of Canada has many other examples of outbreaks.[60]

National database of notifiable diseases (Public Health Agency of Canada): This database includes information on diseases that all provinces consider notifiable.[61] The Public Health Agency of Canada also provides case definitions for these diseases, an extremely useful resource for communicable disease control in the field.

PulseNet Canada: Canada's National Microbiology Laboratory is also involved in surveillance through PulseNet Canada, an information-sharing system. Clinical cases of enteric infectious diseases receive molecular subtyping at PulseNet and a network of laboratories across the country. This allows surveillance for molecular patterns across provinces that might indicate outbreaks.

Chronic Disease Surveillance System (Public Health Agency of Canada): This system synthesizes administrative data collected by the provinces. *Administrative data*—a very common term in Canadian epidemiology—includes information collected during physician billing, drug claims, and other administrative procedures. For example, physicians typically seek payment for their services by submitting "bills" to their provincial health care insurance plan. A bill usually specifies a diagnosis (generally an International Classification of Disease code). In addition, provinces collect data to administer their health care systems. For example, some provinces cover certain drug claims. All of them cover hospital costs in public hospitals (in Canada, almost all hospitals are public hospitals)—so they need to figure out, for example, how much a hospital should get paid for a particular inpatient stay.

National Ambulatory Care Reporting System (Canadian Institute of Health Information), also known as NACRS: This records emergency-department and ambulatory-care data. For example, Bethell et al[62] used NACRS data from Ontario to identify self-harm among youths presenting to emergency departments. Since NACRS contains postal codes, the authors were able to characterize the community size and neighborhood income quintile of these youths by linking the NACRS records to census data using the Statistics Canada Postal Code Conversion File.[63]

This is by no means a comprehensive list. National surveillance systems are also in place for blood safety, congenital anomalies, antimicrobial resistance, and many more issues that require monitoring. The website of the Public Health Agency of Canada[64] provides a summary of national surveillance systems, which has links to more detailed information and, in some cases, to reports and data tables.

Key point: Both provincial and territorial as well as federal public health officials participate in health surveillance activities.

Age- and sex-specific mortality rates

It is relatively easy to calculate a mortality rate, but interpreting rates for an entire population can pose challenges.

Here's an important interpretive factor: different causes of death affect people more or less prominently depending on their age, so it is often important to examine mortality rates for particular age groups. This involves identifying the population size within a particular age range and the number of deaths in the population within that age group.

For similar reasons, there may be value in calculating sex-specific rates, or province-specific rates.

In general, such rates are referred to as *specific mortality rates*, although it is always important to label them in ways that clarify what exactly they are being specific about—e.g., age-specific mortality, sex-specific mortality, and so on.

Age and sex are strong determinants of mortality, and they are also classically nonmodifiable determinants. For these reasons, it is very common to make comparisons of mortality within, rather than across, age and sex groups. Due to the importance of these figures, they are routinely tabulated in tables available on the Statistics Canada web page.[65]

PERINATAL MORTALITY

Several specified rates have wide use because they function as indicators of economic development, general living conditions, social well-being, performance of health systems, and the quality of the environment. These are considered sentinel indicators because they reflect factors relevant to the health of an entire population even if, on the surface, they concern a single age range.

The perinatal mortality rate, also called the perinatal death rate, is a sentinel indicator. In Canada, a perinatal death is defined as the death of a child less than 1 week of age (0 to 6 days) or a stillbirth of 28 or more weeks gestation. Of course, to calculate a perinatal mortality rate, you need both a numerator and a denominator. The denominator here is the number of total births, which consists of live births and late fetal deaths.

A birth counts as a live birth if any sign of life is present after birth (e.g., breathing). To be registered as a stillbirth, there must be no signs of life present, and the fetus must be more than 20 weeks gestation or have a birth weight of at least 500 grams. (A few minor interprovincial differences exist on these points).

Statistics Canada defines the perinatal death rate as the number of perinatal deaths during a given year per 1000 total births (live births plus late fetal deaths) in the same year, where late fetal deaths are defined as stillbirths of 28 weeks or more gestation. Statistics Canada produces a regularly updated data table for perinatal mortality.[66] This data table provides perinatal mortality, both as a count and as a rate, and also provides the underlying constituent counts: late fetal deaths and early neonatal deaths.

INFANT MORTALITY

Infant mortality refers to the death of an infant younger than 1 year. It is usually expressed as a frequency, calculated using the infant death count during a given year divided by the live birth count for the same year. Statistics Canada calculates this statistic irrespective of birth weight, but because prematurity and associated birth weight is an important contributor to infant mortality, the infant mortality rate is reported separately (see Table 13-10-0368-01[67]) for all birth weights and for birth weights over 500 grams.

According to the Conference Board of Canada, Canadian infant mortality rates are shockingly high, even though they have diminished from 27 to 5.1 per 1000 between 1960 and 2007. Of 17 peer nations included in the Organization for Economic Cooperation and Development (OECD), Canada was found to be the second worst (the only nation performing more poorly was the US). However, the rate has continued to drop: a 2017 update of Table 13-10-0368-01 reported the rate for 2013 as 5.0 per 1000 live births, which had declined to 4.5 per 1000 live births by 2017.[67] Among infants with a birth weight of 500 grams or more, the rate in 2017 was 3.4 per 1000 live births.[67]

NEONATAL, POSTNEONATAL, AND UNDER-5 MORTALITY RATES

The neonatal period is the first 28 days of life. The neonatal mortality rate is calculated by dividing deaths occurring in the neonatal period by the number of live births. Postneonatal deaths are those that occur after the neonatal period (age < 28 days) but within infancy (age < 1 year), with the associated rate also being denominated by the number of live births. The under-5 mortality rate has a self-evident meaning. These parameters are most commonly calculated per 1000 live births.

Note that all of these parameters are actually frequencies rather than rates, since they are calculated as proportions. They do not need units in the way that a true rate does, and are called *rates* merely for ease of language. Chen et al worked with these parameters to study health disparities in Indigenous and non-Indigenous residents of Quebec.[68] They found that perinatal and infant mortality rates were elevated in First Nations and Inuit births when compared to non-Indigenous births.

In 2015, the United Nations adopted 17 sustainable development goals with an implementation deadline of 2030.[69] Goal 3 is "good health and well-being," which aims, among other things, to reduce neonatal mortality to 12 per 1000 live births or lower, and under-5 mortality to 25 per 1000 live births or lower. According to UNICEF, Canada has already achieved these goals.[70] For example, Canada's neonatal mortality rate is 4 per 1000 live births and its under-5 mortality rate is 8 per 1000 live births.[70] A leading cause of early life mortality is preterm birth, which is defined as babies born alive before 37 weeks gestation. In 2013, nearly 30 000 births in Canada were preterm births, representing 7.8% of all live births. The highest proportion of preterm births was in Nunavut (12.6%) and the lowest was in PEI (7.1%).[71]

MATERNAL MORTALITY RATIOS

The WHO defines *maternal death* as the death of a woman while pregnant or within 42 days of termination of pregnancy, from any cause related to, or aggravated by, the pregnancy or its management, but not from causes that are accidental or incidental.[72] The maternal mortality ratio is the ratio of maternal deaths to live births. This ratio is increasingly being used as a health indicator in the international context, although it is not yet widely used in Canada. The definition cannot be used without good information on the cause of death, which is not always available or accurate in all countries. For this reason, the WHO has suggested another indicator, pregnancy-related death, which is death within 42 days from the end of pregnancy regardless of the cause.[72] Currently available tabulations from Statistics Canada report maternal mortality from all obstetric causes, and those that occur from obstetric causes during pregnancy or within 42 weeks of the end of pregnancy.[73]

Case-fatality rates

Case-fatality rates are really proportions—another example of using *rate* for ease of language. A preferable term is *case-fatality proportion*, but this is rarely used.

In case-fatality rates, the denominator of the proportion consists of people who have a disease. The numerator consists of those who die while they have this disease. This particular type of mortality measure is unique because the risk interval is not necessarily an interval of time, as is usually the case in the calculation of an incidence proportion or cumulative incidence. Case-fatality rates quantify how many people die when they get sick with a disease, so the fact that they are sick is often more important than any specific time interval.

A 2003 paper published in the *Canadian Medical Association Journal* provides a good example of calculating a case-fatality rate. The paper was written during the outbreak of severe acute respiratory syndrome (SARS) in Toronto. The authors reported that 105 cases of probable SARS had been identified and 13 of these had died, leading to an estimated case-fatality rate of 12.4%.[74,75]

More recently, there have been many estimates of the case-fatality rate for COVID-19 in association with the pandemic of this disease. For example,

Abdollahi et al[76] calculated a COVID-19 case-fatality rate in the usual way, by dividing the total number of deaths due to COVID-19 by the total number of cases, expressing this as a percentage. This led to a case-fatality rate estimate of 4.9%. However, they were concerned that, due to underreporting, the denominator of the estimate may have been underestimated (leading to an inaccurately high case-fatality estimate). After making an adjustment for underreporting, they estimated the case-fatality rate as 1.6%.

Key point: A case-fatality rate is a special type of incidence proportion in which the risk state is characterized by having an illness state rather than a specified time interval.

Observed survival proportions and relative survival ratios

There is often interest in calculating an index of survival similar to a case-fatality rate, but for a disease that does not have an easily definable duration.

Cancer, for example, may go into remission and then recur. In such instances, case-fatality proportions are calculated over defined time intervals, typically 5 years. The Canadian Cancer Society calls the complement of this type of proportion an *observed survival proportion.*[77]

Consider, however, that people might die from a variety of causes over a 5-year period, particularly since many cancers afflict elderly people. In elderly age groups, mortality related to other causes may not be negligible. (This is different than for SARS, for example, where it may be reasonable to assume that everyone dying during their illness with SARS died of SARS.) For this reason, the Canadian Cancer Society recommends an alternative parameter—the 5-year relative survival ratio, which is the ratio of observed survival in a group of people diagnosed with a cancer to the expected survival in a comparable group of people in the general population.[78] Ideally, the comparable group would be a cohort of the same age and sex without cancer, but this is usually approximated using general population mortality. In recent publications, this has been called *net survival.* A relative survival ratio, or net survival, could be calculated over any duration of observation, but 5 years is typically reported in Canadian cancer statistics.

For all cancers, net survival is 63%, meaning that a person diagnosed with cancer has a 63% chance of surviving for at least 5 years, relative to their counterparts in the general population. This ratio is highest for thyroid cancer (98%) and testicular cancer (97%), and lowest for esophageal (15%) and pancreatic cancer (8%).[78]

Key point: The cancer literature contains some different terminology and addresses the issue of case fatality somewhat differently than the infectious disease literature.

Potential years of life lost (PYLL)

Basic mortality parameters, such as overall (or crude) mortality rates, do not factor for age. Age of death, though, affects the impact of death. Deaths that occur in advanced age disrupt families and society less than deaths that occur earlier in life. For example, a death at age 90 may not deprive society of as many person-years of healthy life and economic productivity as a death at birth or age 20.

The parameter of potential years of life lost (PYLL—also YPLL: years of potential life lost) accounts for the age at which various causes of death occur. PYLL can be reported as years lost or it can be reported as a rate. If it is calculated as a rate, the numerator is the number of years "lost" when people die.

To calculate years of life lost due to a particular cause of death, you need some standard of reference. For example, you could use life expectancy at birth, or some ideal, or hoped for, life expectancy. Or, you could use an age judged to be economically significant, such as the typical age of retirement (before and after which deaths may have a different economic impact). In Canada, PYLL is usually calculated using age 75. In other words, a death at age 70 causes 5 years of lost life, and a death at age 20 causes 55 years of lost life. Note that deaths occurring after age 75 do not count at all.

PYLL can be expressed as a rate using a person-time denominator. When this is done, the person-time in the rate is the midyear population of those under age 75.

Key point: PYLL is a strategy for estimating the impact of various sources of cause-specific mortality. The advantage of PYLL is that it accounts for the different ages at which people die from various causes of death.

In Canada, malignant neoplasms are the leading cause of death and heart disease is the second leading cause of death in both men and women.[52] These same causes are the leading causes of PYLL, but other causes of death such as unintentional injuries and intentional self-harm are much more prominent.[79]

Internationally, the use of PYLL as a health indicator has largely been superseded by a composite measure, the disability adjusted life year (DALY), which is discussed later in this chapter. Statistics Canada continues to occasionally report PYLL as an overall population health indicator,[79] but no longer reports cause-specific PYLL.

Avoidable premature mortality

Another way to classify deaths is according to their avoidability. The Canadian Institute of Health Information (CIHI) produces a list of avoidable causes of premature death.[80] As usual in Canada, deaths occurring before age 75 are considered premature. Avoidable premature mortality arises from

2 categories. The first category is preventable deaths and the second is deaths from treatable causes. Preventable deaths are those that could have been avoided by all levels of prevention (primary, secondary, and tertiary). Deaths due to treatable causes are those that could potentially have been prevented by secondary or tertiary prevention. A subset of causes of death comprises both preventable and treatable causes. Overall avoidable mortality, and its 2 subgroups (preventable deaths and deaths due to treatable causes) are reported annually by Statistics Canada in a customizable table.[81] The table is publicly accessible and provides both mortality rates and PYLL rates for these avoidable causes.

LIFE EXPECTANCY

Life expectancy seeks to produce an estimate of the future survival experience of a contemporary cohort. Unlike basic parameters such as prevalence proportions and incidence proportions (which are real quantities), life expectancy is a projection. It is an artificial parameter.

The most commonly calculated type of life expectancy is life expectancy at birth. Imagine that a large group of babies were born today. Now ask the question: How many years, on average, can they expect to live? Stated this way, life expectancy represents the projected average duration of life for a cohort of babies born today.

The challenge is to project this average. There is no perfect solution to this challenge. The mortality rates experienced by a cohort of babies born today are unknown, since this mortality will occur in the future, much of it in the very distant future. The imperfect solution is to take current age-specific mortality rates and use them to form a best guess about how many will die at any given age in the future. (This is why these calculations are best considered projections rather than parameters.) From this, it is possible to calculate life expectancy at birth for a fictitious cohort of newborns.[82]

Life expectancy offers an intuitively accessible means of summarizing a large number of age-specific mortality rates into a single index that people can relate to. Statistics Canada reports estimates for life expectancy that can be accessed through data tables.[83] Estimates of life expectancy for various countries are also reported by the World Health Organization. In Canada, life expectancy at birth is 84.1 years in women and 80.2 years in men.[84] According to Statistics Canada summary tables,[83] from 1920 to 1922, life expectancy was 59 in men and 61 in women. In Canada, the gap in life expectancy between the sexes was less than 2 years in 1921 but subsequently the gap gradually increased, reaching 7 years in 1976.[85] Since then the gap has been gradually narrowing and is currently about 4 years.

Health-adjusted life expectancy (HALE) is an indicator of the average number of years that an individual in a population is expected to live in full health, taking into account years lived in a suboptimal state of health. This is an extension of the concepts applied in the calculation of life expectancy. The HALE approach refines life expectancy by adjusting for years of life lived in less than full health. The World Health Organization developed this approach, although its recent burden-of-disease reports use a different measure: disability-adjusted life-years (DALYs).

A 2013 burden of disease study in Ontario[86] used HALE to assess mental illness and addictive disorders. People tend to live for many years with these conditions, so it is not surprising that the impact of mental disorders and addictions on HALE is very large. The study identified 5 mental disorders producing the greatest burden of disease: major depression, bipolar disorder, alcohol use disorders, social phobia, and schizophrenia. The burden of major depression alone was found to be more than the combined burden of Ontario's 4 most common cancers. The Public Health Agency of Canada has also produced a HALE report for Canada.[87]

Fatal discontinuities

The determinants of health and mortality usually change slowly, producing long-term trends in mortality rates. However, extraordinary events such as epidemics, wars, civil unrest, and natural disasters can produce temporary spikes in mortality called *fatal discontinuities*.[88]

Composite parameters

In a perfect world, everyone with a disease would receive the best treatment possible. In the real world of limited health care dollars, we have to set priorities. Epidemiological data should guide priority setting, but it means putting different diseases onto a single scale of comparison—a challenging task.

For example, how do you compare the significance of migraine and cancer? According to a 2012 Statistics Canada survey,[89] the prevalence of migraine in the Canadian household population is 8.3% (11.8% in women versus 4.7% in men). The 2-year prevalence of all cancers in Canada at roughly the same time[90] is 720.7/100 000, which is less than 1%. Migraine is a long-term recurrent condition that causes pain and disability; cancer is associated with intense treatment needs and high mortality. Comparisons of migraine and cancer must use composite measures capable of quantifying the negative impact of these diseases on individuals' health and duration of life, all on the same scale.

Quality-adjusted life-years (QALYs)

While survival is important, not all survived time is equal. In some cases, disease survivors may have poor quality of life, so a composite parameter of survival time and quality of life during the survival time is useful. This approach is particularly popular in the health economics literature. The World Health Organization defines quality of life as "an individual's perception of their position in life in the context of the culture and value system in which they live and in relation to their goals, expectations, standards and concerns."[91]

It can be challenging, though, to assess quality of life: it involves attaching personal judgements to different health states. A popular approach involves health utilities. Instruments that assess health utility put many different health issues onto a single scale. They do so by assessing the value that people (usually samples of people from population surveys) assign to diverse sets and combinations of health states using specialized techniques (e.g., standard gamble methodologies).

Internationally, the EQ-5D, a 5-item scale developed by the EuroQoL Group,[92] is among the most common health utility instruments. In Canada, the Health Utilities Index (HUI)[93,94] is also popular. The HUI consists of sets of utility weights, meaning that researchers use other instruments to classify a person's health state and then use the HUI to convert the health-state categories into utility scores. The HUI has several versions: recent Canadian studies mostly use the HUI Mark 3. However, even the HUI Mark 3 is now becoming dated. By contrast, the EQ-5D has been actively updated and is taking over as the most important health utility measure in Canada.

Some health-utility weighting schemes assign 1 to indicate perfect health and 0 to indicate states comparable to death. These utility scores can be incorporated into the calculation of quality-adjusted life-years (QALYs). Since health-utility scales place different illnesses on the same scale of population-based preference, such studies can identify opportunities to improve health at a known unit cost—for example, by comparing the cost effectiveness of different treatments, or by determining whether the costs of a gain in health utility are within an acceptable range. Marra et al[95] applied this approach to a systematic review of a vaccination program for human papillomavirus (HPV). HPV, which is sexually transmitted, causes cervical cancer in women: vaccination programs targeting HPV prevent this type of cancer, and so prevent the loss of QALYs that would occur in the absence of vaccination. Marra et al reported generally favourable costs per QALY for HPV vaccination. This suggests that HPV vaccination programs would deliver improved health at a rate per unit cost that is usually considered acceptable in the Canadian health system.

Key point: QALYs attempt to quantify the impact of an intervention on quality of life outcomes and are widely used in health economic evaluations.

Disability-adjusted life-years (DALYs)

Disability-adjusted life-years (DALYs) are another composite measure used to quantify the loss of health associated with diseases and injuries. They are the flagship measure of a major international initiative called the Global Burden of Disease Study.

DALYs are often regarded as a measure of disease burden. Disease burden accounts for both premature mortality (years of life lost, which is conceptually equivalent to PYLL) and years lived with disability due to a disease or injury. These 2 aspects of health are melded using a disability weight, such that DALYs are the sum of the following elements:

- years of life lost
- number of years lived with disability multiplied by a disability weight that reflects the extent of health loss experienced due to the disease

Disability weights reflect health state preferences determined by the Global Burden of Disease investigators using data collected in population surveys.[96] If a disease has a disability weight of 0.5, living with that disease for 10 years is considered equivalent to dying 5 years prematurely. The Global Burden of Disease Study (GBD) uses DALYs to rank the burden caused by a comprehensive set of diseases, injuries, and risk factors on population health in different countries[44,97]—information that can assist those countries with setting priorities for population-health initiatives.

DALYs are useful because they deal with an age-old problem in descriptive epidemiology. Death is an easy thing to measure and almost every country measures it. This creates a tendency to see the impact of diseases from that particular perspective. DALYs make sure that the contribution of disabling conditions is recognized in the assessment of disease burden.

While the GBD publishes reports of DALYs due to various causes in all countries, including Canada, the first country-specific report for Canada, by Lang et al, was published in the Canadian Medical Association Journal in 2018.[98] This paper reported disease burden using DALYs for each year from 1990 to 2016. In 2016, the leading causes of disease burden were (in order of ranking): neoplasms, cardiovascular diseases, musculoskeletal diseases, and mental and substance use disorders, which as a group accounted for about 56% of disability-adjusted life years in Canada in 2016. The biggest contributors to premature mortality (years of life lost, or YLL) were neoplasms and cardiovascular disease; the biggest contributors to years lived with disability (YLD) were musculoskeletal disorders, closely followed by mental and substance use disorders. The major causes of mortality showed declining age-standardized mortality rates over time (with cardiovascular mortality declining faster than that associated with neoplasms, leading to a reversal in rank during the studied time interval). However, age-standardized rates for mental and substance use disorders, for all measures of burden, tended to be stable or to increase slightly. An important contributor to the latter trend was increasing mortality related to the opioid epidemic in the form of overdose deaths. In their Global Burden of Disease report, Lang et al[98] also reported a 2016 estimate of life expectancy for Canada: 82 years. Health-adjusted life expectancy, according to their analysis, was 71 years. Each of these parameters had increased slightly from 10 years earlier in 2006, when life expectancy was 81 and health-adjusted life expectancy was 70.

The Global Burden of Disease methodology has an interesting feature: it can take risk factors into account by calculating the amount of disease burden attributable to specific exposures—a concept called *attributable burden*. Attributable-burden results for Canada were reported by Alam et al in 2019,[99] based on Global Burden of Disease data for 1990 to 2016. In 2016, the 10 risk factors accounting for the largest percentage of disability-adjusted life years in Canada, in order of ranking, were: tobacco, diet, high body mass index, high fasting plasma glucose, high systolic blood pressure, alcohol and drug use, occupational risks, high total cholesterol, impaired kidney function, and air pollution. These authors described changes over time in age-standardized DALY rates attributable to specific risk factors. The overall risk-factor ranking did not change very much between 1990 and 2016, and, although the burden attributable to tobacco diminished during this period, tobacco remained the top-ranked risk factor. Reductions in age-standardized attributable burden also diminished for elevated blood pressure and total cholesterol, whereas burdens attributable to high body mass index, high fasting glucose, and drug and alcohol use all increased.

Key point: Epidemiologists often use rates and proportions to quantify disease impacts and outcomes, but their toolbox also includes composite measures such as QALYs and DALYs that can provide additional sophistication for capturing the impact of diseases and injuries.

Proportional mortality ratios

Since mortality databases record cause-of-death information when people die, the counts in such databases must normally be linked to population-denominator data (such as a midyear population count) to calculate a cause-specific death rate. A simpler, albeit less informative, way of using mortality data is to calculate a proportional mortality ratio. This is the number of deaths due to a specific cause divided by all deaths during the same interval of time. For example, Sadovnik et al[100] reported that the proportion of deaths due to suicide in a multiple sclerosis cohort was 7.5 times that of the age-matched general population. Unfortunately, this type of ratio does not represent any meaningful risk in the population. As the capacity to link databases has become more advanced, this parameter has been declining in use and is considered an obsolete approach to assessing mortality.

Thinking deeper

Calculating central tendency

Often, you can describe the behaviour of a variable with statistical parameters that identify the variable's central or typical values: its central tendency. You can combine these measures of central tendency with a measure of dispersion to describe the distribution of that variable. Chapter 2 introduced the standard error of the prevalence proportion, which is a measure of dispersion for prevalence estimates (see page 21).

The 3 most common ways of quantifying central tendency are the mean, the median, and the mode. The mean is the average value of a variable, calculated by adding all the observed values for the variable and dividing this total by the number of observations. The median is the middle value—a value at which one-half of the observations are higher and one-half are lower. The mode is the most-often-occurring value of a variable.

Table 6 presents the ages of 10 people. Let's use this small data set to illustrate how to calculate the mean, median, and mode.

TABLE 6. A DATA SET WITH THE AGES OF 10 PEOPLE

Identification number	Age
1	48
2	35
3	1
4	43
5	31
6	30
7	26
8	46
9	26
10	50

The mean is the sum of each person's age divided by the number of people. The sample size is $n = 10$, and the identification number provides an index that identifies the individual people from the first (i = 1) to the last (i = 10). In the following formula for mean age, the uppercase Greek letter sigma (Σ) denotes *sum*:

$$\text{Mean Age} = \frac{\sum_{1}^{10}\text{Age}}{n}$$

This kind of statement is a more efficient way of saying this:

$$\text{Mean Age} = \frac{48+35+1+43+31+30+26+46+26+50}{10}$$

The mean is 336/10 or 33.6.

The median is the value that divides the observations in the sample into 2 parts: the half above the median (in this case, 5 observations) and the half below (the remaining 5). The median is easiest to see if the observations are sorted by age. Table 7 contains the same data as Table 6, but sorts the observations by age.

TABLE 7. A DATA SET WITH THE AGES OF 10 PEOPLE, SORTED BY AGE

Identification number	Age
3	1
9	26
7	26
6	30
5	31
2	35
4	43
8	46
1	48
10	50

You can identify the median by counting up to the midpoint (in this case the fifth observation). Here it falls between the values of 31 and 35, and it is traditional to report it as the average of these 2 values, in this case (31 + 35)/2 = 33.

The mode is the value that occurs most often in the data set. In this case, each observed value occurs once with a single exception: 26 occurs twice. Since this is the most-often-occurring value, it is the modal value for age in this data set. The mode is not used very often in epidemiology, but some related terminology is frequently encountered. A distribution with a single central tendency is unimodal, and a distribution with 2 "humps" suggesting 2 central tendencies is bimodal.

Questions

1. Approximately 300,000 people die in Canada each year. Roughly speaking, what is the crude mortality rate in Canada?

2. About 70 Canadians die each year from tuberculosis and about 70 000 die from malignant neoplasms. Roughly speaking, what are the cause-specific mortality rates for these conditions?

3. Calculate the PYLL contributed by the following deaths:
   a. a motor vehicle collision in which 2 people die, aged 20 and 22
   b. a death due to pneumonia in a 95-year-old

4. Identify the 3 main contributors to the following parameters in Canada:
   a. crude mortality
   b. premature mortality
   c. years lived with disability

5. Johansen et al[101] identified first admissions for stroke (people with no admission for stroke within the preceding 5 years) and examined their in-hospital survival in the 28 days following their admission. They reported that 16.7% died during that interval. What type of "rate" is this?

6. List 3 differences between surveillance and research.

7. List 2 limitations of cause-specific mortality as an indicator of population health.

8. PYLL has largely been supplanted by DALYs. Why do you think DALYs have become a preferred measure?

9. DALYs and QALYs can put a diverse set of health problems and diseases onto a single scale, which is an advantage of such composite measures of health status in general. For example, DALYs attributable to sense organ diseases can be compared to infectious diseases, injuries, and noncommunicable diseases. For this reason, DALYs are often promoted as a way to set priorities in health policy, and QALYs are often used to assess the cost-effectiveness of treatments. For example, a treatment that produces 1 QALY for a cost of $50,000 is sometimes arbitrarily considered to be cost-effective.[102] Can you identify any problems with using this kind of parameter for this purpose?

10. Why does Canada not have a single comprehensive source of health surveillance data?

PART III

Vulnerability to error of descriptive studies

Epidemiologic research can go wrong in many ways, but most errors fall into 3 main categories: random error; systematic error leading to bias; and confounding. The next 5 chapters look at these categories of error in the context of descriptive studies and estimates of fundamental descriptive parameters.

Random error from sampling

- Identify and differentiate the 2 main sources of error in epidemiologic research: random error and systematic error.
- Describe the relationship between sampling and random error.
- Define confidence intervals and how to calculate an approximate confidence interval for a proportion.
- Describe the relationship between sample size and precision in a prevalence study.
- Differentiate estimation and statistical testing.
- Describe statistical testing and define key related concepts: significant versus nonsignificant tests, type I and type II error, and statistical power.
- Explain the influence of sample size on statistical power.

Random error, systematic error, and confounding

Estimates of basic parameters are right or wrong, and they can be wrong because of random (stochastic) error or systematic error—in other words, by chance or because of defects in study design. In addition, if 2 basic parameters are compared, they may mix together (confound) the effects of several different factors.

This chapter focuses on errors due to chance. If you understand the role of chance in epidemiological research, you can take steps in your own research to minimize errors due to chance, and you can stay alert to these errors in the research of others.

SOURCES OF ERROR AND CRITICAL APPRAISAL

Critical appraisal is about identifying vulnerabilities and weaknesses in research.

It's an important task: research leads to conclusions that affect people's lives.

It's also a complicated task. It requires a solid framework for approaching the vast amount of information—in words, methods, and numbers—reported in the typical study. Understanding random error and systematic error is a good place to start. A critical reader of a study will accept its conclusions only if the study survives critical appraisal—an attack on its design and methods that aims to identify ways in which a study is likely to be wrong.

Two provisos are in order concerning critical appraisal. First, critical appraisal involves attacks of a sort, but not personal attacks. The process of criticism and defence against criticism in science is not a destructive conflict. It is more like a life-giving force in research. It creates a context of rigour and fosters excellence. Researchers usually seek critical internal reviews of their grant proposals and research papers from colleagues before submitting them to funding agencies and journals. They do this because they understand the value of critical appraisal. Second, in epidemiology at least, the perfect study doesn't exist. If critical appraisal were solely about finding imperfections, it would draw every result into question. Critical appraisal aims to identify potentially important flaws—flaws that threaten the value of the reported information for the goals of clinical practice and public health.

FIGURE 1. A SIMPLE SCHEMATIC FOR CRITICAL APPRAISAL

Assume that the study is wrong
(a "critical" stance)
⇓
Is it wrong because of bias?
⇓ No
Is it wrong because of random error?
⇓ No
Accept that the result may be right
⇓
Interpret the result

Figure 1 shows that critical appraisal begins with questions about systematic error. There is good reason for tackling systematic error first and random error second. But, a clear definition of systematic error comes from a clear understanding of what is meant by random error—which is why we start with this chapter on random error.

The relationship between random error and sampling

Basic parameters such as prevalence and incidence are real: they actually exist in populations. Random error arises when estimates of these parameters are inaccurate due to chance.

We know population parameters are real for the following reason: if we could count every person in a population, and identify exactly who did and did not have a particular disease, we could determine exactly the true (actual, real) prevalence of the disease. By contrast, an estimate of that parameter is not real in the same way: it is an educated guess about the true population parameter.

Chapter 2 covered ways to represent in symbols the difference between true prevalence and estimated prevalence, where *PREVALENCE* stood for the true parameter, and *prevalence* stood for a sample-based estimate.

$$PREVALENCE = \frac{A}{A+B}$$

where A is all the members of a population with disease and B is all the members of a population without disease

$$Prevalence = \frac{a}{a+b}$$

where a is the members of a population sample with disease and b is the members of a population sample without disease

A characteristic of a true population parameter such as PREVALENCE is this: if the parameter were measured multiple times (selecting every member of a population, classifying them with perfect accuracy into diseased and nondiseased groups) the results would always be exactly the same. This lack of variability reflects that a true population parameter is not subject to random error.

To reflect the underlying true parameter, an estimated parameter such as (lowercase) prevalence needs to come from a random sample or, less desirably, some facsimile of a random sample. If not, there is no particular reason to believe the sample-based estimate has any coherent relation to the true parameter. Random samples provide information about true parameters because each observation in the sample is governed by the long-run probabilities that exist in the underlying population through the law of large numbers.

If you were to sample a population several times to repeat the estimate of the parameter, you would likely get a different estimate from each sample. Each sample would almost certainly select a different group of people from the population, and this would deliver different estimates from sample to sample. This variability reflects that estimated parameters are subject to random error: parameters estimated from samples will not always exactly equal the true parameters in a population.

Key point: A parameter (such as prevalence, incidence, etc.) calculated from a population is a real thing with a real definite value, but often such parameters can only be estimated using data collected from samples. The resulting estimates are not real in the same sense. Repeating the process of estimation will lead to different values each time.

Random samples

The samples used to estimate parameters are subsets of larger populations, but they are not just any subsets. The "magic" of the law of large numbers only works if each member of a sample embodies an event (e.g., diseased or not) independent of other events.

The best kind of sample is therefore a random sample—a sample in which the question of who will be selected into the sample cannot be answered. In other words, selection for a random sample is unpredictable. In the sample, each person's disease status is an independent observation that (together with the other observations) reflects the true prevalence in the population.

PROBABILITY SAMPLE, SELECTION PROBABILITY, AND SAMPLING FRAME

A sample for estimating a parameter should also be a probability sample. This means the probability of selecting a person from the population should be known. A simple random sample is the most common and basic form of a probability sample: each member of the population has the same probability of selection.

Imagine that you are conducting a study of the prevalence of smoking in a high school containing $N = 1000$ students. Let's assume your study will have a sample size of $n = 100$. (Note the convention of an uppercase N to represent the number in the population and a lowercase n to represent the number in the sample.) To select your sample, you might list all the students and use some sort of random process to choose 100 from the list. For example, you could assign a number to each student based on the roll of a 10-sided dice, and then choose all the students assigned the number 1 (or any other number up to 10). More likely, you would want to use a computer to automate this task. For example, using a spreadsheet, you could generate a random integer with values 0 to 9 for each member of the target population and then select each respondent with a particular integer value to be a member of the sample.

This selection process would result in a simple random sample. The sample would also be a probability sample, since the selection probability is known (0.1 or 10%). The list of students would be called a *sampling frame*: a list of population elements that serves as the basis for the selection of a sample.

INFERENCE AND TARGET POPULATION

Inference describes the process of gaining information about a population based on data collected from a sample. Estimation is the most important way of making inferences in epidemiology.

Key point: Probability samples are a type of random sample that serve as the basis for making inferences about populations.

In estimation, the true underlying parameter is called the *target of estimation* and the population to which the estimate applies is called the *target population*.

The process of inference ideally has the following straightforward step at its foundation: a random sample used for inference about a target population must come from the target population. However, very often the target population (e.g., all women of childbearing age) is not suited to enumeration in a sampling frame—which acts against the goal of collecting a probability sample. In this case, a specific population may be identified (e.g., all women of childbearing age in a city or province) as a practical way of representing the larger target population. This produces a conceptual distinction between the target population and the sampled population. These are subtle distinctions. Some studies aim to make inferences of broad significance—for example, "smoking cigarettes during pregnancy causes low birth weight." This kind of statement is intended as fact: there is no reason to believe that it would apply in St. John's and not in Vancouver. Other studies are concerned with more focused inference about a fully specified population—for example, "17% of adult residents of Toronto smoke." So, epidemiological studies can have more-strict and less-strict ways of conceptualizing (and labelling) target populations.

SOURCE POPULATION

When the target population is not fully enumerated in a sampling frame, the population from which the sample is actually drawn may be called a *source population* rather than a *target population*. For example, the target population may be all pregnant women and the source population for a particular study may be all women receiving prenatal care in Halifax at a point in time.

Some researchers refer to the sample drawn from a source population as a *study population*. This is confusing, since the distinction between a sample and a population is critical for epidemiological reasoning. But it's a term you will likely see in the literature—just remember that it's not a population, it's a sample.

Random error

Normally, a researcher would not care very much about the prevalence of a disease in a sample. The estimated prevalence is just a tool to learn about a true population parameter. Data from random samples are necessary for inference, but the data collected from such samples are merely the raw material for making inferences. Researchers calculate parameters from data and use statistics to generate inferences about populations.

Key point: Data from samples are the raw materials from which inferences derive. The tools used to derive and refine those inferences are statistical tools.

Understanding random error requires imagination. Think back to the hypothetical study of smoking in a school with $N = 1000$ students. Suppose you have randomly selected $n = 10$ for inclusion in the study. Here's the part that requires imagination. Imagine that you conduct the same study 100 times, drawing a random sample of $n = 10$ each time. For each sample, you measure how many students smoke (for now, let's assume that you can do this with perfect accuracy) and calculate an estimate of prevalence from the resulting proportion. Prior studies have shown that approximately 1 in 10 youths between the ages of 12 and 17 smoked,[103] so for purposes of illustration we will assume that 0.10 is the underlying population prevalence. Figure 2 shows a simulation of what you would expect to see in this scenario. The value for the estimated prevalence peaks at the true value—which in this case is 0.10. So far, so good. But notice that it is possible, if somewhat unlikely, that some of these studies might come up with estimates that are far from the true value, such as 4 times too high.

Of course, in the real world, studies are never repeated many times in this way. Researchers do studies once and they don't know the underlying true parameter. So, in the real world, investigators face the possibility that their estimates may, by chance, fall far from the true parameter. When selection is perfect (as in the simple random sample imagined here) and measurement is perfect, the expected value of a sample-based estimate is exactly the target parameter in the population. But, as Figure 2 shows, chance plays a role in estimation, and an estimate, even from a perfect study, can be wrong. This is the concept of random error (also known as stochastic error and sampling variability).

FIGURE 2. SIMULATED DISTRIBUTION OF 100 PREVALENCE ESTIMATES WHERE TRUE
PREVALENCE = 0.10 AND N = 10

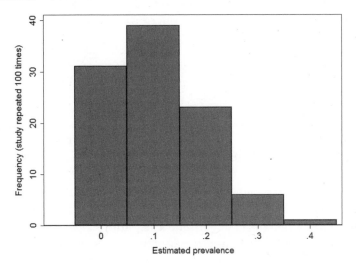

Estimated prevalence

RANDOM ERROR AND THE LAW OF LARGE NUMBERS

Figure 3 repeats the scenario from Figure 2—so, a study done 100 times in a
school with a population of 1000 students—but this time with a sample size of
n = 100 instead of n = 10. The figure shows that a serious error would be less
likely. The range of study outcomes is now much narrower.

FIGURE 3. SIMULATED DISTRIBUTION OF 100 PREVALENCE ESTIMATES WHERE TRUE
PREVALENCE = 0.10 AND N = 100

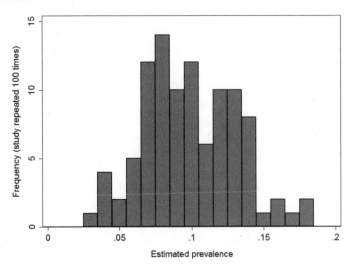

Estimated prevalence

The distributions of the hypothetical study results presented in Figure 2 and Figure 3 are simulations of sampling distributions, and they show the effect of the law of large numbers on random error: larger samples lower the probability that estimates will differ problematically from target parameters.

Key point: Random error in an estimate of an epidemiological parameter gets smaller as the sample size gets larger.

POOLING ESTIMATES TO INCREASE SAMPLE SIZE

There is a way to salvage studies that have a low sample size (and so have a high probability of random error). This involves combining estimates from several studies using meta-analysis. Meta-analysis is usually a component of a systematic review, which is a type of study that applies systematic research methods to better understand a literature of published or unpublished studies. For example, a systematic review uses carefully crafted and clearly documented literature-review strategies to find published studies, and makes careful efforts to find unpublished estimates. It involves carefully examining the literature for evidence that particular types of studies were more likely to be published than others—a phenomenon called *publication bias*. For example, publication bias would happen if positive studies (those with statistically significant results—the concept of statistical significance is discussed later in this chapter) were more likely to be published than negative studies. Systematic reviews also employ careful techniques to assess the quality of studies and to extract the study results accurately.

As the number of journals and number of studies increases, systematic reviews are becoming increasingly important as a way of summarizing available evidence. Meta-analysis and systematic reviews are not the same thing. A systematic review may use meta-analysis to statistically combine estimates from different studies as a means of gaining precision, but not all systematic reviews use meta-analytic methods. Some systematic reviews describe evidence in a literature without seeking to combine estimates statistically, a process called *narrative synthesis*. The Cochrane Collaboration is an international project seeking to produce high quality systematic reviews of important topics. Canadian researchers have been important contributors to this work.[104] Systematic reviews and meta-analysis are increasingly being applied to epidemiological studies, and guidelines for reporting them are available in the Preferred Reporting Items for Systematic Reviews and Meta-Analyses (PRISMA) statement.[105] The PRISMA statement includes a checklist of 27 characteristics that should be included in a report of a systematic review.[106] Because these characteristics need to be reported, they also need to be included in the design of a systematic review, so while intended as a description of how to report a systematic review, the PRISMA checklist also provides a partial guide for how to conduct a high quality systematic review.

In meta-analysis, estimates are only pooled if their differences are small enough to justify pooling. How much difference is "small enough"? If the variation among studies is consistent with the effect of random error, the estimates are said to be *homogeneous*, and pooling is considered justified. If they differ to a greater degree—a situation called *heterogeneity*—the implication is that the studies are estimating different population parameters. This could occur because the studies were conducted in populations with different population parameters, or the studies were of differing quality, or they used different measures, or they have other methodological differences. In such situations, it makes more sense to describe and understand the basis of the differences than to pool the estimates. Because the amount of heterogeneity is so important for deciding when to pool estimates, a statistic for describing it in meta-analysis is available. This statistic is called the *I-squared* (or I^2) value and represents the percent of variability in a set of study results that cannot be explained by random variation. If the I-squared value is low (usually, a value less than 30% or less than 50% is accepted as showing low heterogeneity), then the results can be pooled as if they were all estimates of the same (fixed) population value, which is called *fixed-effects meta-analysis*. If there is some heterogeneity, but not too much, meta-analysis also provides specialized techniques for pooling estimates using what is called *random-effects meta-analysis*. Rather than assuming that all of the estimates are estimating the same population value, random-effects meta-analysis assumes that all of the estimates come from the same distribution of underlying values. The whole idea of pooling is to find the underlying true value (or, in the case of random-effects meta-analysis, a distribution of values) that the studies are estimating. Pooling study results leads to a more precise estimate.

A good example of a systematic review and meta-analysis is a study of depression prevalence in epilepsy conducted by Fiest et al.[32] The literature contained several imprecise estimates of the prevalence of depression in epilepsy. Fiest et al used meta-analysis to combine the results from 9 studies reporting on a total of 29 891 people with epilepsy, leading to an estimated prevalence of "active depression" of 23.1%.

Systematic reviews are usually published in health science journals in a way that is similar to other scientific reports. However, in situations where synthesis of a rapidly evolving literature is urgently needed, a living systematic review may be conducted. Rather than implementing a protocol at a point in time, a living systematic review uses an ongoing process of literature searching, quality assessment, data abstraction, and analysis, continually incorporating new evidence as it becomes available.[107]

At the onset of the COVID-19 pandemic, resources were quickly directed towards researching this new disease. There was an urgency to synthesize this deluge of evidence, leading to the initiation of living systematic reviews. These reviews have since been producing constantly updated evidence synthesis for diverse topics such as ventilation techniques,[108] treatments for the COVID-19 infection,[109] and mental health during the pandemic.[110]

POOLING DATA (RATHER THAN ESTIMATES) TO INCREASE SAMPLE SIZE

Meta-analysis is one approach to improving the precision of epidemiologic estimates. Most commonly, meta-analysis is used to pool estimates of parameters from published studies based on a systematic review. Another approach to meta-analysis involves pooling study data rather than study estimates. This approach is called an *individual person data meta-analysis* (or sometimes an individual patient data meta-analysis). To conduct such a study, the investigator must obtain access to the data sets collected during each study, which can be difficult. If this task can be accomplished, however, there are many advantages to having individual-level data. The most important advantage is that the approach to data analysis can be uniform across the different studies, as the meta-analyst can work independently of the approaches to analysis of original authors. More informative analyses of individual person-level data are often possible.

Until recently, individual person data meta-analyses have been uncommon since scientists have been hesitant to share their data. This hesitancy is one of several factors that have led to a movement called the Open Science Movement, which favours greater availability and accessibility of publicly funded scientific research outputs, rigorous peer review, and greater transparency, all of which magnify the impact of scientific research.[111] An example of application of these principles is an open data platform set up by the federal government to enhance access to data about the COVID-19 pandemic.[112] Internationally, the Open Science Framework has become a popular tool to facilitate research collaboration.[113]

NETWORK META-ANALYSIS

A typical meta-analysis makes pairwise comparisons—for example, it may synthesize evidence about whether a drug works better than placebo. In this case, the pair of exposures under comparison are exposure to a drug versus placebo. In a meta-analysis of observational data, a pairwise comparison may examine whether people with a risk-factor exposure have higher risks than those without. However, in some situations there is value in synthesizing knowledge about a larger number of exposures—for example, when several treatments are available. Typically, the literature contains studies making some, but not all, of the possible head-to-head comparisons of these treatments. In some situations, such a literature allows formulation of indirect comparisons. Consider a situation in which 2 drugs have been compared to placebo, but not directly to each other. The performance of the drugs against placebo may provide indirect evidence of each drug's effectiveness. For example, if drug A performs much better than placebo compared to drug B, which is only modestly more effective than placebo, the indirect evidence suggests that drug A is the more effective of the 2 drugs. Network meta-analysis is a technique for evidence synthesis that uses network-analysis techniques to synthesize evidence from a literature that includes both direct and indirect evidence.

As systematic reviews of various types have become more common, the same, or closely related, questions often become the focus of more than one review. This has created a need to synthesize the findings of systematic reviews. An approach to doing this, called an *umbrella review*, has been proposed and is becoming increasing popular. Umbrella reviews began to appear in the mid-2000s, and methodological approaches to conducting them are beginning to be standardized.[114] In 2020 alone, more than 100 umbrella reviews were published.

As an example, Veronese et al[115] conducted an umbrella review to examine whether chocolate consumption conferred health risks or benefits. They identified 10 systematic reviews of this topic, 8 of which included meta-analysis. Collectively, the observational studies from these systematic reviews reported data from more than a million people. The umbrella review found evidence of reduced risk of cardiovascular disease, acute myocardial infarction, stroke, and diabetes. However, the umbrella review found that the credibility of the evidence was weak.

Quantifying random error

Epidemiology has 2 statistical strategies for dealing with random error: confidence intervals and statistical tests.

Confidence intervals

If you are designing a prevalence study, you want a sample size large enough to give you confidence in your estimates. If you are reading a study, you want to know how much confidence you can have in the study's results. Confidence intervals are the preferred statistical method for answering questions about confidence.

Here's a simple way to interpret confidence intervals: when working with sample-based data to generate estimated parameters, confidence intervals define a range of plausible values for true population parameters.

Two numbers called *confidence limits* demarcate confidence intervals: a number at the lower end of an interval's range (the lower confidence limit) and a number at the upper end (the upper confidence limit).

The best types of confidence intervals are exact confidence intervals, which are based on exact probabilities. These are difficult to calculate by hand, but easy to calculate with statistical software packages.

ESTIMATING CONFIDENCE INTERVALS

Many formulas can calculate approximate versions of confidence intervals. Under the assumption that a sampling distribution conforms to a normal distribution—which is a symmetrical bell-shaped distribution (roughly seen in Figure 3)—these formulas often take the following form: the point estimate (the value calculated from the study data) plus or minus the standard error multiplied by a number representing the desired level of confidence for the estimate.

Most investigators seek 95% confidence in their research, which makes the multiplier (based on a normal distribution) 1.96. So, you can approximate a 95% confidence interval (95% CI) as plus or minus 1.96 times the standard error of the parameter being estimated.

A formula for calculating standard error is presented on page 21. For now, let's revisit our hypothetical student-smoking study and assume a standard error of 0.04 for an estimated proportion from a sample of $n = 100$ in which the true population prevalence is 0.10. Multiplying the standard error by 1.96 gives us a value of 0.078, such that an approximate 95% CI is the estimated prevalence (whatever that might be in an individual study—remember that it is not going to be exactly 0.10 very often due to sampling variability) plus or minus 0.078. This provides a range of values within which it is possible to be 95% confident that the true population value lies.

You can also understand confidence intervals as long-run frequencies. For example, you could say that if a study were repeated many times, 95% of the time the confidence interval would include the true value.

PRECISION

The concept of precision is closely related to confidence intervals. Precision refers to the width of a confidence interval. Wide intervals mean low precision and narrow intervals mean high precision.

Precision is inversely related to the risk of random error. It is a key factor to consider in study design, and is directly relevant to critical appraisal of a study's vulnerability to random error. Epidemiological studies need designs that allow them to achieve adequate precision. When planning a study, the size of the sample must be decided. The sample size is the study-design issue that is most important for controlling or preventing random error. In practice, this means epidemiological studies must have large sample sizes, but sample-size calculations are needed to determine how large a sample is necessary. Precision-based sample-size calculations estimate the precision achievable in a study with a given sample size.

Key point: Epidemiological studies must provide adequate precision if their estimates are to be useful. In practice, this means that they must have large sample sizes.

FOREST PLOTS IN META-ANALYSIS

An interesting example of the use of confidence intervals is a type of plot seen in meta-analyses. Recall that meta-analysis is used to pool estimates from studies uncovered in systematic reviews, with the goal of increasing precision. Figure 4 shows a series of 20 studies, each having a sample size of 100 and each estimating a fixed prevalence of 0.5. Each of the 20 studies has similar precision, and the true population value usually falls within the 95% confidence limits seen in the figure, as expected. The diamond-shaped indicator at the bottom of the figure is the pooled value, according to a fixed-effect meta-analysis. In this case, the fixed-effects model combines the study estimates into a weighted average, weighted by the inverse of the variance associated with each study-level estimate. Variance is the standard error (introduced in the previous section) squared, so variance gets smaller as the sample size gets larger. These weights are presented on the right-hand side of the figure. Since there are 20 equally sized studies in this example, each study contributes about 5% to the pooled estimate. The I^2 value is small, indicating that there is little heterogeneity (as expected, since the underlying population prevalence has a fixed value of 0.5). Note that the pooling leads to greatly increased precision. The pooled estimate has a much narrower confidence interval than any of the individual studies.

A contrasting forest plot is presented in Figure 5. Here, the first 10 studies are estimating a prevalence of 40% and the next 10 studies are estimating a prevalence of 60%. The I^2 value suggests a lot of heterogeneity is present and the overall pooled estimate provides a poor description of both groups. In this situation, it would make most sense to evaluate the 2 sets of studies separately, as depicted in Figure 6.

FIGURE 4. FOREST PLOT SHOWING 20 SIMULATED STUDIES (*N* = 100 EACH), PREVALENCE (LABELLED ES) = 0.5

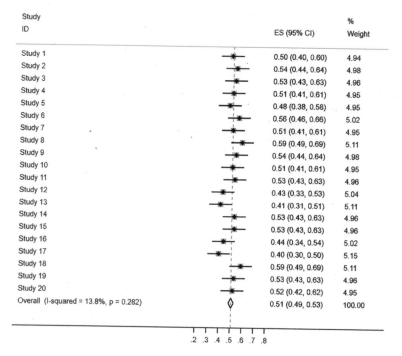

Study ID	ES (95% CI)	% Weight
Study 1	0.50 (0.40, 0.60)	4.94
Study 2	0.54 (0.44, 0.64)	4.98
Study 3	0.53 (0.43, 0.63)	4.96
Study 4	0.51 (0.41, 0.61)	4.95
Study 5	0.48 (0.38, 0.58)	4.95
Study 6	0.56 (0.46, 0.66)	5.02
Study 7	0.51 (0.41, 0.61)	4.95
Study 8	0.59 (0.49, 0.69)	5.11
Study 9	0.54 (0.44, 0.64)	4.98
Study 10	0.51 (0.41, 0.61)	4.95
Study 11	0.53 (0.43, 0.63)	4.96
Study 12	0.43 (0.33, 0.53)	5.04
Study 13	0.41 (0.31, 0.51)	5.11
Study 14	0.53 (0.43, 0.63)	4.96
Study 15	0.53 (0.43, 0.63)	4.96
Study 16	0.44 (0.34, 0.54)	5.02
Study 17	0.40 (0.30, 0.50)	5.15
Study 18	0.59 (0.49, 0.69)	5.11
Study 19	0.53 (0.43, 0.63)	4.96
Study 20	0.52 (0.42, 0.62)	4.95
Overall (I-squared = 13.8%, p = 0.282)	0.51 (0.49, 0.53)	100.00

.2 .3 .4 .5 .6 .7 .8

FIGURE 5. FOREST PLOT SHOWING 20 SIMULATED STUDIES (*N* = 100 EACH), PREVALENCE (LABELLED ES) = 0.4 OR 0.5

Study ID	ES (95% CI)	% Weight
Study 1	0.37 (0.28, 0.46)	5.06
Study 2	0.46 (0.36, 0.56)	4.75
Study 3	0.31 (0.22, 0.40)	5.51
Study 4	0.43 (0.33, 0.53)	4.81
Study 5	0.35 (0.26, 0.44)	5.18
Study 6	0.41 (0.31, 0.51)	4.87
Study 7	0.29 (0.20, 0.38)	5.73
Study 8	0.39 (0.29, 0.49)	4.96
Study 9	0.35 (0.26, 0.44)	5.18
Study 10	0.37 (0.28, 0.46)	5.06
Study 11	0.57 (0.47, 0.67)	4.81
Study 12	0.59 (0.49, 0.69)	4.87
Study 13	0.67 (0.58, 0.76)	5.33
Study 14	0.55 (0.45, 0.65)	4.76
Study 15	0.51 (0.41, 0.61)	4.72
Study 16	0.57 (0.47, 0.67)	4.81
Study 17	0.59 (0.49, 0.69)	4.87
Study 18	0.60 (0.50, 0.70)	4.91
Study 19	0.59 (0.49, 0.69)	4.87
Study 20	0.60 (0.50, 0.70)	4.91
Overall (I-squared = 83.5%, p = 0.000)	0.48 (0.45, 0.50)	100.00

.2 .3 .4 .5 .6 .7 .8

FIGURE 6. FOREST PLOT SHOWING 20 SIMULATED STUDIES (*N* = 100 EACH), PREVALENCE (LABELLED ES) = 0.4 OR 0.5, META-ANALYZED AS SUBGROUP

Study ID		ES (95% CI)	% Weight
1			
Study 1		0.33 (0.24, 0.42)	10.71
Study 2		0.42 (0.32, 0.52)	9.72
Study 3		0.46 (0.36, 0.56)	9.53
Study 4		0.38 (0.28, 0.48)	10.05
Study 5		0.43 (0.33, 0.53)	9.66
Study 6		0.43 (0.33, 0.53)	9.66
Study 7		0.40 (0.30, 0.50)	9.86
Study 8		0.42 (0.32, 0.52)	9.72
Study 9		0.29 (0.20, 0.38)	11.50
Study 10		0.44 (0.34, 0.54)	9.61
Subtotal (I-squared = 21.0%, p = 0.250)		0.40 (0.37, 0.43)	100.00
2			
Study 11		0.63 (0.54, 0.72)	9.92
Study 12		0.63 (0.54, 0.72)	9.92
Study 13		0.65 (0.56, 0.74)	10.16
Study 14		0.61 (0.51, 0.71)	9.72
Study 15		0.59 (0.49, 0.69)	9.56
Study 16		0.57 (0.47, 0.67)	9.43
Study 17		0.60 (0.50, 0.70)	9.63
Study 18		0.57 (0.47, 0.67)	9.43
Study 19		0.75 (0.67, 0.83)	12.33
Study 20		0.63 (0.54, 0.72)	9.92
Subtotal (I-squared = 24.7%, p = 0.216)		0.63 (0.60, 0.66)	100.00

.2 .3 .4 .5 .6 .7 .8

Statistical tests

Epidemiologists use statistical tests less often than confidence intervals. Statistical tests do not have much value in the context of prevalence estimates, so we will use an analytical question to discuss them: whether or not a risk factor (an exposure) is associated with a disease.

Statistical tests begin by formulating a null hypothesis. This amounts to a conjecture that an exposure has no effect on a disease. Of course, in an analytical study, a researcher is likely conducting the study for the opposite reason: because they suspect a particular exposure does, in fact, affect a disease. However, it is much easier to refute a hypothesis than to prove a hypothesis—you only need 1 piece of evidence to refute, but a mountain of evidence to prove (and some say no amount of evidence will entirely prove a hypothesis). So, if a researcher wants to evaluate whether an exposure is associated with a disease, they assume there is no association. In other words, they adopt the null hypothesis for the purpose of trying to disprove it.

Key point: A statistical test can only seek to disprove a hypothesis. These tests cannot directly support a hypothesis.

The next step is to analyze the data collected in the study using an appropriate statistical test. The statistical test assumes the null hypothesis is true, and calculates the probability that what was observed in the data (or something more extreme) would arise given the null hypothesis. This probability is the P value associated with the statistical test, and 5% is the typical critical value against which a determination is made. If a set of findings, or more extreme findings, would occur less than 5% of the time, it is concluded that the findings are unlikely under the null hypothesis, so that the null hypothesis is rejected and the alternative hypothesis—that there is an association between exposure and disease—is accepted. If the P value is less than 5%, the null hypothesis can be rejected with 95% confidence, and the statistical test is said to be significant. Another name for critical value is *alpha value*.

TYPE I ERROR AND TYPE II ERROR

A statistical test provides a binary outcome. It either rejects, or fails to reject, a null hypothesis, and thereby finds, or fails to find, evidence of an association.

There are 2 ways in which a statistical test can be wrong.

If the null hypothesis really is true, but the results of the statistical test are significant, a type I error has occurred. The probability of type I error is preset by the statistical testing procedure. Since 5% is usually the chosen cut point for assessment of significance, it can be expected that 5% of significant results will be due to chance and therefore represent type I errors.

If the null hypothesis really is false, but a statistical test is not significant, a type II error has occurred. Type II errors are related to the concept of statistical power. Statistical power is the probability of (correctly) rejecting a null hypothesis that is false. The risk of type II error in a study is the complement of power. If the power of a study is 80%, it has an 80% chance of detecting (with a significant test result) that the null hypothesis is false, assuming that the null hypothesis actually is false. Consequently, this level of power signifies a 20% chance that a type II error will occur. Sometimes, the probability of a type II error is called the *ß probability*, such that power = 1 minus ß.

Figure 7 summarizes the types of error associated with statistical tests.

How can statistical errors be avoided? Type I error is best avoided by limiting the number of tests. If a study evaluates a single hypothesis, the risk of type I error is correctly quantified by the specified critical value, usually 5%. However, if many tests are done, then it is very likely that 1 or more of the significant results will be erroneous. Type II error is best avoided by ensuring an adequate sample size. Sample size is a key determinant of statistical power—just as in the area of estimation it was the key determinant of precision. Modern statistical software usually includes commands for calculating power according to different assumptions and at different sample sizes. Such calculations are indispensable in the planning of an epidemiological study.

FIGURE 7. ERRORS THAT CAN ARISE FROM STATISTICAL TESTS

	An association exists in the population (null hypothesis is false)	No association exists in the population (null hypothesis is true)
Statistical test is significant	No error	Type I error
Statistical test is not significant	Type II error	No error

A worrisome feature of errors in statistical tests is that they can be used to distort scientific results—an unethical practice informally known as *p-hacking*. For example, an unethical or incompetent investigator could repeatedly conduct analysis during an ongoing study, and stop collecting data when a significant *P* value is achieved. Or, they could analyze measures, or use the same measures in multiple ways, and only report the significant results—a process knows as a "fishing expedition."

The best protection against p-hacking is the prior publication of a study protocol that includes an analysis plan. If this protocol is published before the data are analyzed, then deviations from the original analysis plan cannot be hidden. The PRISMA checklist, described on page 68 as a reporting guide for systematic reviews, requires authors to indicate if a review protocol exists and where it can be accessed. This helps to protect against p-hacking. The archiving of study protocols before studies are conducted is standard procedure for systematic reviews and randomized controlled trials. They are equally valuable for observational studies, and they are increasingly seen in the observational literature.

Clearly formulated research questions are another protection against p-hacking. The most widely used approach to formulating clear questions is "PICO," originally proposed by Richardson et al. PICO is an acronym for key components of a research question, which Richardson et al describe as: 1) the patient or problem being addressed; 2) the intervention or exposure being considered; 3) the comparison intervention or exposure, when relevant; and 4) the clinical outcomes of interest.[116] Some epidemiologists add "population" as the *P* in PICO to make this system fully applicable to epidemiologic research.

Theory may also give protection. A theory is a set of ideas or concepts that provides a system for explaining a phenomenon. If there is a strong theory, it may provide strong ideas about key questions to be asked, allowing a detailed analysis plan to focus on a small set of hypothesized outcomes. Disciplined adherence to such a plan can help prevent type I errors and p-hacking.

Finally, statistical tests can be 1-tailed or 2-tailed. When the null hypothesis states that there is no difference between 2 groups, a 2-tailed test evaluates the probability that the observed outcomes (or more extreme outcomes) could arise by chance, without specifying the direction of the difference. In a 1-tailed test, the direction is specified. For example, a 1-tailed test might be done if an exposure could only increase, and never decrease, the risk of a disease. By contrast, a 2-tailed test would allow for the exposure to increase or decrease the risk of disease. Almost always, 2-tailed tests are preferred in epidemiological research.

Confidence intervals versus statistical tests

Why are confidence intervals preferred over statistical tests in epidemiology?

One reason is that some of the goals of epidemiology are better accommodated by confidence intervals. Descriptive epidemiologic research often has the goal of estimating a parameter such as prevalence, which has no meaningful null hypothesis to reject. Analytical studies have the explicit goal of evaluating a hypothesis, so in theory statistical testing is a better fit with analytical studies.

However, the goal of evaluating associations is usually done by estimating parameters that embody the comparison of interest (e.g., a comparison between 2 incidence proportions). These parameters have null values built into them. For example, an analytic parameter called *relative risk* is calculated as a ratio: the risk for people exposed to a risk factor (numerator) and the risk for those not exposed to the risk factor (denominator). Under the null hypothesis, the relative risk would be 1.0. As it turns out, if a 95% confidence interval for the null hypothesis fails to include this null value, then a statistical test of the null hypothesis would have been significant at the 5% level of confidence. Therefore, confidence intervals provide all of the information that statistical tests provide, but also much more: they also provide an estimate of the strength of association and identify a range of plausible values for that parameter in the population.

Thinking deeper

Calculating confidence intervals

Chapter 2 presented a formula for estimating the standard error of a proportion:

$$\text{Standard Error} = \sqrt{\frac{p \times (1-p)}{n}}$$

where p is any proportion estimated from a sample of size n

You can use this general formula to calculate an approximate 95% confidence interval (95% CI) in situations where you can reasonably expect a normal distribution for p. You can use the prevalence calculated from a sample to estimate standard error. The following formula gives this general approach, substituting *prevalence* for the unspecified proportion (p):

$$\text{Lower 95\% Confidence Limit} = \text{Prevalence} - 1.96\sqrt{\frac{\text{Prevalence} \times (1 - \text{Prevalence})}{n}}$$

$$\text{Upper 95\% Confidence Limit} = \text{Prevalence} + 1.96\sqrt{\frac{\text{Prevalence} \times (1 - \text{Prevalence})}{n}}$$

Think about our hypothetical student-smoking study again. Table 8 presents data for an iteration of this study where $n = 100$.

TABLE 8. 1 × 2 TABLE DEPICTING SMOKING STATUS IN A SAMPLE OF $N = 100$ STUDENTS

Smokes	Does not smoke	Total
11	89	100

This is how you would calculate the approximate 95% confidence interval for the data in Table 8:

$$\text{Lower 95\% Confidence Limit} = \text{Prevalence} - 1.96\sqrt{\frac{0.11 \times (1 - 0.11)}{100}}$$

$$\text{Upper 95\% Confidence Limit} = \text{Prevalence} + 1.96\sqrt{\frac{0.11 \times (1 - 0.11)}{100}}$$

This approximates the 95% CI (rounded to 2 decimal places) as 0.05–0.17, which means you can be close to 95% confident that the true population value is within this range.

Of course, in research, it's better to calculate exact confidence intervals with statistical software, and you should always do exact calculations for work that appears in presentations or publications. For the data in Table 8, statistical software calculates the exact confidence interval as 0.06–0.19, which is fairly close to the formula-derived approximation.

The confidence-interval formula is useful for designing studies that aim to estimate a parameter such as prevalence. Researchers might have a strong idea of the true prevalence—for example, in the case of the hypothetical student-smoking study, we knew 0.10 was likely the true prevalence.[103] They can then estimate the standard error based on the confidence-interval formula, using the expected prevalence and the anticipated sample size. Such a calculation allows prediction about the extent of precision achievable with a particular sample size. If a researcher knows the level of precision required to achieve the objectives of a study, they can evaluate the adequacy of different sample sizes through a series of such calculations. This strategy is called *precision-based sample-size calculation*. See the paper by Johnston et al, "Do clinicians understand the size of treatment effects?", for an example of using this strategy.[117(p27)]

Questions

1. What are the key features of critical appraisal? To what extent are these features applied in media reports covering health issues?

2. Describe the defining characteristic of random error in epidemiology.

3. A study by Thege et al[118] reported the prevalence of self-reported sex addiction as 3%, with a standard error of 0.42%. What is an approximate 95% CI for this estimate of the prevalence of sex addiction?

4. The study by Thege et al used a survey conducted over the telephone. Some randomly reached respondents might have been hesitant to disclose information about their sex lives over the phone. Would this have resulted in random error?

5. Bonaparte et al[36] reported that the age-adjusted incidence rate for amyotrophic lateral sclerosis in Newfoundland in 2003 was 2.13 per 100 000, and reported an associated 95% CI of 0.11–4.15 per 100 000. Provide an interpretation for this confidence interval.

6. Why is the critical value for statistical significance most often set at 5%?

7. Setting the critical value for statistical significance at 5% implies a 5% chance of type I error. Power is often set at 80% when studies are designed, suggesting a 20% chance of type II error. Why is it acceptable that the chance of type II error should be 4 times higher than the chance of type I error?

8. Some authors report the statistical significance of study results approximately (e.g., $P < 0.05$), whereas others prefer to report the exact P value (e.g., $P = 0.037$). Which approach do you feel is superior?

9. Statistical software programs sometimes report P values that are equal to zero (e.g., $P = 0.00$). Do you think it makes sense to report P values in this way?

10. State 3 advantages of confidence intervals over tests of statistical significance.

Measurement error that leads to misclassification

OBJECTIVES

- Define measurement error, and distinguish it from selection error.
- Distinguish among nominal, ordinal, ratio, and interval data, and continuous and discrete data.
- Define and explain strategies for describing classification errors: sensitivity and specificity; positive and negative predictive value; Bayes' theorem; likelihood ratios; and reliability.

Measurement error in context

Chapter 5 covered random error in epidemiological research.

Chapters 6, 7, and 8 focus on systematic error. Unlike random error, systematic error does not diminish with larger sample size. It comes from defects in study design that remain unchanged no matter how large the sample. Systematic error leads to bias in epidemiological research—in other words, estimates that systematically over- or underestimate the true values.

For descriptive parameters such as prevalence, there are 2 types of study-design defects that can introduce systematic error: measurement error and selection error.

This chapter and the next look at measurement error: first, at its sources and at ways to quantify its extent; and then, at its effect on parameter estimation.

Chapter 8 looks at selection error and its effects on parameter estimation.

What is measurement error?

Epidemiological estimates are precisely that: estimates of underlying epidemiology, not direct representations. To calculate an epidemiological estimate, you need to assign values to 1 or more variables for all members of the sample that forms the basis of your estimate. Assigning these values requires measurement.

In a prevalence study, each member of a sample is assigned a variable that can take on different values depending on the member's disease status. Once assigned, these values are recorded as pieces of information collectively referred to as data, and are stored in a data set for analysis.

But, assigning values to variables is not always a perfect process. It is possible that a person with a disease may be incorrectly classified as not having that disease and vice versa.

Epidemiologists are often concerned with classification into categories (especially disease and exposure categories), so errors of classification—misclassification—are a particularly important type of measurement error in epidemiology.

Measurement error compromises the accuracy of epidemiological estimates. It is important to understand how such errors occur so that they can be avoided during study design and, if not, detected during critical appraisal.

Types of data

There are several distinct types of data (all of which provide information). Different types of data require different ways of thinking about measurement. Also, different statistical techniques are appropriate for different types of data. You need to understand data types to do good data analysis, and to understand statistical analyses reported in studies.

Nominal, ordinal, ratio, and interval data

Nominal data are an important data type for epidemiology. As the name suggests, nominal data conform to categories that can be named, such as sex (male and female), marital status (married, unmarried, divorced. widowed), race (Asian, Métis, Caucasian, etc.), and country of origin (Canada, Uganda, Peru, etc.). There is no ordering of these categories. Usually, a diagnosis is a nominal category, as is exposure to a risk factor.

Ordinal data provide information about ranking. Some studies use rating scales to assign numbers to otherwise abstract concepts such as self-esteem, distress, or quality of life. These data have no physical meaning as numbers, and therefore cannot usually be treated as real numbers. For example, many of Statistics Canada's national surveys use the Kessler-6 or K-6 scale (named after its developer, Ron Kessler of Harvard University) to assess nonspecific psychological distress.[119] This scale provides scores on a range of 0 to 24. Because these are numerical scores, it is tempting to give the numbers real meaning—for example, to view a score of 10 as "twice" a score of 5, or to view the difference between scores of 5 and 10 as equivalent to the difference between scores of 15 and 20. However, these scores do not possess mathematical properties, except that a higher score is greater than a lower score.

Here's an example of rating that results in ordinal data. A questionnaire asks, "During the past month, about how often did you feel nervous?" A subject can respond, "all of the time" (which is scored 4), "most of the time" (scored 3), "some of the time" (scored 2), "a little of the time" (scored 1), and "none of the time" (scored 0). The numbers rank narrative statements. Clearly, a score of 4 is greater than a score of 2, but nothing says it's 2 times greater. Normal operations of arithmetic, such as calculating ratios, do not apply to this kind of data.

Types of data to which mathematical concepts such as ratios and differences apply can be called *numerical data*. This term requires careful use, however, since numbers are sometimes assigned arbitrarily to ordinal (or sometimes even nominal) data.

Ratio data are data for which ratios are meaningful. Height is an example of ratio data. A person 2 metres tall is twice as tall as a person 1 metre tall.

Interval data are data for which differences are meaningful. Height is again an example: it is a real physical quantity and, so, has meaningful intervals. The difference in the height of a person 2 metres tall and a person 1 metre tall is exactly the same as the difference in height between people who are 2 and 3 metres tall.

It is possible for a scale to have interval properties but not ratio properties. For example, the Celsius temperature scale does not allow you to say that 15 degrees is only half as warm as 30 degrees—because 0 on this scale is arbitrary, chosen for convenience (the temperature at which water freezes under specified atmospheric conditions). By contrast, the Kelvin scale has a real 0 (absolute zero) and therefore is a ratio and an interval scale.

Discrete versus continuous data

Height and temperature are also examples of continuous variables. Any values for height or temperature have, at least in theory, an infinite number of values between them, although in reality there is a limit to the level of precision with which such variables can be measured.

By contrast, a discrete variable has a limited and countable number of possible values. Note that nominal and ordinal variables are not discrete, since such variables do not have real numerical values. A typical example of a discrete variable is a count, such as the number of people in a city or the number of diagnoses assigned to a person. Counted data of this type is sometimes called *cardinal data*. There are interrelationships between these types of data. Having a disease or not is a nominal distinction that has no real relationship to a number. However, if the number of people with a disease is counted, this count becomes a numerical variable having discrete values.

A note about the word data

Epidemiologists, and others, use the word *data* sometimes as a singular term ("the data has a normal distribution") and sometimes as a plural term ("the data have a normal distribution"). This causes a degree of acrimony.

Data derives from Latin: it is a second declension noun of the neuter type. This means that the singular form is *datum* and the plural is *data*. So, by origin, *data* is plural, but its use as a singular term has more and more currency. Some researchers regard the plural usage as a deliberate archaism that serves no purpose.

Other second declension neuter nouns from Latin—those that have not come into common use among the general public—have not evolved in the same way. A good example from epidemiology (and geology) is *stratum* (singular) and *strata* (plural).

This book uses *data* as a plural.

Categorizing continuous variables

In the social sciences, researchers often frown on categorizing continuous variables—variables that are not inherently categorical. Researchers in epidemiology, however, frequently categorize continuous variables. In epidemiology, continuous variables often have meaningful ranges that translate into meaningful categories.

Body mass index, used as an indicator of body composition, is an example. Body mass index is calculated as body weight (in kilograms) divided by height (in metres) squared. This index could theoretically divide into an infinite number of categories—so, it is a continuous variable. However, it is often divided into categories defined by ranges of value, such as underweight, normal weight, overweight, and obese.

Blood pressure is another example. Blood pressure is inherently a continuous variable, but it is often made into a binary variable: normotensive (normal blood pressure) and hypertensive (high blood pressure). Such categorization inevitably results in the loss of some information. For example, if a diastolic blood pressure greater than 90 millimetres of mercury (mmHg) is regarded as hypertensive in a binary categorization, then 89 mmHg will be treated differently than 91 mmHg, even though the actual values are nearly identical. The binary categorization also means that 91 mmHg will be treated the same as 120 mmHg, even though these values are very different.

A lot of categorization occurs in epidemiology despite this obvious loss of information. There is a reason. Epidemiology is a health research discipline, and its methods are closely tied to real-world decision making in professional practice, health service planning, and health policy. Categories often facilitate real-world decisions. They provide guidelines to practitioners about which patients require treatment; they help service planners determine how many people need treatment; and they help policy makers anticipate the preventive value of interventions.

You could say the concept of diagnosis itself imposes categories onto what are sometimes graduated or continuous departures from a physiologic norm. Take blood pressure again. Even though blood pressure is inherently a continuous variable, we know that blood pressure above certain thresholds has impacts on health and requires treatment.

> *Key point:* Artificial categorization is a theoretically problematic manoeuvre, but it often makes sense in epidemiology.

Quantifying classification errors

As a result of the predominant use of categories in epidemiology, the most important forms of measurement error are those that involve classification into the wrong categories, or misclassification. Fortunately, a set of parameters exists that quantify the likelihood of misclassification and thereby the accuracy of measurement.

Sensitivity and specificity

There are 2 key parameters that quantify the extent of misclassification: sensitivity and specificity.

Both these parameters quantify the performance of a classification method or instrument in relation to a gold standard. A gold standard is a measurement that does not make classification errors. Table 9 shows a way of dividing a group of people according to their true status (the columns, according to a gold standard) and the way in which they are classified by a potentially error-prone test or classification procedure. Until recently, this type of 2 × 2 table didn't have its own name. However, a term from the computer science literature is beginning to be used: *confusion matrix*. The table refers to a diagnostic test, so the column titles refer to a gold standard designation of disease status. Note, however, that you could use a table of this type for any type of attribute.

> *Key point:* Determining the performance of a diagnostic test requires comparison to a gold standard.

TABLE 9. 2 × 2 TABLE DESCRIBING THE PERFORMANCE OF A CLASSIFICATION PROCEDURE

	Has the disease	Does not have the disease
Test positive	True positive (*tp*)	False positive (*fp*)
Test negative	False negative (*fn*)	True negative (*tn*)

As with many other epidemiological parameters, sensitivity and specificity can be conceptualized as either a frequency or probability. The labels contained in Table 9 (tp, *fp*, *fn*, *tn*) offer a means of producing formulas to estimate sensitivity and specificity from a sample:

$$\text{Sensitivity} = \frac{tp}{tp + fn}$$

$$\text{Specificity} = \frac{tn}{tn + fp}$$

Note the use of lowercase letters in these formulas, in keeping with the conventions for sample-based estimates.

VALIDATION STUDIES

The sort of study from which sensitivity and specificity are calculated is called a *validation study*. Validation studies involve a series of steps. First, researchers obtain a sample of people with and without a disease (according to a gold standard assessment instrument). They then administer a test or classification procedure to each member of the sample, which allows them to classify each respondent into one of the 4 groups identified in Table 9: tp, fp, fn, tn. From these counts, they can estimate the sensitivity and specificity as a frequency that—if the study is conducted properly and has a large enough sample—provides information about the probabilities of correct and incorrect classification.

Stated in the language of probability, sensitivity is the probability that a person with an attribute is classified correctly by a test (or other classification procedure). Specificity is the probability that a person without the attribute is correctly classified by a test (or classification procedure). Of course, in an epidemiological study, the attribute could be exposure or disease.

Sensitivity and specificity describe test characteristics: they reflect the performance of a test itself, rather than the characteristics of the population in which the tests are used.

Key point: Sensitivity and specificity are characteristics of a test or classification procedure, and do not depend very much on characteristics of the population in which the test is used.

THE CONCEPT OF VALIDITY

Sensitivity and specificity quantify the performance of a test or classification procedure in relation to the truth (a gold standard classification). In other words, they provide an assessment of the truthfulness of the results of that test or procedure.

Validity—a term with various uses commonly encountered in the epidemiological literature—refers to the same issue of truthfulness one way or another. So, an epidemiological study is valid if its results provide an accurate reflection of an epidemiologic reality, and a diagnostic test is valid if it accurately identifies the disease status of those who are tested. The term *validity* appears in other contexts as well. It always refers to whether a result is truthful or correct, such as the validity of interpretations or judgements of investigators.

Complements of sensitivity and specificity

Many of the proportions and probabilities encountered in epidemiological studies have complementary proportions and probabilities. The term *complementary* means these probabilities add up to 1. For example, if prevalence is the proportion of a population that has a disease, the complementary proportion consists of those who do not have the disease.

In classification, complementary proportions and probabilities are especially important, and have their own names. The complement of sensitivity is the false-negative rate. (Here, unfortunately, is another questionable use of *rate*. The name for this complement would be better as *false-negative proportion*, but this is rarely used.) The false-negative rate is the proportion of those with the disease who are classified incorrectly as not having it.

$$\text{False-Negative Rate} = 1 - \text{Sensitivity}$$

Considering the terminology, it seems perfectly reasonable to call sensitivity the *true-positive proportion*.

The complement of specificity is the false-positive rate (or, preferably, proportion). This is the proportion of people without the disease who end up being classified as having it.

$$\text{False-Positive Rate} = 1 - \text{Specificity}$$

Both sensitivity and specificity are determined by comparing the classification provided by a test or classification procedure to a true gold standard—in other words, by comparing the performance of the test to a criterion that determines whether the test's classification is correct or not. This means that both sensitivity and specificity are examples of criterion validity.

Predictive value

Sensitivity and specificity are the most important parameters for quantifying the validity of a testing procedure, but they have a notable limitation. Both parameters are conditional probabilities—necessitating the term *given* in their probability-based definitions. For example, sensitivity is the probability of a positive test given the presence of disease. Specificity is the probability of a negative test given the absence of a disease. However, both probabilities are conditional on a status that is unknown—whether a person has the disease (or other attribute) or not. Obviously, if disease status were known, there would be no need for the test. Because of this limitation, 2 other important classification parameters are needed: positive and negative predictive values.

Positive predictive value is the probability of disease given a positive result on a test or classification procedure. Negative predictive value is the probability of no disease given a negative test result. The advantage of these parameters is immediately apparent: they are still conditional probabilities, but they are conditional on something that is known (test status) rather than something that is unknown (disease status). Again, these are frequencies that can be estimated from samples, but which represent probabilities.

A frequency-based formula for positive predictive value, calculated from a sample, is as follows:

$$\text{Positive Predictive Value} = \frac{tp}{tp + fp}$$

Here is a frequency-based formula for negative predictive value, calculated from a sample:

$$\text{Negative Predictive Value} = \frac{tn}{tn + fn}$$

These parameters are very helpful to clinicians who have performed diagnostic tests and need to interpret the results. They are also very important for screening—where a brief test is administered to populations in an effort to increase early detection of a disease.

Positive predictive value and negative predictive value address a problem with sensitivity and specificity, but these parameters come with their own difficulty—namely, they do not describe test characteristics (unlike sensitivity and specificity). They depend partially on the performance of the test or classification procedure in question, and partially on the frequency of disease in a population. In other words, the same test or classification procedure, with the same sensitivity and specificity, can lead to extremely different predictive values in different populations.

Key point: Predictive values of diagnostic tests and other classification procedures partially reflect the performance of the tests, but partially reflect the characteristics of the population in which the tests are administered.

Bayes' theorem

Bayes' theorem, which is a theorem of conditional probability, provides a formula for understanding the relationship among predictive value, sensitivity, specificity, and the prior probability of disease:

$$\text{Positive Predictive Value} = \frac{Se \times \text{Prior Probability}}{\left(Se \times \text{Prior Probability}\right) + \left[\left(1 - Sp\right) \times \left(1 - \text{Prior Probability}\right)\right]}$$

where Se is sensitivity and Sp is specificity

Prior probability, sometimes also called *pretest probability*, is the probability that a person being tested has the disease before the test results are known. For example, if testing is performed in a clinic where a known proportion of patients has the disease, this proportion is a tangible baseline frequency—often called a *base rate* in the clinical epidemiology literature (yet another unfortunate use of *rate*). The proportion could also represent a clinician's judgement of the probability of disease in a particular patient, given the patient's signs and symptoms. In the case of a test used for population screening, the prior probability—again, often called the *base rate*—is the prevalence of disease in the population being screened.

Key point: Predictive value can be calculated from characteristics of a test (sensitivity and specificity) and the pretest probability or prevalence of a disease.

A similar formula can be used to calculate the negative predictive value of a test:

$$\text{Negative Predictive Value} = \frac{Sp \times \left(1 - \text{Prior Probability}\right)}{\left[Sp \times \left(1 - \text{Prior Probability}\right)\right] + \left[\left(1 - Se\right) \times \left(\text{Prior Probability}\right)\right]}$$

where Se is sensitivity and Sp is specificity

These formulas may look complicated, but they are similar to the frequency-based formulas presented earlier in this chapter. If you look carefully, you will see the similarities. The numerator of the Bayesian formula for negative predictive value is the product of the frequency of people who do not have the disease (the complement of the frequency of those who do) multiplied by the frequency with which they are correctly classified as not having the disease (specificity). So, the numerator is the expected proportion of true negatives in the sample. The left-hand term in the denominator is identical to the numerator, aligning with the frequency-based definition. The right-hand term in the denominator equates with the expected proportion of false-negative results— given the false-negative rate (1 − sensitivity) associated with the test—multiplied by the frequency of disease. As in the formulas for positive and negative predictive value, the denominator represents both true-negative and false-negative results.

Likelihood ratios

A likelihood ratio is another important way to quantify the meaning of tests or classification procedures. It can be expressed in positive or negative terms, but the positive version—the likelihood ratio positive—is most common. In fact, *likelihood ratio* generally means the likelihood ratio positive.

The parameter can be calculated using the sensitivity and specificity of the test:

$$\text{Likelihood Ratio} = \frac{\text{Sensitivity}}{1 - \text{Specificity}}$$

Conceptually, this is the probability of a positive test when disease is truly present divided by the probability of a positive test when disease is truly absent (or, the true-positive rate divided by the false-positive rate). This likelihood ratio can be used to calculate the impact of a positive test on the best estimate of whether a person has a disease. The relationship is as follows:

$$\text{Posttest Odds} = \text{Pretest Odds} \times \text{Likelihood Ratio}$$

Clearly, this is similar to the Bayesian approach, but it uses odds rather than proportions. The pretest odds are akin to the pretest probability (or a base rate expressed as odds). This is, perhaps, a quicker and more straightforward way to estimate the likelihood of disease, given a test result, than the Bayesian formula. Odds, however, are less familiar to most people than frequencies and proportions. Fortunately, as noted in chapter 3 (see page 31), it is very easy to calculate odds from proportions and vice versa.

$$\text{Odds} = \frac{\text{Proportion}}{1 - \text{Proportion}}$$

$$\text{Proportion} = \frac{\text{Odds}}{1 + \text{Odds}}$$

The specific parameters mentioned above are the most important indices of measurement validity used in epidemiology: they are all examples of criterion validity when the criterion is a gold standard. However, in your reading you may encounter additional terminology describing validity, especially in situations in which there is no available gold standard, or where one seems unnecessary. *Face validity* means that the measure seems (on its face) to be measuring what is intended. For example, a common questionnaire item asks,

"In general would you say your health is excellent, very good, good, fair, or poor?" This item seems, on its face, to be measuring perceived health. *Concurrent validity* (a type of criterion validity) means that the test agrees with something else (a criterion), but adds the additional proviso that agreement is assessed at a point in time. *Predictive valdity* means that the measure can predict something that it should predict in the future. For example, the intelligence quotient (IQ) is intended to predict performance in school. It would not be considered valid unless it did so.

Reliability

Interrater and test-retest reliability

Reliability refers to the repeatability of a measure. In epidemiology, there are 2 key types of reliability: interrater reliability and test-retest reliability.

Often, measurement requires a "rater"—for example, a clinician who decides (rates) whether a patient has a disease. If the procedure for diagnosis is reliable, 2 clinicians assessing the same patient should come to the same conclusion. This concept of agreement between different raters is the concept of interrater reliability.

The concept of test-retest reliability applies if a clinician were to assess the same patient more than once—if the procedure for diagnosis is reliable, the clinician should come to the same conclusion each time.

When used in research, these terms do not always apply to assignment of a diagnosis. They may refer to the repeatability of any type of measure of any type of attribute.

Coefficients for quantifying reliability

Where ratings consist of nominal classifications, such as diagnoses, reliability is often quantified with kappa coefficients. Where ratings consist of ordinal or numerical classifications, reliability is quantified with correlation coefficients.

Correlation coefficients include the Pearson product moment coefficient, the Spearman rank correlation coefficient, and the intraclass correlation coefficient (ICC). The Pearson and Spearman coefficients both compare pairs of measures: the Spearman coefficient uses rankings and is considered more appropriate for ordinal data, whereas the Pearson coefficient is usually more appropriate for continuous data. The ICC compares groups of measures.

Correlation coefficients have a range of values between 1 and -1, where 1 indicates perfect positive linear relationship, -1 indicates perfect negative linear relationship, and 0 indicates no linear relationship. The kappa coefficient has a similar interpretation, although the "linear" part does not apply because the kappa coefficient quantifies agreement between nominal ratings.

Oremus et al[120] published an interesting assessment of reliability statistics. These investigators examined the reliability of scales used to rate the quality of published studies. This type of quality rating is used to guide the selection of studies for systematic reviews of the health science literature. The investigators noted that students often do the work of quality rating, so they used student ratings to assess the interrater and test-retest reliability of 2 numeric scales, and of ratings based on categorical indicators (e.g., excellent, mediocre, poor). They used correlation coefficients to assess agreement of the numeric scales and kappa coefficients for the categorical indicators. They found generally poor interrater reliability, but better test-retest reliability. They hypothesized that better training of student raters would enhance the quality of systematic reviews of the literature.

With self-rated measures (e.g., where study subjects rate some aspect of themselves), the concept of interrater reliability does not apply. However, test-retest reliability is still an important characteristic of such measures. For example, Kassam et al developed a scale to measure stigmatizing attitudes about mental illness held by health care professionals. This study was a component of the antistigma work of Mental Health Commission of Canada.[121] Kassam's scale—called the OMS-HC—is a 20-item scale that produces ordinal scores with potential values between 20 and 100. Because this scale produces dimensional ratings rather than nominal ones, kappa coefficients were not appropriate as measures of agreement. Instead, the study used ICCs to quantify test-retest reliability. The study reported an ICC of 0.66, which was interpreted as adequate test-retest reliability.

Another metric related to testing, called the *positivity rate* (or, sometimes, the percent positive) has become widely used during the COVID-19 pandemic. This is the overall proportion of test results that are positive. In the pandemic, this has come to mean the percentage of COVID-19 tests that are positive. Unlike the parameters discussed so far, the positivity rate is not a measure of test performance. Neither is it a test of disease prevalence—however, during the pandemic, the positivity rate has come to be interpreted as an indicator of trends in prevalence. If the positivity rate is increasing, this might mean that prevalence is increasing under the assumption that the increased positivity rate is not merely due to diminishing specificity or improving sensitivity of the test itself. In other words, the positive test results include both true positives and false positives, and increasing prevalence is likely to be represented by an increasing proportion of true positive tests, and, thereby, also overall positive tests.

However, the positivity rate could also reflect the mix of people who seek or receive testing. For example, if COVID-19 tests are widely available to people who are asymptomatic, the positivity rate is likely to be lower than if testing is restricted to people with symptoms suggestive of COVID-19. Positivity rates have been reported as a surveillance parameter in a variety of contexts apart from COVID-19. For example, the positivity rate for cannabis tests has been suggested as a possible measure of trends in cannabis use since legalization.[122] However, the positivity rate is not a true epidemiological parameter, because it depends both on prevalence and the targeting of diagnostic tests. Consequently, it is rarely used in epidemiologic research.

Thinking deeper

Equivalence of Bayes' theorem and likelihood ratios

Bayes' theorem and likelihood ratios accomplish the same goal: to anticipate the probability of a disease (or other attribute) when a test result is known. They (and other formulas in this chapter) derive from the same 2 × 2 table.

A paper by Joseph et al[123] reported the following 2 × 2 table (Table 10) to test for *Strongyloides* infection in 162 Cambodian refugees arriving in Montreal in the 1980s.

TABLE 10. 2 × 2 TABLE FROM JOSEPH ET AL[123]

	Stool exam positive	Stool exam negative	Total
Serology positive	38	87	125
Serology negative	2	35	37
Total	40	122	162

If the serology results are treated as a gold standard in this table (although Joseph et al did not treat them this way), the stool examination is seen to be insensitive (38/125 = 30.4%) but highly specific (35/37 = 94.6%). This means that the likelihood ratio positive (sensitivity divided by 1 − specificity) is 5.6.

Imagine you are using the stool examination test in a population with a base rate of 5%. Using Bayes' theorem, the positive predictive value is:

$$\text{Positive Predictive Value} = \frac{0.304 \times 0.05}{(0.304 \times 0.05) + \left[(1-0.096) \times (1-0.05)\right]} = 0.228 = 22.8\%$$

Note that you can convert a base rate of 0.05 into odds using the formula on page 31 (it becomes a pretest odds of 0.053). The posttest odds of disease can be calculated as the product of the likelihood ratio positive and the pretest odds: 0.053 × 5.6 = 0.296. Converting this back to a proportion (proportion = odds divided by 1 + odds), the result is 0.228 or 22.8%, which is identical to the result attained through the Bayesian calculation.

This example illustrates a general principle: the approach using the likelihood ratio positive and the approach using Bayes' theorem are identical. They are just different ways of looking at the same thing.

Questions

Davidson et al[124] examined the performance of colour Doppler ultrasound in the diagnosis of deep vein thrombosis (DVT) in patients undergoing elective surgeries, with disappointing results. They reported the following 2 × 2 table (see Table 11) showing the results of the ultrasound tests versus the gold standard of venography.

TABLE 11. COLOUR DOPPLER ULTRASOUND VERSUS VENOGRAPHY IN THE DIAGNOSIS OF DVT[124]

	Venography positive	Venography negative
Colour Doppler ultrasound indicates DVT	8	23
Colour Doppler ultrasound indicates no DVT	13	275

1. What is the sensitivity and specificity of the ultrasound tests versus venography as a gold standard?

2. What are the odds of DVT in the sample? From these odds, calculate the prevalence.

3. What is the likelihood ratio positive for the ultrasound test?

4. Calculate the posttest odds and positive predictive value for those who are ultrasound positive.

5. If the pretest probability is 50% (pretest odds = 1), what is the positive predictive value?

6. To describe the ability of a diagnostic test to classify disease status, would it make sense to compare the odds of a positive test in those with a disease to the odds of a positive test in those without a disease? For example, by dividing 1 of these odds by the other?

7. Imagine that you are designing a new diagnostic test for a disease. Your motivation is to detect the disease early in its course so that it can be treated more effectively. The disease must be treated surgically and the surgical procedure used for this disease is itself very risky. Based on this information, would you prefer that your new diagnostic test be highly sensitive or highly specific?

8. Epidemiologists tend to like categorical measures, such as (nominal) diagnostic categories. Nominal categories can be criticized for the loss of information that occurs when they are applied to continuous variables. For example, blood pressure is a continuous variable, but it can be used to classify people into 2 groups: hypertensive (high blood pressure) and normotensive (normal blood pressure), which are nominal categories. Suppose that a systolic blood pressure of 140 mmHg is used to divide people into these 2 groups. A loss of information seems to occur: 141 mmHg is considered different than 140 mmHg, but 180 mmHg is considered the same as 141 mmHg. In view of this problem, can you state a justification for categorizing a variable that is inherently continuous? Can you think of other inherently continuous variables that could be changed into nominal categories?

9. An incompetent clinician becomes bored with diagnostic testing and unethically decides to flip a coin to assign a diagnosis. What would the expected sensitivity and specificity of this "testing" procedure be?

10. The "testing" procedure in question 9 is obviously completely useless. Or is it? Suppose that you decided to assign diagnoses using coin tosses (with heads meaning that the disease is present and tails meaning it is absent) in a population in which everybody (100%) has the disease. What will the positive predictive value of this "test" be in this context? Do you still think that the test is useless?

7

Misclassification bias in descriptive studies

OBJECTIVES

• Define misclassification bias as a type of systematic error.
• Describe sources of misclassification bias in terms of sensitivity and specificity.
• Explain the concept of direction of bias when misclassification bias occurs.
• Describe situations in which misclassification bias may result in over- or underestimation of a descriptive parameter.

Misclassification bias in context

Chapter 6 introduced the first of 2 types of systematic error in epidemiological research: measurement error. Specifically, it focused on measurement error that leads to misclassification.

This chapter describes misclassification bias: the effect of misclassification—measurement error—on estimating parameters. (*Bias* means the effect of systematic error.) Since erroneous measurement leads to misclassification, the resulting type of bias could be called *measurement bias*. Another name is *information bias*. However, due to the emphasis of epidemiology on categories and classification, this chapter will use the term *misclassification bias*.

Understanding misclassification bias involves understanding how errors in classification translate into systematic over- or underestimation of parameters such as prevalence and incidence. This chapter will focus on prevalence, but the same principles apply to the estimation of any type of proportion, including incidence proportions.

Sources of misclassification bias

Misclassification bias results from systematic error in measurement—in other words, from flawed disease-detection tests, diagnostic algorithms, classification protocols, and so on. These flaws come from the design of these tests, algorithms, and protocols.

Flawed tests, algorithms, and protocols are like incorrectly calibrated rulers: every time you use them, they give you erroneous measurements. The error they generate does not come from chance (unlike random error), so increasing the number of measurements you make (the sample size) doesn't help. The more things you measure with a flawed ruler, the bigger your pool of erroneous data.

To understand the bias in measurement generated by a flawed ruler, you look at its calibration compared to an accurate ruler. To understand the bias generated by flawed tests, algorithms, and protocols, you look at their sensitivity and specificity.

Low sensitivity

A measurement (e.g., a diagnostic test, a classification protocol) with low sensitivity will not detect disease in all study subjects with disease. Imagine conducting a prevalence study where the measurements (tests, protocols) for identifying the disease are insensitive. You collect the data and classify disease according to the results of the (insensitive) measurements. After data collection, you enter the data into a study database from which prevalence can be calculated. Since only the subjects who tested positive appear in this data set as cases of disease—and since the insensitive measurement did not identify all cases of disease—the numerator of the estimated prevalence proportion will be smaller than it should be. However, all members of the sample, regardless of their disease status or classification, will be present in the denominator. Therefore, low sensitivity (at least when there is perfect specificity) will lead to an underestimation of prevalence.

> *Key point:* Measurements (e.g., tests, protocols) that are insensitive will tend to bias frequency estimates such as prevalence away from the true population parameter in the direction of producing estimates that are too low.

Low specificity

A measurement with low specificity will mistakenly classify some disease-free subjects as diseased. These are false positives. These misclassified subjects will end up in the numerator of the calculated frequency—but again, the denominator of the calculated parameter does not change. This will make the estimated prevalence too high.

Key point: Methods of disease classification that are nonspecific will tend to bias frequency estimates such as prevalence toward values higher than the true population value.

Low sensitivity and specificity

In some situations, a trade-off could exist between sensitivity and specificity, such that the tendency to underestimate due to low sensitivity and the tendency to overestimate due to low specificity would cancel out. This would lead to an unbiased prevalence estimate, but it does not often occur. Most diseases afflict only a small proportion of the population, so prevalence studies contain far fewer people with disease than without. As a result, many more false positives than false negatives tend to occur when sensitivity and specificity are comparable. Specificity needs to be very high in most cases to avoid a substantial overestimation of prevalence.

Describing the direction of misclassification bias

Descriptive parameters such as prevalence and incidence proportion always have values between 0 and 1 because the contents of their numerators are included in their denominators. As a result, the direction of bias can be anticipated given the effect of misclassification on the numerator of the proportion. Misclassification bias can result in an estimate that is too high (positive bias) or too low (negative bias). The idea of using these particular words to describe the direction of bias derives from a formula for relative bias.

This formula depicts bias in relation to the true value of the parameter being estimated. Here is the relative bias formula:

$$\text{Relative Bias} = \frac{e(\text{Prevalence}) - \text{PREVALENCE}}{\text{PREVALENCE}}$$

where *e(Prevalence)* is the expected value of sample-based estimates and *PREVALENCE* is the true parameter

The expected value of the sample-based parameter (the central tendency of the distribution of estimates were the study to be repeated many times)—in the absence of bias—is the same as PREVALENCE. If the distribution of estimates centres around a value that is too low, the formula will produce a negative value. If the distribution of estimates centres around a value that is too high, it will produce a positive value. This demonstrates the value of *positive* and *negative* for describing the direction of misclassification bias. However, while the formula has some conceptual value in understanding the direction of bias, it has little practical value since PREVALENCE is unknown. Indeed, were it known, there would be no need to estimate it.

Other terms for misclassification bias

Unfortunately, the literature uses a variety of terms for misclassification bias.

For example, if diagnosticians are overzealous—counting suspected cases of a disease as disease—the resulting false-positive rate (a lack of specificity) produces a positive bias and an overestimation of prevalence. *Misclassification bias* would be a good term to describe this, but some epidemiologists call it *diagnostic suspicion bias* or *interviewer bias*. These terms attempt to describe the study defect that is causing bias. However, it is always best to articulate an actual mechanism through which bias might occur, and this usually involves more than just assigning a mechanism.

Compare these statements:

- "This study is vulnerable to diagnostic suspicion bias."
- "Diagnostic suspicion may have lowered the specificity of classification of disease status, leading to an inflation of the numerator of the prevalence proportion with false positives, causing misclassification bias and leading to an overestimation of prevalence."

The first statement is less wordy, but the second statement is much more informative and precise.

Key point: There are many terms to describe different forms or mechanisms of bias that might occur in specific studies, but it is not necessary to know these terms.

THE RELATIONSHIP BETWEEN BIAS AND RANDOM ERROR

What should be considered first, random error or bias? This is an important question in study design and in critical appraisal.

You can make a case for considering bias first. In the absence of bias, a study's results remain vulnerable to random error. In the presence of bias, however, it is difficult to say what random error means. In unbiased studies, confidence intervals quantify the extent of vulnerability to random error. However, if an estimate is systematically biased, it is difficult to say what the confidence intervals are quantifying.

If you calculate a conventional confidence interval for a biased estimate, the interval will centre on the biased estimate rather than the true population value. As the sample size increases, the width of those confidence intervals will become narrower, but still centre on the wrong thing. With increasing sample sizes, confidence intervals for a biased estimate will actually be less likely to incorporate the true parameter value. Any interpretation of those confidence intervals (such as a statement of confidence that the true population value lies within the range specified by the 2 confidence limits) is untrue.

Bias results from study-design flaws: careful study design can usually avoid them. Where misclassification bias is concerned, this means making sure that study variables are measured accurately. In reviewing a study with serious design flaws, such as inaccurate measurement, a thoughtful critical appraiser will not pay much attention to the statistics (knowing these to be wrong) and will instead focus on the effects of systematic error.

Thinking deeper

Exploring the magnitude of misclassification bias

An estimate of prevalence is based on a 1 × 2 table (see Table 12). You can generate this kind of table if you have classified a sample into diseased and nondiseased groups.

TABLE 12. 1 × 2 TABLE WITH SAMPLE-BASED DATA FROM A PREVALENCE STUDY

Disease	No disease	Total
a	b	n

On page 20, we described the calculation of prevalence from a table such as Table 12 in a way that did not acknowledge classification errors: the formula for prevalence was simply $a/(a + b)$ or equivalently a/n. If, however, a study is vulnerable to misclassification bias, the numbers in the table do not actually represent people with or without the disease. Instead, they partially represent a flawed way in which the study has classified its subjects as having or not having disease.

To anticipate the effect of misclassification, you can break down each of the columns in this table. You can divide subjects identified as having the disease—denoted a in the table—into 2 groups: those correctly classified as having the disease (the true positives, tp) and those incorrectly classified as having the disease (false positives, fp). You can similarly divide those identified without the disease (denoted b) as correctly classified (true negatives, tn) and incorrectly classified (false negatives, fn). This is a sobering thought. The law of large numbers is the driving force behind epidemiological research and of course it is still operating—but, where misclassification bias enters in, the law no longer operates in the service of valid estimation. A prevalence estimate is calculated as:

$$\text{Prevalence} = \frac{a}{a+b} = \frac{a}{n}$$

This is actually estimating an entity expressed in the next formula (below). Note that, because the denominator of a prevalence proportion contains the entire sample regardless of how classified, the possibility of misclassification does not affect the denominator and it can therefore be written simply as n rather than $tp + fp + fn + tn$.

$$\text{Prevalence} = \frac{tp + fp}{n}$$

The expected number of true positives is the proportion of those who actually have the disease and are classified correctly (sensitivity $\times$ a), and the expected number of false positives is the number without the disease multiplied by the false-positive rate: $(1 - \text{specificity}) \times b$. Pulling it all together, the result is a strange looking formula:

$$e\left(\text{Prevalence}\right) = \frac{\left(\text{Sensitivity} \times a\right) + \left[\left(1 - \text{Specificity}\right) \times b\right]}{n}$$

where $e(Prevalence)$ is the expected value of the estimated prevalence

Note that if sensitivity and specificity are both perfect (having values of 1), this equation reduces to the following form (a way of saying that measurement is perfect and that the estimated prevalence is not subject to misclassification bias):

$$\text{Prevalence} = \frac{a}{n}$$

Let's return to our formula for $e(prevalence)$:

$$e\left(\text{Prevalence}\right) = \frac{\left(\text{Sensitivity} \times a\right) + \left[\left(1 - \text{Specificity}\right) \times b\right]}{n}$$

Consider what would happen to estimated prevalence if sensitivity or specificity were less than perfect. Suppose that specificity is perfect and sensitivity is less than 1. In this instance, the formula reduces to the following (since specificity is 1, the right-hand term in the numerator disappears):

$$e\left(\text{Prevalence}\right) = \frac{\left(\text{Sensitivity} \times a\right)}{n}$$

So, if there is perfect specificity, imperfect sensitivity will always lead to an underestimation of prevalence.

What happens when sensitivity is perfect and specificity is less than 1? In this circumstance, the equation reduces to:

$$e(\text{Prevalence}) = \frac{a + \left[(1 - \text{Specificity}) \times b\right]}{n}$$

Whenever specificity is less than 1, the numerator of the prevalence equation will be inflated by false positives, and the expected value of the sampling distribution for this parameter will be systematically higher than that of the true population value.

You can use these formulas to anticipate the direction of bias—and also the magnitude of bias. You could, for example, consider the impact of a sensitivity or specificity of 0.5 versus 0.9 on the expected value of the estimated prevalence by replacing sensitivity and specificity with these values and calculating the expected value of the estimate.

Questions

1. The Canadian Longitudinal Study on Aging (CLSA) is a 20-year prospective study. The study includes measurement of a set of chronic medical conditions. The scope of the CLSA (which has a sample size of 50 000) is too large to have each participant assessed by a clinical diagnostician, so it uses self-reported diagnoses. Because self-reported diagnoses may be inaccurate, the investigators sought to develop algorithms based on self-report data. They calculated the sensitivity and specificity of proposed algorithms in relation to high-quality clinical assessments, which served as a gold standard.[125] There were 20 people with 1 of several chronic conditions included in the algorithm-study sample.

   a. One assessment involved an algorithm for symptoms of Parkinson disease (parkinsonism). The algorithm had excellent sensitivity and specificity: both were 100%. Does this mean that studies using the algorithm (especially the CLSA) would be free of misclassification bias?

   b. One of the algorithms for diabetes was 100% sensitive but only 70% specific. Do you think that application of the algorithm would lead to over- or underestimation of the population prevalence of diabetes?

2. Foebel et al[126] investigated the validity of a rating instrument called interRAI to diagnose neurological conditions. InterRAI was intended for use in people receiving home care, long-term care, and mental-health care. The investigators compared the data they collected through interRAI with data from—presumably accurate—patient records. They reported excellent specificity but variable sensitivity, depending on the diagnosis. For example, for traumatic brain injury the specificity was 99% and the sensitivity was 22%.

   a. Would you anticipate bias in a prevalence estimate of traumatic brain injury?

   b. If so, in what direction?

3. Kassam et al[121] developed a scale to assess mental-illness-related stigma in health professionals. Several studies have used this scale to assess the level of stigma held by members of various health professions and their trainees.

    a. People who hold negative beliefs (stigma) toward people with mental illness may not admit to their beliefs. Do you think this could make studies estimating the mean level of stigma vulnerable to bias?

    b. If so, in what direction?

4. Mothers whose newborn babies have malformations often think hard about possible causes of those malformations. Drugs and medications are often suspected of increasing the risk of fetal malformations.

    a. Would a tendency of mothers whose babies have malformations to think hard about drugs or medications they may have taken during pregnancy introduce bias into an estimate of the frequency of use of those drugs and medications?

    b. What would be the best way to control such bias?

5. A major source of data for epidemiological research in Canada is administrative data. These data are collected during the process of administering the health system during tasks such as reimbursing hospitals for the care they provide or paying fees to physicians for services that they perform. Marrie et al[127] have developed algorithms for the detection of comorbidity in neurological patients using linked administrative databases in Manitoba. As a validation standard, they conducted chart reviews, allowing calculation of sensitivity and specificity for alternative algorithms. Do you agree that a chart review can be used as a gold standard?

6. It can be difficult for people to distinguish migraine headaches from tension headaches. People sometimes think, erroneously, that a severe tension headache must be a migraine (in fact, the syndrome of migraine has unique features). Despite this, some prevalence studies rely on self-report to identify migraine.[128] In your opinion, which is likely to be most affected by the difficulty in differentiating between these 2 types of headaches: sensitivity or specificity? Would this likely result in an over- or underestimate of the prevalence?

7. A study uses an "excellent" diagnostic measure with nearly perfect measurement properties (e.g., specificity = 99%) to assess the prevalence of a rare disease (prevalence: 5 per 100 000). Would you be concerned that even this "excellent" test could produce an inaccurate prevalence estimate?

8. Many Canadian epidemiological studies use case definitions to identify specific conditions in the administrative data that is collected by the Canadian health system. For example, studies identify conditions based on the billing codes that physicians submit to provincial health care insurance plans. The diagnostic code G35 under the ICD-10 system—a system used in most provinces—indicates multiple sclerosis (MS). Some case definitions require this code to appear once to count as an identified case of MS. Others require it to appear twice at least 6 months apart—indicating that the code was assigned by a physician seeking to be paid for a visit with a relevant patient on at least 2 occasions over a 6-month period. Which type of definition is more sensitive? Which do you think is more specific?

9. Canadian studies seeking to document the validity of case definitions from administrative data often do not have access to a gold standard, so they rely on demonstrating that a particular definition produces a plausible value for prevalence. Can you identify a potential flaw in this approach? Could an inaccurate classification procedure produce a plausible prevalence estimate?

10. Based on what you know about sensitivity and specificity, and the effects of low sensitivity and specificity on prevalence estimates, would you expect studies using self-reported assessments of body weight to produce over- or underestimates of obesity prevalence?

Selection error and selection bias in descriptive studies

OBJECTIVES

- Define selection bias as a type of systematic error arising from participation or nonparticipation in a study.
- Identify sources of selection bias: selection itself, nonconsent, attrition, and (in some respects) missing data.
- Describe the mechanism by which defective selection can introduce bias into an estimated frequency such as prevalence.
- Describe the direction of bias in a defective prevalence study in which selection depends on disease status.

Selection bias in context

So far, we have covered random error (chapter 5), and 1 of 2 types of systematic error and bias in epidemiology: measurement error leading to misclassification (chapter 6) and misclassification bias (chapter 7).

This chapter covers the second type of systematic error and bias in epidemiology: selection error and bias.

For clarity, the breakdown that follows compares: random error; misclassification error and bias; and selection error and bias.

Type of error	Sources of error	Type of bias
Random error	Chance	N/A
Systematic error		
• Measurement error	Flaws in study design (flawed measurement leading to misclassification)	Misclassification bias
• Selection error	Flaws in study design (flawed sampling procedures that choose participants)	Selection bias
	Other factors related to participation (e.g., subjects withdrawing from a study)	

In selection error, all sources of error are related to participation, so some researchers call the bias that results *participation bias*. In other classifications, bias arising from sampling and from attrition have separate labels.[129] Note that only 1 of the sources of error in selection error really counts as a defect in selection (in the strictest use of the word): flawed sampling procedures, which determine who researchers choose as study participants. We use *selection error* as shorthand for other factors related to participation, even if sampling procedures are not flawed, because they all lead to bias through a similar mechanism. These factors include, for example, decisions by subjects not to participate in a study, or not to participate fully.

Key point: Selection bias is a type of systematic error that results from study-design defects, and other factors, that affect who participates in an epidemiologic study.

Selection error from sampling procedures
To understand flawed sampling procedures, you need to understand ideal sampling procedures. Ideal sampling procedures deliver probability samples, where the probability of selection for each member of the sample is known.

Ideal sampling: probability samples
Chapter 5 discussed the concept of random sampling (see page 64). In simple random sampling, each member of a population has the same chance of being selected into a sample. In other words, the selection probability for each member of the population is the same. With random sampling (assuming perfect measurement), the law of large numbers ensures that the proportions observed in samples closely reflect the true population values, at least when samples are large.

Simple random sampling belongs to a broader category of sampling procedures called *probability sampling*.

In probability sampling, there is a known probability of selection for each member of the population, but each member doesn't necessarily have the same probability of selection. Stratified sampling—another type of probability sampling—involves differing (but known) probabilities of selection for members of a population. Researchers use stratified sampling to make estimates within population subgroups. To limit the imprecision of these estimates, they ensure adequate numbers of subjects from target subgroups in their study samples.

For example, national surveys conducted by Statistics Canada, such as the Canadian Community Health Survey,[130] use stratified sampling. Because these surveys are federal initiatives, they are designed to provide useful estimates to all the provinces. However, some provinces are much larger than others. A simple random sample of the Canadian population would lead to small sample sizes in small provinces such as Prince Edward Island—which would make estimates made for this province imprecise. As a result, the design of the study ensures that selection probabilities for small provinces are larger than they would be in a simple random sample. These surveys often also oversample the 12-to-17 age range to provide adequate precision for this important age group.[130]

Stratified sampling also played a role in a mental health survey conducted in New Zealand: the probability of selection for Maori people was doubled, and for Pacific people quadrupled, to allow estimation in these subgroups.[131]

Most studies using stratified sampling have overall estimates as a goal, in addition to estimates for subgroups. For example, the surveys conducted by Statistics Canada aim for national estimates as well as provincial estimates. In making national estimates, researchers offset the unequal selection probabilities with sampling weights. These ensure that national estimates do not overrepresent subgroups.

In stratified sampling, researchers deliberately alter selection probabilities to make them unequal in known ways, and use sampling weights to prevent these unequal probabilities from introducing bias in overall estimates.

By contrast, unequal selection probabilities due to defective study design introduce bias in ways that cannot be corrected after the fact.

The discussion in this section has focused on probability samples. Samples in which the probabilities of selection are unknown are called *convenience samples*. As the name implies, convenience samples are convenient to collect. Unfortunately, the absence of probability in sampling means that there is no strong reason to believe that any estimate arising from the sample is providing information about the target population.

The real world of imperfect sampling

Even if researchers intend to obtain a probability sample, in reality they may not achieve equal probability of selection for all study subjects, or they may not know the exact probability of each subject's selection. Either of these problems can lead to selection bias, and they can occur at different steps of the sample-selection process.

The first step in sampling is to identify a sampling frame (chapter 5 also discusses sampling frames—see page 64). This is sometimes easy. For example, if you want to study the population of students at a particular university, a list of all registered students would provide a logical and straightforward sampling frame. But what if you want to make inferences about the population of a city or town? In this case, a list of residents may not exist. The only list, in theory, would be a census. Census lists do exist, but they are not usually accessible to researchers for reasons of privacy—in Canada, federal census data are protected by the Statistics Act.

The next step is selecting a sample from the sampling frame. If a real sampling frame is available (i.e., a list of all people in a population of interest), you can obtain a true probability sample fairly easily. For example, if you want a 10% simple random sample from a list of university registrants, you could enter the list into a spreadsheet or database, and then randomly generate an integer in the range of 0 to 9 (all with equal probability) for each entry. You could then choose all of the entries with a specific value as a means of randomly selecting 1 in 10.

The Canadian Community Health Survey now uses 3 sampling frames: an area frame, based on the location of a household; a telephone frame, based on a list of residential telephone numbers; and a frame that uses data from the Canadian Child Tax Benefit program to select 12-to-17-year-old respondents.[130]

When a list of an entire population is not available, probability sampling is not possible.

STRATEGIES FOR REPRESENTATIVE SAMPLING

Without a real sampling frame, the best you can do is to collect a representative sample—a sample, in other words, that you believe represents the real population.

Many studies use area frames and telephone frames as the basis for representative sampling.

Key point: While probability sampling is always the preferred procedure, researchers must often devise other ways to obtain representative samples.

AREA FRAMES

Area frames define populations geographically. To obtain a representative sample from an area frame, you would typically do the following: first use maps to define geographical areas, then identify households within those areas, and finally select individuals from those households. Statistics Canada uses area frames for a variety of national surveys, including the Canadian Community Health Survey.

TELEPHONE FRAMES

Telephone frames come from lists of telephone numbers, such as Internet telephone directories or old-fashioned paper telephone directories. Telephone directories, however, have never provided reliable sampling frames because people can choose to keep their numbers unlisted. Historically, this problem was addressed by random digit dialing (RDD), which involves randomly manipulating telephone numbers to equalize the probability of reaching listed versus unlisted numbers. Random dialing often uses single digit substitution: you select a telephone number from a list of telephone numbers and substitute 1 of its digits (usually the final digit) with a randomly generated number between 0 and 9. Presumably, using the random-digit phone number makes the chance of reaching an unlisted number or a listed number the same.

Telephone frames usually involve phone numbers that connect to households, not to individuals. If a research team reaches a household through telephone sampling, they must typically select 1 person from that household to participate in their survey. This is not a trivial matter. The most common procedure is to select 1 person randomly, or to use a nonrandom procedure, such as selecting the person with the most recent birthday.[132] Random selection in a household with 2 people results in a 50% chance of each person being selected; in a household with 10 people, it results in a 10% chance. The number of phone lines coming into a household also changes selection probabilities (the more phone lines to a household, the higher the selection probability for members of that household). Sampling weights can be used to offset these problems.[133]

Some problems, though, limit the usefulness of telephone surveys in less manageable ways.

Telephone surveys worked quite well before the 1990s, at which point their usefulness began to decline. In general, they show a trend toward declining response rates. Telephone fraud and telemarketing may have contributed to this trend: people are more cautious about providing personal information over the phone, and they use call-blocking and call-screening technologies—all of which can affect response rates to RDD surveys. An RDD survey conducted in Alberta had to call 36 068 telephone numbers to obtain a sample of 3304 participants.[134]

An even greater threat to telephone sampling comes from the rise of mobile phones over landlines. Mobile phones are not usually listed in directories, so you can't use them to produce a representative sample through digit substitution. You could try calling large numbers of randomly generated phone numbers, but many of these numbers would be nonworking, or would reach businesses or fax machines: you might call hundreds of them before connecting to a potential participant.

Finally, not everybody owns a telephone. If the target population is a community population, investigators want an equal chance of reaching each person—something that cannot happen by phone if not everybody has a phone.

Key point: Telephone survey methods are of declining importance in epidemiology due to difficulties in obtaining a representative sample in this way.

OTHER SAMPLE FRAMES

Mail surveys were once a mainstay of epidemiological research, but they are also becoming less and less useful.[135] People are using mail less and show an increasing tendency not to respond to mailed survey requests. Furthermore, stamps are very expensive.

The decline in telephone and mail strategies for sampling has generated a lot of interest in Internet-based sampling. However, the Internet does not provide a good foundation for representative samples: there is no enumeration of people with Internet access or any way to systematically enumerate a sampling frame consisting of those people.

Internet surveys are also popular. Unfortunately, these surveys rarely use probability sampling. Instead, the sample is usually "recruited" from users of social media, or sent out to a mass email list. Typically, such surveys have no definable target population and are essentially recruiting volunteers. Often, they cannot even report a response rate. None of mechanisms by which the laws of probability link estimated parameters to population values apply in such surveys. Consequently, the estimates they produce are often of little interest.

TRENDS IN SAMPLE FRAMES

Major data collection platforms have increasingly become the foundation for epidemiological research. These platforms include registries of disease. For example, cancer registries are very important sampling vehicles in cancer epidemiology.[77] Registered diseases are growing in number, and registries now exist for neurology,[136] muscular dystrophy,[137] and trauma.[138,139] The establishment of a cerebral palsy registry at McGill University has made Canada a leader in this area.[140] In addition, provinces have registries of persons insured for health care—and since Canada has universal health care, these can prove useful for sampling. An example of this approach is a survey looking at rates of West Nile virus infection in Alberta.[141]

National surveys conducted by Statistics Canada are another important source of data for epidemiological research. The most important health survey is the Canadian Community Health Survey, which collects data from approximately 65 000 Canadians every year on a continuous data-collection cycle. These surveys collect extensive and far-reaching data using high-quality sampling and data collection procedures. Statistics Canada has procedures in place for epidemiologists to access these data, with safeguards to ensure compliance with the Statistics Act. The procedures require research to take place inside regional data centres—a set of secure data-analysis facilities with locations at many of Canada's major universities.[142] Statistics Canada calculates sophisticated sampling weights for these data, which it also makes available to researchers. You can access these data files through a portal operated by the Canadian Research Data Centres Network, which first requires you to complete an application and review process.[143]

Selection error from other factors: consent, attrition, and missing data

Obtaining a sample is obviously a very challenging aspect of selection in epidemiology, but the challenges don't stop there. Just because a person has been selected for participation in a study doesn't mean they will participate.

Unlike the national census, people are not legally obliged to participate in research. To participate, people must provide consent for participation. Rather than a legal principle, consent reflects an ethical principle called the *respect for persons principle*. This principle recognizes the intrinsic respect and consideration that is always owed to peoples' autonomy. People must be able to decide for themselves whether they wish to participate in a research study. To make such a decision, people must know the implications of their participation (what it would mean to agree to participate) and they must be free of coercion so that their choices about participation are fully autonomous.

People hold different opinions about health related topics, and some have more trust than others in health research and health researchers. Some people selected into a study sample decline to participate. Others may agree to participate, but may refuse to answer certain questions—this results in missing data, which in turn may result in selection bias (due to these respondents' lack of participation in the calculation of an estimate). In longitudinal studies, participants may lose interest and drop out, resulting in sample attrition. Attrition can also occur because participants move out of the study area, or because researchers fail to track changes in participant contact information, and for many other reasons.

Key point: Any factor affecting participation in a study that is related to the condition being studied has the potential to introduce selection bias.

The mechanism of selection bias in prevalence estimates

Suppose that a study's sampling procedure is flawed in the sense that people with disease are more likely to be selected into the study than people without disease. This means that the numerator in the prevalence calculation (denoted *a*) will be too large.

$$\text{Prevalence} = \frac{a}{a+b}$$

Let's assume prevalence is estimated from a simple random sample and classification has been free of error. The observed proportion of people with disease has an expected value—*e(prevalence)*—related to the proportion of people in the population that have the disease (the true population value). The expected value of the count represented by a is the population value (A) multiplied by the selection probability $p_{selection}$.

$$e\left(\text{Prevalence}\right) = \frac{A \times p_{selection}}{\left(A \times p_{selection}\right) + \left(B \times p_{selection}\right)}$$

Clearly, if there is only 1 selection probability ($p_{selection}$), which is the case for a simple random sample, there will be no bias since the expected value of the estimate will be the population prevalence. So, $p_{selection}$ cancels out and the equation reduces as follows:

$$e\left(\text{Prevalence}\right) = \frac{A}{A+B} = \text{PREVALENCE}$$

However, if there were 2 different selection probabilities—1 for people with the disease and 1 for people without the disease—then systematic error will result. The expected value of the estimated parameter would not be the true value of the population. If people with the disease had a higher probability of selection, the numerator of the prevalence equation would be too large and prevalence would be overestimated. If people without the disease had a higher probability of selection, the denominator would be too large and the prevalence would be underestimated. The same principles apply to other barriers to participation, such as nonconsent, attrition, and failure to provide necessary data. If any of these barriers correlate with disease status, they will systematically skew prevalence estimates from true values. Missing data, if it means that some people with missing data cannot be included in the 1 × 2 table from which the estimate is made, can also cause selection bias. However, in each case, if the reason for nonparticipation is unrelated to disease status, bias will not occur, since the numerator and denominator of the prevalence will be equally affected.

Selection bias in systematic reviews

Systematic reviews select studies from the literature rather than selecting people from a population. Their goal is to identify 100% of studies addressing a particular question (a selection probability of 1). However, their procedures for selecting studies can be imperfect, so, if they use meta-analysis to calculate pooled estimates, the resulting meta-analytic estimates are also subject to bias. The biggest concern is that studies reporting negative results would be less likely be published than studies reporting positive results. This could occur for several reasons. Investigators who are excited about a new treatment may pursue its publication less vigorously if they are disappointed by a negative result. Peer reviewers may not find negative results as interesting as positive results, and may be less supportive of publication than they would be for positive results. Editors of journals may want to improve what are called the *impact factors* of their journals by selecting papers for publication that they feel will be more often cited, so they may be hesitant to publish negative findings. Studies that are never published cannot be identified in systematic literature searches. The resulting bias is called *publication bias*. A funnel plot is a type of graphic used to detect publication bias. In a funnel plot, each study in the meta-analysis is represented by a point in a scatterplot of a measure of precision on the y-axis and study effect on the x-axis. One expects that large studies will have high precision and therefore be quite similar to one another, whereas smaller studies will have lower precision and the estimates of effect will be more variable. This leads to a funnel-shaped pattern, as seen in Figure 8. In this figure, the measure of effect is the log odds ratio and the measure of precision is the standard error of the log odds ratio. If small studies in particular are less likely to be published when their results are negative, studies will be selectively missing from the left-hand portion of the plot, creating an asymmetrical appearance, as seen in Figure 9.

FIGURE 8. FUNNEL PLOT: ALL STUDIES EQUALLY LIKELY TO BE PUBLISHED

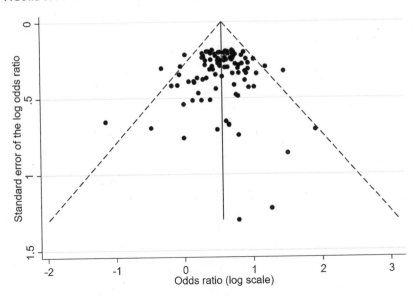

FIGURE 9. FUNNEL PLOT: NONSIGNIFICANT STUDIES LESS LIKELY TO BE PUBLISHED

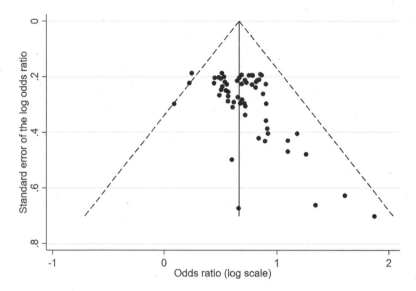

ETHICS IN EPIDEMIOLOGICAL RESEARCH

In this chapter, we have touched on an ethical consideration—the principle of respect for each person's autonomy. However, the ethics of conducting epidemiologic research is broader than this. Canada's 3 main research-funding agencies have mapped out a framework for ethical research. This framework is called TCPS2—the *Tri-Council Policy Statement: Ethical Conduct for Research Involving Humans*, now in its second edition.[144] TCPS2 requires ethical decisions to be made at the local level by ethics review boards, which are officially constituted to bring the right mix of perspectives and expertise to ethical deliberations.

> *Key point:* Health research in Canada is guided by a national tri-council policy statement, but administered at a regional or institutional level through duly constituted ethics review boards.

Many principles are involved in health research ethics. These principles form part of complex decisions to allow or disallow studies—decisions that also engage different priorities, perceptions, and beliefs. Ethical principles important to epidemiological research include:

Respect for persons: Researchers must recognize the intrinsic value of human beings and respect the autonomy of research subjects.[144]

Beneficence: Research must aim to do good rather than harm.

Nonmaleficence: Research should avoid doing harm wherever possible. Of course, there is almost always some potential for harm and some potential for benefit in research. TCPS2 stipulates that ethical research must safeguard the welfare of research participants.[144]

Utilitarian principle: The possibility of good should outweigh the possibility of harm.

Confidentiality: Research must have safeguards in place to ensure personal information does not fall into the wrong hands—for example, safe data storage and strict protection of information collected during research.

Privacy: Research must respect people's inherent right to keep their personal information to themselves. Research almost always involves collecting personal information of some type and therefore always entails a degree of invasion of privacy. This negative aspect of research must be minimized by appropriate limits (only collecting information that is needed by the study) and by the hope that this harm will be offset by useful results that lead to positive changes in health.

Justice: This term refers to an obligation to treat all people fairly and equitably.[144] Research should benefit those who bear the harms of research. It is unjust to exploit a group—for example: students, prisoners, or the socioeconomically disadvantaged—to obtain knowledge that does not directly benefit the group. In the past, some health researchers coerced participation from vulnerable groups such as psychiatric patients[145] and vulnerable members of Canada's First Nations.[146] Such activities transgress the ethical principle of justice.

The Panel on Research Ethics, which is a federal government agency, offers an online tutorial about TCPS2 called the Course on Research Ethics (CORE).[147] Some academic institutions in Canada require their researchers to take this course.

Thinking deeper

Selection bias in symbols

The rules governing the occurrence and direction of selection bias are intuitive:

- If people with the attribute whose frequency is being estimated are more likely to participate, the estimated frequency will be biased upwards (positive bias).

- If people with the attribute are less likely to participate, the estimate will be biased downwards (negative bias).

Note that each scenario represents a departure from the ideal of a simple random sample (where every person in the population has the same probability of selection into a study). To understand how this type of bias unfolds, a new concept is required: conditional selection probability.

Recall the 1 × 2 table—restated below as Table 13—from which prevalence for a target population could be calculated assuming that we had complete data on each person in that population (and also assuming perfect measurement):

TABLE 13. 1 × 2 TABLE FOR A POPULATION

Disease	No disease	Total
A	B	N

To calculate an estimated prevalence for this population, some members of the population will be selected. Table 14 restates the 1 × 2 table for calculating estimated prevalence from a sample population (denoted as usual with lowercase letters):

TABLE 14. 1 × 2 TABLE FOR A SAMPLE

Disease	No disease	Total
a	b	n

Recall the concept of selection probability ($p_{selection}$). Selection probability is the probability that a member of the target population is selected into the sample.

In a simple random sample, there is a single selection probability that applies to each member of the population. In a sample influenced by selection errors, however, the selection probability for those having the disease differs from the selection probability of those who do not have the disease—so, 2 probabilities are at work. To think through the precise mechanism of selection bias in a prevalence study, it is necessary to define these 2 probabilities.

The conditional nature of these probabilities is depicted by a vertical line that can be read as "given." The probability of selection given disease is $p_{selection|disease}$ and that for nondisease is $p_{selection|nondisease}$.

The expected value for the number of people with disease in a study sample is the number of people in the target population with the disease (A) multiplied by the probability of selection given that they have the disease. Depicting this as an expected value using the letter e:

$$e(a) = A \times p_{selection|disease}$$

And the expected value for the number of people without the disease is similarly:

$$e(b) = B \times P_{\text{selection}|\text{nondisease}}$$

This allows an expanded version of the formula for an estimated prevalence that incorporates the idea of a selection probability:

$$e(\text{Prevalence}) = \frac{A \times P_{\text{selection}|\text{disease}}}{\left(A \times P_{\text{selection}|\text{disease}}\right) + \left(B \times P_{\text{selection}|\text{nondisease}}\right)}$$

Imagine that each selection probability is 0.1 (in other words, that 1 in 10 members of the population are selected into the study—a simple random sample). In this case:

$$e(\text{Prevalence}) = \frac{A \times 0.1}{\left(A \times 0.1\right) + \left(B \times 0.1\right)}$$

Factoring out the selection probability in the denominator:

$$e(\text{Prevalence}) = \frac{A \times 0.1}{0.1 \times \left(A + B\right)}$$

Or:

$$e(\text{Prevalence}) = \frac{A}{A + B}$$

This is another way of saying that, for any simple random sample, the expected value of the prevalence will be the true population prevalence—in other words, it will not be biased.

If the selection probabilities for diseased and nondiseased subjects are unequal, the expanded equation makes clear that bias will result. It also makes clear that, in this event, increasing the sample size (which essentially means increasing the selection probabilities) will not fix this problem. Recall that this features helps to distinguish bias from random error: increasing the sample size does not fix the problem.

As with all types of bias, selection bias casts a shadow over all statistical analyses based on the biased samples.

Questions

1. The Canadian Community Health Survey is a large-scale initiative that includes both general health surveys and surveys that have more specialized content. In 2012, a mental-health-focused survey was conducted.[148] This survey used a combination of an area frame and a random digit dialed (RDD) telephone

frame. The survey collected data by interviewing some subjects face to face, and some subjects via telephone. Alcohol and drug dependence (among other disorders) were assessed in the survey. The greater social distance associated with telephone interviewing means that respondents were more willing to disclose their use of alcohol and drugs, thereby leading to a higher estimated prevalence of alcohol and drug dependence.

   a. Do you think that this could be an important cause of selection bias?

   b. Mental disorders tend to be stigmatized conditions. Stigmatization consists of negative attitudes and behaviours. Could fear of stigma result in selection bias in a study of this type? How?

   c. The response rate in this survey was about 70%. If the response rate had been 100% instead of 70%, could selection bias occur?

2. Another feature of the Canadian Community Health Survey (CCHS) is that its target population consists of household residents. People with severe dementia tend to live in institutions, rather than at home. People with dementia are therefore less likely to be selected into the CCHS than people without dementia. Will this cause selection bias in an estimate of dementia prevalence?

3. A study used physician-billing claims and hospitalization data (a type of administrative data) to estimate the prevalence of autoimmune inflammatory myopathy in the province of Alberta, both in the general population and in aboriginal populations.[149] To be coded as having this condition, it was necessary to see a physician or be admitted to hospital. Could this have caused selection bias?

4. Several iterations of the CCHS have sought to measure schizophrenia prevalence using self-report items included in an interview.[150] People with schizophrenia, when they are ill, can develop delusions that cause them to feel that they are in danger (a persecutory delusion). Conceivably, some people with this illness, if they were ill at the time of the interview, might have refused to participate.

   a. Could a lower response rate among people with schizophrenia lead to selection bias in an estimate of schizophrenia prevalence?

   b. If so, in what direction?

5. A longitudinal study followed a community sample of 3304 for 3 months to assess their risk of depression.[134] Those who were not depressed at baseline were tracked prospectively with telephone interviews every 2 weeks to estimate their incidence of depression. Those who became depressed may have felt tired or hopeless, which may have increased their rate of attrition from the study. Would this have resulted in a biased incidence estimate?

6. Socioeconomic status (a concept combining several indicators of social status such as occupation and income) is a determinant of many health outcomes. Yet, socioeconomic status is also often associated with lower response rates in survey research. Describe at least 1 mechanism by which socioeconomic status could introduce selection bias into a prevalence estimate.

7. Prevalence studies often rely on self-reported or professionally diagnosed chronic conditions to identify people that have a disease. For example, many surveys include the question "Have you been diagnosed by a health professional with diabetes?" Diseases that are not well known, or that are poorly

understood, may not be reported by the people afflicted or by physicians. Would lack of awareness and reporting cause selection bias?

8. A study aims to estimate the prevalence of glaucoma, an eye disease. Some people with glaucoma have visual impairments. In this study, potential participants who cannot read the consent form cannot provide consent, and are therefore not allowed to participate. Would this cause selection bias? What could you do to deal with this problem?

9. A study seeking to estimate the prevalence of carpal tunnel syndrome in the general population is based on a sample of data-entry personnel from an information technology company. The plan is to interview these personnel in their homes and assess them for the syndrome using portable diagnostic technology. People with carpal tunnel syndrome (caused by overuse—e.g., by too much typing on a keyboard) are more likely to be off work on disability, and consequently are more likely to be at home when the survey interviewer arrives. Do you think this would cause selection bias? What direction would the bias be? What is the defect in the study design responsible for this problem? What could you do to avoid the occurrence of bias in this study?

10. You have conducted a study of the prevalence of risky sexual behaviours in young adults. You obtained a perfect simple random sample and achieved a 100% response rate among your 100 selected participants. Unfortunately, 10% of the respondents refuse to answer questions about their risky behaviours. As a result, when you calculate the prevalence, your analysis is based on 90 respondents. The respondents that had engaged in risky behaviours were twice as likely not to answer the questions, so prevalence is underestimated. What is the source of this bias? Is it misclassification or selection bias? Defend your answer.

9

Confounding in descriptive studies

OBJECTIVES

- Define confounding.
- Define and describe strategies to adjust for confounding in descriptive studies: stratification, direct standardization, and indirect standardization.
- Describe the concept of weighting.

Confounding in context

So far, this book has discussed 2 categories of error in epidemiological research: random error, and defective study design leading to misclassification bias and selection bias. We have explored these in the context of descriptive studies and basic parameters, particularly prevalence.

This chapter looks at the third key category of error: confounding. In descriptive studies, confounding results in a failure to accurately assess important (useful, actionable) variables from a variety of variables at play in a population.

The problem of confounding: intermixing of effects

If a determinant cannot be changed, it is of little interest. Classic examples of nonmodifiable determinants are age and sex. They contribute strongly to the risk of many conditions, yet they cannot be changed. Populations often differ in terms of such nonmodifiable determinants. Descriptive epidemiologic comparisons of different populations are therefore complicated by the fact that potentially interesting differences might merely reflect underlying differences in nonmodifiable determinants. For this reason, there is a lot of interest in determining whether health outcomes differ among populations apart from the effects of certain nonmodifiable determinants. If differences remain after adjustment for nonmodifiable determinants, those differences are more interesting and more likely to result from modifiable factors.

Key point: Modifiable determinants of health outcomes are much more important than nonmodifiable determinants. Only modifiable determinants can lead to effective preventive interventions.

The intermixing of more and less interesting effects when populations are compared is called *confounding.* In descriptive epidemiology, the main procedures to handle confounding involve standardization. Procedures for standardization adjust for the nonmodifiable, and therefore less interesting, effects of (most commonly) age and sex in 2 populations. This allows unconfounded comparisons. While standardization for age and sex is commonplace, the same procedures can be used, in principle, to adjust for almost any variable that might confound more interesting comparisons.

After such adjustments, persistence of a difference between 2 populations poses the question of why that difference exists. A persistent difference most likely arises from the effects of modifiable risk factors. At this stage, the focus of epidemiological inquiry shifts from description to analysis—from descriptive studies to analytical studies. Descriptive studies tend to generate hypotheses about etiology, whereas analytical studies often address specific hypotheses about disease etiology.

A note about terminology

Terminology for variables that influence health status can take a variety of forms. A cause of a disease, in epidemiology, is usually referred to as a *risk factor.* A variable associated with increased risk in a way that is not due to a cause-effect relationship may be called a *risk marker* or *risk indicator.* Because most diseases have multiple contributing causes, questions of causation often assume a nuanced meaning in epidemiology—a meaning not adequately captured by a simplistic single-cause-leading-to-single-effect logic. As a result, some epidemiologists prefer to regard risk factors as component causes (a concept explored in more detail later).

An example of a nonstandardized difference in mortality

Standardization procedures most often apply to the interpretation of mortality data, which is a form of incidence data.

Unadjusted mortality rates reveal large differences between Canada's provinces and its northern territories. Another note about terminology: *crude mortality* is another name for an unadjusted mortality rate.

Key point: In epidemiology, rates and frequencies can be presented as adjusted or unadjusted (crude) parameters.

Chapter 4 discussed the reports of mortality in Canada's provinces and territories that Statistics Canada regularly updates and publishes (see page 42). Let's look at that data again.

To find data on the Statistics Canada website, it's often best to browse by subject, starting from the main page, and follow the links to what you need. (Another option is to run a search on the website using a search term such as "mortality," but you may find that this returns a large number of resources.) Click "access our data" on the main page, which provides a subject list. From that list, click "population and demography," and then "mortality." This leads to a list of resources that includes both summary tables and detailed data tables for mortality. Additional population data may be found on the open government website—for example, the population estimates for the past several decades.[151]

The Statistics Canada website data tables allow you to manipulate and download data. When you open up a data table on the website, you will see tabs for "add/remove data," which allow you to customize a table by selecting the information and format that you need, such as geographical areas of interest and specific data elements (e.g., numbers of deaths or death rates).[65] In a data table for deaths and age-specific mortality rates, by selecting Ontario and Nunavut under "geography, place of residence" you can see the mortality rates in these 2 areas. In 2019, the mortality for Ontario is 7.4 per 1000 years^{-1}; the mortality rate for Nunavut is considerably lower at 5.6 per 1000 years^{-1}.

On the surface, this would appear to be an important descriptive epidemiologic finding. Why are the rates higher in Ontario? Might there be significant environmental differences or perhaps psychosocial or lifestyle factors accounting for this difference? In keeping with the general role of epidemiology in public health, the finding might motivate a search for such causes in the hope that modifiable determinants might be identified, leading to public health interventions capable of preventing the apparent excess mortality in Ontario.

However, many factors differ between Nunavut and Ontario, which could account for the difference in mortality rates, and some of these factors are more interesting than others. These factors are not evident in a simple consideration of crude mortality rates—indeed, they are intermixed, or confounded, in these crude rates. Two of these factors are age and sex. If the apparent difference in mortality rates were due exclusively to differences in age or sex, then the difference in mortality rates would not be useful for identifying preventive opportunities, because age and sex cannot be changed.

A proviso, of course, is that the difference in crude mortality does say something. A greater proportion of Ontario residents die each year than Nunavut residents. This may be important information for some purposes, such as planning health services for end-of-life care. To identify opportunities for prevention, however, you would want to know whether the difference in mortality is due to something more than differences in age or sex.

Strategies to adjust for confounding in descriptive studies

Stratification

Stratification is the simplest type of adjustment to unconfound variables.

If a difference in a mortality rate is due to sex or age, or both, then those differences will not be apparent within sex or age strata. A difference that is due to sex cannot explain a difference between women in 2 populations, for example. Similarly, a difference between 2 populations that is due to age cannot explain a difference seen within the same age groups when the 2 populations are compared.

The Statistics Canada website has links to data tables that report age- and sex-specific mortality rates. Table 15 shows the mortality rates by sex for Nunavut and Ontario in 2019 from a Statistics Canada data table (Table 13-10-0701-01, "Mortality Rates by Age Group"[65]). As opposed to crude mortality, these estimates reflect sex-specific mortality rates in each locality. They can also be referred to as *sex-stratified mortality rates*. Data tables available on the Statistics Canada website make it particularly easy to extract data from its national tables and create customized tables like Table 15. In this case, starting from the main Statistics Canada page for its table on mortality rates by age group, click "add/remove data" and then the tab labelled "sex" in order to customize the table for sex. To customize the table to provide sex-stratified mortality rates, deselect "both sexes" and instead select "male" and "female." Now, you can click the "download" tab at the top of the title (be sure to download the data "as displayed," not the entire table). This provides the customized table as a comma-delimited data file, which you can import into almost any spreadsheet, database, or statistical software.

TABLE 15. SEX-STRATIFIED MORTALITY RATES PER 1000 YEAR^{-1} FOR ONTARIO AND NUNAVUT[65]

	Ontario	Nunavut
Male	7.6	6.2
Female	7.1	4.9

Table 15 shows that mortality rates are higher in men than women in each location. The sex-specific mortality rates continue to be higher in Ontario than Nunavut. Table 16 presents the same data, stratified this time by age group.

TABLE 16. AGE-STRATIFIED MORTALITY RATES PER 1000 YEAR[-1] IN ONTARIO AND NUNAVUT[65]

	Ontario	Nunavut
< 1 year	4.6	16.1
1 to 4 years	0.1	0.9
5 to 9 years	0.1	0
10 to 14 years	0.1	1.3
15 to 19 years	0.3	4
20 to 24 years	0.5	2.3
25 to 29 years	0.6	4.3
30 to 34 years	0.8	3.9
35 to 39 years	0.9	1.9
40 to 44 years	1.2	1.8
45 to 49 years	1.7	5
50 to 54 years	2.8	7.2
55 to 59 years	4.5	8.3
60 to 64 years	6.9	22.8
65 to 69 years	10.7	23.3
70 to 74 years	16.3	33.6
75 to 79 years	26.4	72.1
80 to 84 years	47.1	151.3
85 to 89 years	86.1	162.2
90 years and over	186.9	80

This age-stratified data presents a very different picture from the crude mortality rates and sex-specific mortality rates, which showed higher rates in Ontario. Almost all of the age-specific mortality rates are higher in Nunavut. There is also a typical pattern of age-specific mortality: fairly high mortality in the first year of life (something almost always seen in age-specific mortality data), low mortality until middle age, and rapidly increasing mortality with increasing age.

The pattern in the age-stratified data indicates that the crude mortality rates were misleading. Nunavut appears to have a higher rate of mortality, once the effect of age is accounted for. The suggestion from the crude data (apparently lower mortality in Nunavut) is not valid within any age category. A possible exception is the 90+ age group, which shows higher age-specific mortality in Ontario. The misleading impression provided by the crude mortality rate must have come from confounding by age. Since age is a strong determinant of mortality, a differing age distribution in Ontario versus Nunavut has created a misleading set of crude mortality estimates. Specifically, people in Ontario tend to be older, so, when the entire population is considered,

TABLE 17. AGE- AND SEX-STRATIFIED MORTALITY RATES PER 1000 YEAR[-1] IN ONTARIO AND NUNAVUT[65]

	Male		Female	
	Ontario	Nunavut	Ontario	Nunavut
< 1 year	4.8	15.7	4.2	16.5
1 to 4 years	0.2	1.1	0.1	0.6
5 to 9 years	0.1	0	0.1	0
10 to 14 years	0.1	1	0.1	1.6
15 to 19 years	0.4	6.7	0.2	1.2
20 to 24 years	0.6	3.2	0.3	1.3
25 to 29 years	0.9	6.8	0.4	1.9
30 to 34 years	1	3.8	0.5	3.9
35 to 39 years	1.2	2.2	0.7	1.5
40 to 44 years	1.6	3.5	0.9	0
45 to 49 years	2.1	7	1.3	2.8
50 to 54 years	3.3	7.5	2.2	6.7
55 to 59 years	5.6	10.6	3.3	5.9
60 to 64 years	8.7	23.2	5.2	22.4
65 to 69 years	13.4	18	8.1	30.2
70 to 74 years	20.2	33.3	12.9	33.8
75 to 79 years	31.9	47.6	21.7	94
80 to 84 years	56.8	130.4	39.7	180
85 to 89 years	104.5	100	73.9	235.3
90 years and over	208.7	153.8	177.1	0

the older population in Ontario leads to the misleading impression that living in Ontario is associated with higher mortality.

Confounding can invalidate epidemiological estimates, just like errors of classification and selection. However, as a threat to validity, confounding falls into a slightly different category than misclassification and selection bias. With misclassification and selection bias, study-design defects lead to systematic error, false data, and, as a result, invalid results. The crude mortality estimates from Nunavut and Ontario are not invalid in the same sense. Crude mortality in a particular case is a valid estimate of the true crude mortality rate in the population. It is not wrong—it is just misleading when a comparison is made between the 2 locations. An adjusted estimate, such as an age-stratified rate, is no longer misleading because it disentangles the characteristics of Nunavut from the age of the people who live in Nunavut.

Key point: Stratified rates are a form of adjusted rates. Stratification is 1 procedure for adjustment.

Table 17 shows the same data as Table 16 with simultaneous stratification for age and sex. This table begins to show some of the weaknesses of stratification as an adjustment technique. While the same general trends are evident, the division of the fairly small Nunavut population into age and sex strata makes the numbers sufficiently small that patterns become more difficult to see.

Direct standardization

Stratification is a perfectly good way to adjust for potential confounding variables, but it has drawbacks. It requires you to look through a data table row by row. Also, stratification magnifies errors of chance within strata, where the numbers can be small and subject to random variability. Since small samples lead to more random error, dividing a large data set into smaller strata increases the random variation typically seen in stratum-specific estimates.

When stratum-specific rates are available, direct standardization is a common way to simplify comparisons between rates. In direct standardization, you choose a standardizing population and use it as a bridge between the 2 rates.

Direct standardization takes a set of stratum-specific rates and weights them by the stratum-specific structure of the chosen standardizing population. In the Nunavut-Ontario mortality-rates comparison, the procedure asks: If both of these populations had the same age and sex distribution (that of the standardizing population), what would their expected mortality rate be?

The choice of a standardizing population is somewhat arbitrary. In the Nunavut-Ontario comparison, it would be possible to use the age and sex distribution of either Nunavut or Ontario. A common choice, however, would be to use the age and sex distribution of the national population. A standardizing population should be roughly similar to the populations being standardized.

In direct standardization, the standardizing population is divided proportionally, and the proportion of the population falling into each age and sex group becomes a means of weighting the stratum-specific estimates. The stratum-specific estimates are multiplied by these weights, and then all the weighted rates are added to produce the standardized rates. Tables 18 and 19 provide an example of standardization for the Nunavut-Ontario comparison for age in males and females, respectively. In each case, the stratum-specific values from Table 17 are presented, along with the proportion of the national population in each age-sex stratum (according to postcensal estimates arising from the 2016 census).[152]

The age-standardized rates from Table 18 and Table 19 show that Nunavut has a higher mortality rate than Ontario once the effect of age is addressed. This is true for both men and women.

Statistics Canada produces a data table for cause-specific mortality that has age-standardized mortality as an output option.[154] In the data table, the

TABLE 18. DIRECT STANDARDIZATION FOR AGE OF ONTARIO AND NUNAVUT MORTALITY DATA FOR MALES[153,65]

Age at time of death	Male mortality rates/1000 person years[-1]		Weights*	Weighted rates (Ontario)	Weighted rates (Nunavut)
	Ontario	Nunavut			
< 1 year	4.8	15.7	0.010195408	0.048937958	0.160067906
1 to 4 years	0.2	1.1	0.042837739	0.008567548	0.047121513
5 to 9 years	0.1	0	0.05582716	0.005582716	0
10 to 14 years	0.1	1	0.055423595	0.00554236	0.055423595
15 to 19 years	0.4	6.7	0.057993125	0.02319725	0.388553938
20 to 24 years	0.6	3.2	0.069209975	0.041525985	0.22147192
25 to 29 years	0.9	6.8	0.072484005	0.065235605	0.492891234
30 to 34 years	1	3.8	0.070625345	0.070625345	0.268376311
35 to 39 years	1.2	2.2	0.068998181	0.082797817	0.151795998
40 to 44 years	1.6	3.5	0.064178845	0.102686152	0.224625958
45 to 49 years	2.1	7	0.063757826	0.133891435	0.446304782
50 to 54 years	3.3	7.5	0.066741148	0.220245788	0.50055861
55 to 59 years	5.6	10.6	0.073249163	0.410195313	0.776441128
60 to 64 years	8.7	23.2	0.066212358	0.576047515	1.536126706
65 to 69 years	13.4	18	0.054466238	0.729847589	0.980392284
70 to 74 years	20.2	33.3	0.043770147	0.884156969	1.457545895
75 to 79 years	31.9	47.6	0.029087817	0.927901362	1.384580089
80 to 84 years	56.8	130.4	0.018633556	1.058385981	2.429815702
85 to 89 years	104.5	100	0.010976841	1.147079885	1.0976841
90 years and over	208.7	153.8	0.005331529	1.112690102	0.81998916
Directly standardized rate/1000 years[-1]				7.563	12.789

*proportion of the national male population in each age category

age-standardized mortality is expressed per 100 000 years[-1], and simultaneously adjusts for age and sex rather than adjusting for age separately in males and females. The results are, however, consistent with the directly age-standardized rates presented in Table 18 and Table 19. They show higher crude mortality in Ontario than Nunavut in 2019 (737.0 per 100 000 population in Ontario versus 556.8 per 100 000 population), but a lower age-standardized rate in Ontario (636.9 per 100 000 population) than Nunavut (1410.6 per 100 000 population), consistent with the direct standardizations presented in Tables 18 and 19.

TABLE 19. DIRECT STANDARDIZATION FOR AGE OF ONTARIO AND NUNAVUT MORTALITY DATA FOR FEMALES[65]

	Female mortality rates/1000 person years^{-1}		Weights*	Weighted rates (Ontario)	Weighted rates (Nunavut)
	Ontario	Nunavut			
< 1 year	4.2	16.5	0.009594	0.04029517	0.158302452
1 to 4 years	0.1	0.6	0.040202	0.00402018	0.024121077
5 to 9 years	0.1	0	0.052777	0.005277666	0
10 to 14 years	0.1	1.6	0.05275	0.005274991	0.084399851
15 to 19 years	0.2	1.2	0.054524	0.010904792	0.065428752
20 to 24 years	0.3	1.3	0.062533	0.018759947	0.081293105
25 to 29 years	0.4	1.9	0.067257	0.02690295	0.127789014
30 to 34 years	0.5	3.9	0.067985	0.033992423	0.265140899
35 to 39 years	0.7	1.5	0.068327	0.047828648	0.10248996
40 to 44 years	0.9	0	0.064673	0.058205517	0
45 to 49 years	1.3	2.8	0.06381	0.082952429	0.178666771
50 to 54 years	2.2	6.7	0.066499	0.146296823	0.445540325
55 to 59 years	3.3	5.9	0.073127	0.24131976	0.43145048
60 to 64 years	5.2	22.4	0.067511	0.35105603	1.51224136
65 to 69 years	8.1	30.2	0.057121	0.462679808	1.725053113
70 to 74 years	12.9	33.8	0.047054	0.606995491	1.590422293
75 to 79 years	21.7	94	0.032857	0.712991041	3.08853262
80 to 84 years	39.7	180	0.023283	0.924353838	4.19102496
85 to 89 years	73.9	235.3	0.016229	1.199305364	3.818627228
90 years and over	177.1	0	0.011889	2.105514095	0
Directly standardized rate/1000 years^{-1}				7.085	17.891

*proportion of the national female population in each age category

An important thing to remember about directly standardized rates is that they are imaginary. Conceptually, in the examples presented, a directly standardized mortality rate represents a mortality rate that is expected to occur in the imaginary scenario where both Nunavut and Ontario have exactly the same age distribution as the national population. Neither of them does. Because it is an imaginary rate, the standardized rate should not be assigned any particular significance other than its intended purpose, which is to facilitate comparisons. Looking at Table 18 and Table 19, the key point is that for both men and women, the Nunavut rate is higher. It would be wrong to compare the sex-specific rates in this case, because the male and female tables use different standardizing weights. (In Table 18, the weights are the proportions of men within the national population in each age group. In Table 19, the weights are the proportions of women within the national population in each age group.) In addition, it would be inappropriate to compare these directly standardized rates to those of other countries since other countries would have different standardizing populations.

Indirect standardization

Indirect standardization is another strategy for increasing the comparability of 2 populations.

A typical scenario involves concern that an occupational group may have an elevated risk of an adverse health outcome. You could address this question by comparing the crude mortality rate in the targeted workers (or some other group, which for ease of language will be called the *exposed group* here) with that of other occupations or the general population. The outcome of interest is usually mortality, but it can be another outcome. In the discussion that follows, *mortality* will be used to simplify the language. Unfortunately, a simple comparison between an exposed occupational cohort and the general population, due to the possibility of confounding, would probably not be a valid comparison. Often, age- and sex-specific incidence or mortality rates are available for the general population, but not for the occupational (or other) cohort in question, so you can't use direct standardization to address this confounding. Another approach—indirect standardization—is necessary.

As with direct standardization, indirect standardization uses a standardizing population. In indirect standardization, stratum-specific (usually age- and sex-specific) rates from the standardizing population are multiplied by (you could say *weighted by*) the proportion of the exposed cohort falling into each of those age-sex categories. This multiplication predicts the expected deaths (or other outcome) in the exposed cohort, under the null hypothesis that the cohort has the same age- and sex-specific mortality rates as the standardizing population.

The next step is to divide the actually observed deaths by the expected deaths, creating a parameter called the *standardized mortality ratio* (SMR). If the expected and observed deaths have very similar values, the SMR will be close to 1. This means that the exposed group does not have an elevated risk of death. On the other hand, if the group has an elevated risk of mortality, the SMR is greater than 1.

$$SMR = \frac{Observed}{Expected}$$

where *observed* means the actual number of deaths that have occurred in the exposed cohort and *expected* is the sum of the expected number of deaths in a series of age- and sex-specific strata

---

Key point: Indirect standardization involves the calculation of an SMR, a parameter that embodies a comparison of an exposed cohort to a general population rate.

The abbreviation *SMR* can also stand for *standardized morbidity ratio* if the outcome of concern is morbidity (having a disease) rather than mortality. The same principles apply. Also, the same procedure can be used to standardize incidence rather than mortality. In this case, the resulting parameter is called the *standardized incidence ratio* (SIR).

Here's an interesting feature of the SMR for exposed occupational groups: intuition suggests that a value of 1 should indicate a lack of effect of the exposure on mortality or morbidity, but an SMR of 1.0 is actually a cause for concern. The reason is an effect called the *healthy worker effect*. People working at a job are expected to be healthier than people who are not working, so when an SMR is calculated for an occupational cohort using the general population as the standardizing population, expectation is that the SMR should be less than 1.

Another point about the SMR is that this parameter is often expressed as a percentage:

$$\text{SMR}\,(\%) = \left[\frac{\text{Observed}}{\text{Expected}}\right] \times 100$$

We'll use the comparison of all-cause mortality in Nunavut and Ontario in 2019 to demonstrate calculating an SMR. Table 20 shows the population of Nunavut in 5-year age strata[155] and age-specific mortality rates for the overall Canadian population.[152] Multiplying the counts in the Nunavut age strata by the national age-specific mortality rates (which are converted to decimal values here to simplify the units, and presented in addition to the 1000 years^{-1} rates recorded in the data table) leads to an expected number of deaths in each age stratum. As with direct standardization, these are imaginary estimates that represent the number of deaths that would be expected to occur within each stratum in Nunavut under the assumption that Nunavut residents have the same mortality rates as the national population. Finally, the actual number of deaths in 2019,[154] which in this case is 215, is used to produce the SMR.

The elevated SMR leads to the same conclusion as the results of direct standardization: age standardized mortality is elevated in Nunavut.

Thinking deeper

The concept of weighting

This chapter has described 2 procedures for comparing populations in the presence of possible confounding variables. These procedures, especially direct standardization, provide an introduction to the concept of weighting.

TABLE 20. STANDARDIZED MORTALITY RATIO FOR NUNAVUT: INDIRECT STANDARDIZATION FOR AGE USING THE NATIONAL POPULATION AS THE STANDARDIZING POPULATION[153,65]

| Age group | National age-specific mortality rates | | Nunavut population | Expected deaths |
	(/1000 person years⁻¹)	(person year⁻¹)		
< 1 year	4.4	0.0044	870	3.828
1 to 4 years	0.2	0.0002	3,389	0.6778
5 to 9 years	0.1	0.0001	4,283	0.4283
10 to 14 years	0.1	0.0001	3,798	0.3798
15 to 19 years	0.3	0.0003	3,269	0.9807
20 to 24 years	0.5	0.0005	3,086	1.543
25 to 29 years	0.7	0.0007	3,232	2.2624
30 to 34 years	0.8	0.0008	3,109	2.4872
35 to 39 years	0.9	0.0009	2,670	2.403
40 to 44 years	1.2	0.0012	2,198	2.6376
45 to 49 years	1.8	0.0018	2,200	3.96
50 to 54 years	2.8	0.0028	2,234	6.2552
55 to 59 years	4.5	0.0045	2,115	9.5175
60 to 64 years	7.0	0.007	1,053	7.371
65 to 69 years	10.8	0.0108	686	7.4088
70 to 74 years	17.1	0.0171	447	7.6437
75 to 79 years	27.9	0.0279	222	6.1938
80 to 84 years	49.1	0.0491	119	5.8429
85 to 89 years	88.8	0.0888	37	3.2856
90 and over	188.4	0.1884	25	4.71
Total deaths expected				79.82
Observed				215
SMR				2.69
SMR (%)				269%

Direct standardization uses the proportion of the standardizing population in a particular age and sex stratum to weight age- and sex-specific rates or frequencies in 2 populations. This facilitates more meaningful comparisons between the populations.

Population surveys often use a similar weighting procedure to approximate simple random sampling (which produces ideal samples).

Think about some of the national surveys that Statistics Canada conducts. These surveys use multiple-stage selection procedures, because obtaining a simple random sample for Canada's large and dispersed population poses many obstacles. A random sample would first require a list of every survey-eligible person in the country (e.g., a list of all household residents who are not members of the armed forces and do not live on reservations or in institutions)—a very long list, and difficult to compile. After selecting a random subset of subjects from this list, researchers would need to contact the subjects—and possibly travel across the country to interview them, which would be prohibitively expensive.

However, by selecting a particular geographical area for a survey, a researcher can travel to that area, obtain a list of households within it, contact those households, and randomly select 1 or more participants from among the residents of each household. This multiple-stage approach is much more efficient than simple random sampling in large-scale population surveys.

A multiple-stage approach to sampling means that different members of the sample have different selection probabilities. For example, imagine the step in a multiple-stage sampling procedure where a researcher randomly selects 1 person from a household into a study: if that household has 2 members, the probability of either of them being selected is 0.5, which is one-half the selection probability associated with a 1-person household and twice the selection probability of a 4-person household. The same problem would emerge with selection of households from areas that contain different numbers of households.

SAMPLING WEIGHTS

The problem of different selection probabilities is addressed by the calculation of sampling weights. A common type of weighting uses the inverse (in other words, the reciprocal) of the sampling probability. If each observation from 2-person households is multiplied by a probability weight (the inverse of the 0.5 sampling probability, $1/0.5 = 2$), and the resulting weight is used in the calculation of an estimate, this corrects the problem of unequal selection probability, and the weighted prevalence estimate will again reflect what would have been seen in a simple random sample.

The calculation of sampling weights is usually more complicated than our example: multiple-stage sampling procedures can have many steps, and studies using them build in stratified sampling as well. Each step may alter the probability of selection, which complicates the calculation of sampling weights.

The calculation of sampling weights can also attempt to address the possibility of selection bias that results from refusal, nonconsent, attrition, and so on. If such "drop-outs" have characteristics in common, sampling weights can adjust for them. These are called *nonresponse weights* or (since they usually amount to an adjustment to another weight calculated to account for broader study-design issues) *nonresponse adjustment to sampling weights.* Think back to the discussion of selection bias in a chapter 8: selection bias occurs when the probability of selection is influenced by disease status. Disease status, of course, is not known when a person drops out or refuses to participate in a study. Adjustments for nonresponse, therefore, must incorporate some guesswork. They must try to make adjustments based on characteristics of those who do not participate, but not on the key characteristic (i.e., whether their participation depended on disease status). For this reason, adjustments for nonresponse are no substitute for the best way to avoid such bias: making sure that the rate of participation is high.

UNEQUAL SELECTION PROBABILITIES, CLUSTERING, AND WEIGHTING

A sampling procedure that results in unequal selection probabilities is an example of a design effect. Design effects result from the ways in which a study was deliberately designed. An example is the effect of a sampling procedure that results in unequal selection probabilities. This design effect can be corrected using sampling weights. Attrition and nonconsent are not design effects since they are not a planned component of the study. These are study-design defects: they represent problems in the way a study was conducted. Design effects are more predictable than the problems that arise from study-design defects and can more easily be corrected using data analysis procedures such as weighting.

Multiple stages of selection produce design effects. In these situations, the members of the sample fall into clusters, such as geographical areas. The problem with clustering is that members of a cluster are likely more similar to each other than randomly selected people in the general population. Failure to account for this design effect results in underestimation of standard error if conventional statistical analyses are used, and, consequently, unrealistically narrow confidence intervals for estimated parameters. Survey-analysis software has special procedures to correct for this design effect and generate accurate confidence intervals.

WEIGHTING IN STATISTICS CANADA DATA

The national surveys conducted by Statistics Canada provide several options for properly addressing the issues of unequal selection probabilities and clustering.

When Statistics Canada conducts a survey, it typically produces 2 data sets, including a public use microdata file, or PUMF. (PUMFs are available for download by researchers and students at major Canadian universities.) PUMFs place continuous variables in categories and remove certain variables as safeguards to protect against the identification of individual survey respondents. These data sets are made available to researchers and students at Canadian universities through a program called the Data Liberation Initiative.[156]

Each survey respondent in a PUMF file has an associated weight. This is a frequency weight and is somewhat different than the type of sampling weight described above (where the weight represents the inverse of the selection probability). A frequency weight specifies the number of people in a population represented by each individual respondent. Statistical software can use this weight to produce valid estimates.

Statistics Canada also has a method for dealing with clustering in PUMF data, based on a replicate bootstrap weighting procedure, the technicalities of which are beyond the scope of this book. Nevertheless, implementing replicate bootstrap weights into data analysis is not difficult using modern software. You can find information about the accessibility of PUMF data at your particular university, including information about who to contact to access it, on the web page for the Data Liberation Initiative.[157]

Statistics Canada's regional data centres, located at most major Canadian universities, house full Statistics Canada data sets. These large and complex data sets allow detailed analysis. Statistics Canada produces replicate bootstrap weights that allow calculation of valid estimates, with accurate confidence intervals for this master file data, similar to that used for PUMF files.

The regional data centres in Canada are an underused resource. Most university-based researchers in Canada are eligible for access to these data sets. Those who check into them are often surprised to find the centres have collected and stored important data related to their areas of interest.[158]

Statistics Canada describes the content and study-design characteristics of the various data sets on its website.

Questions

1. Zablotska et al[159] studied the long-term mortality and cancer incidence experienced by uranium workers and mill workers employed in Port Radium, NWT, and Beaverlodge, Saskatchewan, and at a radium and uranium refining and processing plant in Port Hope, Ontario. They linked the workers' records to the Canadian Mortality Database (CMDB) and the Canadian Cancer Database to ascertain cancer-related mortality to 1999. They observed 42 cases of deaths due to non-Hodgkins lymphoma in their cohort, compared to 46.28 expected deaths determined using statistics from the general population.
   a. What type of standardization is this?
   b. What is the SMR for mortality due to non-Hodgkins lymphoma?
   c. Provide an interpretation of the result.

2. As a component of the Vancouver Injection Drug Users Study (VIDUS), Spittal et al[160] monitored 520 female intravenous drug users, 68 of whom died during follow-up. Using the female population of British Columbia as a standardizing population, they calculated an SMR for this group of 47.3.
   a. What does this SMR mean?
   b. What are some possible explanations for an SMR of this magnitude?

3. Karamanis et al[161] used Swedish health data to evaluate whether women treated for anorexia nervosa might have a lower cancer incidence. Their rationale was that caloric restriction lowers cancer incidence in some animal models. Using the general population as a standardizing population, they reported an SMR of 2.5 for lung cancer mortality. Can you think of a possible explanation for this finding?

4. Callaghan et al[162] followed a cohort of patients discharged from California hospitals after admissions for alcohol- and drug-related diagnoses. The patients were followed for 16 years, after which the investigators calculated age-, sex-, and race-adjusted SMRs for deaths due to motor vehicle accidents. These SMRs ranged from 2.3 for cannabis to 3.8 for cocaine. The SMR for alcohol was 4.5. In your opinion, what are the implications of these SMRs?

5. Nijjar et al[163] wanted to investigate whether different ethnic groups have different risk of acute myocardial infarction (AMI) in the province of British Columbia. Using hospital administrative data, they attempted to identify all patients with incident AMI in BC during a defined time interval. Ethnicity was determined by analyzing surnames. The investigators used direct age standardization to support comparisons of incidence among 3 groups. Among men, those of South Asian ethnicity had the highest age standardized incidence rate (SIR), followed by those of Caucasian and Chinese ethnicity. The investigators found a similar ranking in women. These investigators were not studying mortality, which is the most common use of direct standardization. In your opinion, is it appropriate to use direct standardization in an incidence analysis like this?

6. You are asked for advice by a health administrator. The administrator is working on a budget for health services and needs to plan for an expected number of investigations of ectopic pregnancies. The population of the area in question has a larger proportion of women of childbearing age than the average health planning district in Canada. For this reason, the administrator is considering the potential advantages and disadvantages of age-standardizing estimates of the need for such investigations. What advice would you offer?

7. For direct standardization, what would generally be the best source of information about a standardizing population?

8. A high rate of mortality is suspected in a particular nursing home. The residents of this nursing home, however, are much older than members of the general population, so indirect standardization is carried out using age- and sex-specific estimates from the general population. The SMR is found to be 2.0. How would you interpret this estimate?

9. What are the advantages and disadvantages of stratification as an alternative to standardization?

10. In comparisons of 2 populations, direct standardization addresses the issue of confounding by using the distribution of potential confounding variables (such as age and sex) in a standardizing population. For example, in this chapter the Canadian national population distribution was used to standardize mortality-rate estimates from Nunavut and Ontario. Would it be more accurate to use the actual population of Nunavut and Ontario to standardize the respective rates?

PART IV

Study designs and their vulnerability to error

So far, we have covered the fundamentals of epidemiology by discussing descriptive studies. Most epidemiological studies, however, are analytical, or at least have some analytical goals.

Descriptive studies measure the distribution and prevalence of disease. By contrast, analytical studies measure association between exposure and disease, and make inferences about causation.

Analytical studies are vulnerable to the same kinds of error as descriptive studies, but sometimes with added complications that require different strategies.

Cross-sectional studies

OBJECTIVES

- Define cross-sectional studies.
- Differentiate between the potential descriptive and analytical goals of cross-sectional studies.
- Describe the following measures of association: prevalence differences, prevalence ratios, prevalence odds ratios, and specific types of linear equations.
- Explain how to interpret measures of association calculated from cross-sectional data.
- List strengths and weaknesses of cross-sectional studies.

CRITICAL APPRAISAL AND CLASSIFICATION OF STUDY DESIGNS

The ability to correctly classify study designs is a useful skill.

Classifying the design of a study facilitates communication: a single label (e.g., "cross-sectional study") conveys information about the study's methodology.

Study-design classification also helps with critical appraisal, because particular methodological vulnerabilities are typically associated with different designs. In addition, the process of classifying a study's design requires close attention to key aspects of its methodology, which helps to bring a conceptual structure to the process of reading papers and critical appraisal.

Study-design classification resembles aspects of clinical assessment, such as taking a history from a patient or conducting a physical examination. It involves an organized series of steps and questions that collect key information. Classification of a study design probes the way in which a study was conducted. As you read a study, you look for evidence. This makes reading a study into a procedure for evaluating that study.

Key point: Critical appraisal is more than just reading a study and intuitively identifying problems with it. Critical appraisal involves asking and answering a series of key questions. It is a more formal way of looking at studies, and seeks clear conclusions about the value of studies. Classification of study design is an early step in critical appraisal.

Approaches to study-design classification

The best approach to study-design classification is to determine the key features studies actually possess.

A common approach, however, is to categorize studies presumptively as either descriptive (concerned with the distribution or prevalence of disease) or analytical (concerned with causal connections between exposure and disease).

This presumptive descriptive-analytic division emphasizes the goals and motivations generally associated with particular study designs. For example, the cross-sectional study design is often considered descriptive, because it cannot usually allow causal inference. Cross-sectional studies measure exposure and disease at a single point in time, so they cannot meet a basic criterion for causal judgement: that causes must temporally precede effects. Therefore, causal inference is usually not possible from a cross-sectional study.

However, there are some instances where exposures can reasonably be interpreted as preceding the onset of disease, even in cross-sectional data. For example, if the exposure is a birth-related event or a gene, and the disease has its onset well after birth—say, in adulthood—cross-sectional data may be sufficient to clarify temporality.

So, cross-sectional studies can be analytic, which makes the descriptive-analytic distinction a risky starting point for classifying study design.

The distinction is also risky because the goals of investigators are not always clearly evident. An investigator may have analytic aims, but may deliver data that are descriptive only. Or, they may have descriptive aims, but nevertheless interpret some of their findings as having causal significance. Because of these ambiguities, it is better to classify study designs on more defensible grounds than the presumptive descriptive-analytic distinction.

> *Key point:* Accurate classification of a study's design should start with documented features of the study, not with the stated or assumed descriptive-versus-analytical motivations of the investigators.

What is a cross-sectional study?

Epidemiological studies fall into 3 main categories: cross-sectional studies, case-control studies, and prospective cohort studies.

Cross-sectional studies are studies in which all data are collected at a single point in time. A study designed to estimate point prevalence (called a *prevalence study*, see page 17) is an example of a cross-sectional study. A prevalence study provides a snapshot of disease status in a population at a point in time. Prevalence studies are generally descriptive in their goals, but they can also have analytical goals involving hypotheses about disease-exposure associations. Most often, such goals involve determining the existence of a disease-exposure association, or generating etiological hypotheses, rather than evaluating etiological hypotheses. In such instances, the key characteristic of a cross-sectional study is that both the disease and exposure variables are measured at a single point in time.

It's important, however, to stay flexible about what is meant by "a single point in time." Obviously, no study can occur in an instant. A prevalence study may take months or even years to conduct. Conceptually, however, these studies take place at a point in time. In addition, the idea of a "single point in time" refers to the study design, not to the timing of events. For example, Afifi et al[164] analyzed cross-sectional data from the national Canadian Community Health Survey (see the information on this survey that follows) to examine associations between child abuse and adult mental health outcomes. The survey collected all of its data during a single interview with each respondent. The fact that the child abuse occurred years before the data collection does not change the fact that this is a cross-sectional study.

Examples of cross-sectional studies

CANADIAN COMMUNITY HEALTH SURVEY

The Canadian Community Health Survey (CCHS) is an ongoing program of cross-sectional surveys carried out by Statistics Canada.

The CCHS survey program has several goals[130]:

- support health surveillance programs by providing health data at the national, provincial, and intraprovincial levels

- provide a single data source for health research on small populations and rare characteristics
- provide timely release of information and easy accessibility to a diverse community of users
- create a flexible survey instrument that includes a rapid response option to address emerging issues related to the health of the population

Data collection for the general health component of the CCHS is continuous, occurring throughout the year, but the data are aggregated into annual and 2-year data sets that describe the health of the Canadian household population at what can be considered points in time. The CCHS collects data on the prevalence of various chronic health conditions, and the prevalence of important risk-factor exposures such as smoking. It also measures certain health status characteristics (e.g., distress, depression, perceived health) using validated instruments and describes the use of health care resources.

ALCOHOL- AND DRUG-IMPAIRED DRIVING AMONG CANADIAN STUDENTS: MINAKER ET AL

In 2017, Minaker et al[165] reported an analysis of the prevalence of risky driving behaviours, such as driving while under the influence of alcohol or cannabis, or being a passenger in a car when the driver had been drinking alcohol or using marijuana. They used data from a study called the Canadian Student Tobacco, Alcohol and Drugs Survey, which included 24 650 students sampled from schools in each of the Canadian provinces. The sampling procedure selected schools within each of the 10 provinces, and then invited all students in those schools to participate in the survey. In addition to estimating the overall prevalence of driving after substance use (for example, 4.7% reported driving after drinking in the preceding 30 days), they also reported characteristics associated with this risky behaviour, including sex (the prevalence was higher in boys than girls, for example) and area-level characteristics (the prevalence was higher in rural than urban areas, for example).

A summary of results from the 2018–2019 Canadian Student Tobacco, Alcohol and Drugs Survey is now available to investigators.[166] The survey provides cross-sectional data on many topics related to substance use in students.

EFFECTS OF DRUGS TO TREAT PARKINSON DISEASE: WEINTRAUB ET AL

In 2010, Weintraub et al[167] used a cross-sectional study to quantify a possible association between drugs for treating Parkinson disease and impulse-control disorders.

Parkinson disease is a progressive neurological disease characterized by tremor, rigidity, slowed movement, and gait problems, as well as cognitive and behavioural changes. These symptoms are believed come from the death of dopamine-producing cells in the brain. Treatment of Parkinson disease often includes drugs—dopamine agonists—that act on the same brain receptors as dopamine. However, due to one of dopamine's other roles in the brain (e.g., neurotransmission in the reward centres of the brain), dopamine agonists may be associated with an increased frequency of impulse-control disorders. When taking dopaminergic medications, people with Parkinson disease may anticipate greater rewards from potentially risky activities such as gambling or sexual activity. To study this association, Weintraub et al conducted a cross-sectional study. They identified dual goals for their study: to estimate the "point frequency" (prevalence) of impulse-control disorders in people with Parkinson disease, and to assess the association of these disorders with dopamine-replacement therapies (a category that includes dopamine agonists and also levodopa, which is converted to dopamine in the brain). The investigators, exemplifying the intermixture of descriptive and analytical motivations that underlie many epidemiological studies, hypothesized that patients treated with dopamine agonists would have a higher prevalence of impulse-control disorders than those not treated with dopamine agonists. Study subjects with Parkinson disease were recruited from movement-disorder centres in the United States and Canada. Their use of medication was recorded, and an assessment with validated instruments was used to identify 4 impulse-control disorders: problem gambling, compulsive sexual behaviour, compulsive buying, and binge eating.

The final study sample included 3090 participants. Dopamine agonists were used in about two-thirds of the sample. An impulse-control disorder was identified in 13.6% of the sample. Those treated with a dopamine agonist had a higher prevalence of 1 or more impulse-control disorders (17.1%) than those not treated with dopamine agonists (6.9%). This translated into an odds ratio (this parameter is discussed in more detail below) of 2.72, which was reported with an associated 95% CI of 2.08–3.54. The authors concluded that these medications were associated with an elevated prevalence of impulse-control disorders in this population.

VITAMIN D INSUFFICIENCY AMONG CANADIAN CREE: RIVERIN ET AL

Riverin et al[168] analyzed data from the Nituuchischaayihtitaau Aschii multicommunity environment and health study, which collected data from 7 of 9 Eastern James Bay Cree communities in the months of May to September from 2005 to 2009. Blood samples were collected by a research nurse to measure vitamin D levels, and bilingual interviewers assessed demographic variables, body mass index, diet, and activity patterns. Deficiency was defined as < 30 nmol/L. The overall prevalence of vitamin D deficiency was 5.7%. The prevalence of insufficiency (< 50 nmol/L) was nearly 50%, and was higher in the following groups: women; obese participants; younger participants; those whose blood sample was drawn in the spring; those with low levels of fish and milk intake; and those reporting lower levels of vigorous physical activity. Note that even though data were collected during several years, the study design involves examining associations at a point in time, so this analysis should be classified as a cross-sectional study.

How cross-sectional studies look at association

When cross-sectional studies go beyond estimation of prevalence to include an assessment of risk factors, the data can be represented by a 2 × 2 table—a version of the table encountered in chapter 6 (see Table 9, page 85). Rather than quantifying the contingency between a test and a gold standard, this 2 × 2 table depicts the association between an exposure and a disease.

The fundamental dichotomy between population and sample are just as important as always. Therefore, it is best to present two 2 × 2 tables: Table 21 displays the exposure-disease contingencies in a population (using the convention of uppercase letters) and Table 22 displays contingencies as observed in a sample drawn from that population (using the convention of lowercase letters).

TABLE 21. 2 × 2 TABLE FOR DATA FROM A CROSS-SECTIONAL STUDY OF AN ENTIRE POPULATION

	Disease	No disease
Exposed	A	B
Nonexposed	C	D

TABLE 22. 2 × 2 TABLE FOR DATA FROM A CROSS-SECTIONAL STUDY OF A SAMPLE

	Disease	No disease
Exposed	a	b
Nonexposed	c	d

Tables 21 and 22, in themselves, are not particularly effective in communicating the contingency. The question of interest in such a cross-sectional study is whether the prevalence of disease differs between the exposed group and the nonexposed group. You can use the tables to calculate a prevalence estimate for each group and then compare the 2 prevalence estimates. Considering the sample data, this reduces 4 numbers to 2 proportions, facilitating comparison:

$$\text{Prevalence}(\text{exposed}) = \frac{a}{a+b}$$

$$\text{Prevalence}(\text{nonexposed}) = \frac{c}{c+d}$$

It would be even better to examine the association with a single number. There are a variety of ways to do this, such as subtracting 1 prevalence from the other (a prevalence difference), or making a ratio of the 2 prevalences (a prevalence ratio), or calculating the prevalence as odds and making a ratio of odds in the exposed group and nonexposed group (a prevalence odds ratio). Such parameters embody a comparison of the 2 prevalences, and are therefore measures of association.

Prevalence differences

Here's how to calculate a prevalence difference for a population:

$$\text{PREVALENCE Difference} = \frac{A}{A+B} - \frac{C}{C+D}$$

For a sample, it is:

$$\text{Prevalence Difference} = \frac{a}{a+b} - \frac{c}{c+d}$$

Differentiating the second equation from the first serves as a reminder that a sample-based estimate is subject to random or stochastic error. If you repeated this study many times, and calculated the prevalence difference many times, a distribution of prevalence differences would emerge. If the sample sizes from these repeated studies were small, this distribution would be broad. By contrast, if the repeated studies had large sample sizes, this distribution would be narrower. If procedures for measurement and selection were perfect, the law of large numbers provides a reason to believe that the distribution will centre around the population value. The estimates arising from such "perfect" studies may sometimes differ quite a bit from the population value, but if the study is sufficiently large, big differences are unlikely.

We say "perfect" as a reminder that imperfect measurement and selection can lead to systematically erroneous prevalence estimates. Measures of association based on prevalence estimates are, like the prevalence estimates themselves, vulnerable to study-design defects that lead to misclassification bias and selection bias.

Key point: A prevalence difference is a measure of association because it embodies a comparison between 2 simpler parameters, which are prevalences in exposed and nonexposed groups.

Prevalence ratios

To calculate a prevalence ratio, you divide the 2 prevalences:

$$\text{PREVALENCE Ratio} = \frac{\dfrac{A}{A+B}}{\dfrac{C}{C+D}}$$

Or, for a sample:

$$\text{Prevalence Ratio} = \frac{\dfrac{a}{a+b}}{\dfrac{c}{c+d}}$$

Note that a ratio is simply 1 number divided by another, which means the prevalence proportion itself is technically a ratio—and sometimes also called a *prevalence ratio*.

Odds ratios

Odds ratios are commonly encountered, and use odds rather than prevalence proportions. (Differences in odds, however, are not used.)

An odds ratio can refer to any ratio of odds. Therefore, when calculating an odds ratio from a cross-sectional study, it is best to explicitly label that parameter as a prevalence odds ratio.

$$\text{PREVALENCE Odds Ratio} = \frac{\dfrac{A}{B}}{\dfrac{C}{D}} = \frac{AD}{BC}$$

Or, for a sample:

$$\text{Prevalence Odds Ratio} = \frac{\dfrac{a}{b}}{\dfrac{c}{d}} = \frac{ad}{bc}$$

Key point: An epidemiological association between exposure and disease can be expressed as the ratio of prevalence in nonexposed and exposed groups (including prevalence odds).

Linear equations

The formulas for prevalence difference, prevalence ratio, and prevalence odds ratio all derive from the classic 2 × 2 contingency tables depicting an exposure-disease relationship, such as Table 21 and Table 22.

The same goal of comparing 2 prevalence estimates can also be accomplished by a linear equation—a simple equation that describes a line using an intercept and slope term.

To see how this works, we can form such an equation using 3 symbols: alpha (α), beta (β) and X_e. Here, α is the intercept term and β is the slope term for the linear equation. X_e is a variable that represents exposure to a risk factor. Suppose that—in addition to being part of the equation for a line—α represents prevalence in the nonexposed group and β represents the risk difference. To make this type of equation work, we also need the indicator variable (X_e) representing exposure. An indicator variable for exposure assumes a value of 0 (meaning not exposed) or 1 (meaning exposed). This leads to a simple form of a linear equation:

$$\text{Prevalence} = \alpha + \beta X_e$$

Note that in its simplest form, as above, this equation doesn't actually describe a line, merely 2 prevalence estimates: a prevalence for the exposed group and a prevalence for the nonexposed group. X_e can have 2 values: 0 to represent nonexposure and 1 to represent exposure. For the group that is not exposed, where the value of X_e is 0, the term to the right of the plus sign disappears: prevalence equals α. For the exposed group, where X_e is 1, the prevalence equals $\alpha + \beta$, which makes sense because this is the baseline prevalence in the nonexposed group plus the amount of extra prevalence (the prevalence difference) that goes along with exposure.

Key point: The same information provided by a 2 × 2 contingency table for disease and exposure can be represented using an equation that has a linear form.

The value of expressing 2 prevalence estimates using a single equation of the type shown above may not be obvious at this stage. The equation doesn't add any information beyond presenting the 2 frequencies themselves. However, equations of this form are important tools for addressing confounding and effect modification, issues of importance in analytic studies that are discussed in later chapters. The relationship described above is a starting point for the use of linear models for epidemiological analysis.

LOG-TRANSFORMED PREVALENCE

There is another interesting relationship that emerges from the general idea of depicting prevalence data for exposed and nonexposed groups using an equation of linear form. This relationship unfolds when the equation describes the natural logarithm (here abbreviated *log*) of the prevalence. Consider the following equation:

$$\text{Log Prevalence} = \alpha + \beta X_e$$

Here, the log prevalence in the exposed group is α + β, and the log prevalence in the nonexposed group is α. In this case, β is the difference in the log prevalence associated with exposure. The log prevalence in the exposed group minus the log prevalence in the nonexposed group is β, so taken together with the rule for subtraction of logarithms (log a – log b = log a/b), you can see that β in this type of equation is actually a log prevalence ratio. Again, the value of this type of equation may not be obvious at this stage, but it is a foundation for important analysis strategies.

LOG-TRANSFORMED PREVALENCE ODDS

Epidemiological studies often use odds ratios (in our current discussion of cross-sectional studies, these would be prevalence odds ratios) to describe association. The study of effects associated with drugs to treat Parkinson disease by Weintraub et al[167] and the study of vitamin D deficiency in James Bay Cree populations[168] are examples (see pages 140–141).

The use of odds to describe association leads to an equation of linear form in which the β coefficient is a log odds ratio, or—more specifically for the purposes of this chapter—a log prevalence odds ratio. This type of equation is the basis of another approach to statistical modelling that is widely used in epidemiology: logistic regression analysis.

$$\text{Log Odds} = \alpha + \beta X_e$$

Key point: Log-transformed models based on linear equations are the basis of several approaches to epidemiological analysis. The coefficients in such models represent the log of ratio-based measures of association.

Strengths and weaknesses of cross-sectional studies

Strengths

Valuable snapshots of disease: Cross-sectional studies provide accurate snapshots of the amount of disease in a population at a point in time. This is very useful for descriptive purposes. Planners and administrators of health services use this kind of information to anticipate the level of services required to meet the needs of populations. Since cross-sectional studies often use probability sampling, they can provide very good estimates of population parameters.

Description of disease occurrence across multiple variables: Cross-sectional studies can describe the occurrence of disease in relation to multiple exposure and disease variables. The Canadian Community Health Survey is an example of a study that measures many exposure and disease variables. It's important to remember, though, that cross-sectional associations (as quantified by prevalence differences, prevalence ratios, or prevalence odds ratios) do not provide comparisons of risk. Prevalence is determined by incidence (a concept closely aligned with risk) and also by duration. Duration, in turn, is influenced by mortality and other aspects of prognosis. This means that cross-sectional associations may (or may not) reflect an impact of exposure on disease etiology, mortality, or prognosis. Nevertheless, such estimates can be informative: they can help specify groups with a high burden of illness and may generate hypotheses for future studies.

Cost efficiency: Cross-sectional studies can be less expensive to conduct than other types of studies because they do not track participants over time, something that usually costs a lot of money.

Invulnerability to attrition: Attrition (loss of participants) is a vulnerability of studies that follow subjects over long periods of time, and can result in selection bias. Attrition does not affect cross-sectional studies, because these studies collect data at a single point in time.

Weaknesses

Lack of causal inference: Cross-sectional studies rarely directly contribute to understanding causation. This is largely because they measure disease and exposure at a point in time, which often precludes determination of the temporal relationship between exposure and disease. Since a cause must logically precede an effect, the point-in-time data of cross-sectional studies is a strong impediment to causal reasoning.

No determination of risk: Cross-sectional studies cannot determine risk. An exposure that increases the incidence of disease will increase prevalence, other things being equal, but an exposure that leads to more rapid death will decrease prevalence by shortening the duration of disease. An exposure that affects the rate of recovery from a disease can increase or decrease the prevalence depending on whether it decreases or increases the rate of recovery.

Inefficiency for rare diseases: Cross-sectional studies can be an inefficient way to study rare diseases or associations with rare exposures. A cross-sectional study might end up collecting a lot of data only to have a small number of respondents in some of the cells of the 2×2 table arising from the data. This will usually lead to wide confidence intervals.

Sensitivity to time-dependent frequency changes: Cross-sectional studies can be misleading when disease frequency changes over time. For example, diseases that occur more often in winter—say, seasonal affective disorders or seasonal influenza—will have different prevalences depending on the season when they are measured.

Key point: Like all study designs, the cross-sectional design is associated with strengths and weaknesses. It is the best design for some purposes and not for others.

Thinking deeper

Confidence intervals for odds ratios

This chapter has made a distinction between sample-based and population-based analyses. Sample-based analyses are subject to random error, so confidence intervals for such estimates are needed. Confidence intervals help to quantify the vulnerability of an estimate to random error. Formulas to calculate confidence intervals are available for all the parameters discussed in this chapter, but the formulas are not always accurate. It is usually better to use statistical software to calculate exact confidence intervals for such parameters.

With this proviso in mind, there is a formula for calculating confidence intervals for an odds ratio that usually works quite well. It is worth understanding this formula for at least 2 reasons. First, it allows such calculations to be made quickly—e.g., while reading a study in which confidence intervals are not reported. Second, practicing this sort of calculation can help to solidify your understanding of confidence intervals. The trick to this particular formula is that instead of being based on the odds ratio itself, which tends not to be normally distributed, the formula is based on the log odds ratio.

Table 23 shows a 2 × 2 table from the Weintraub et al study.

TABLE 23. 2 × 2 TABLE FOR DATA FROM A CROSS-SECTIONAL STUDY[167(P592)]

	Impulse-control disorder	No impulse-control disorder
Exposed to dopamine agonists	348	1692
Nonexposed to dopamine agonists	72	978

The odds ratio from Table 23 is:

$$\text{Prevalence Odds Ratio} = \frac{\dfrac{a}{b}}{\dfrac{c}{d}} = \frac{ad}{bc} = \frac{348 \times 978}{72 \times 1692} = 2.8$$

Note that this odds ratio is slightly different from what the study reported. In the study, the data were stratified by country (US versus Canada) and a more complex type of odds ratio, the Mantel-Haenszel odds ratio, was used for the calculation while accounting for this stratification.

Odds ratios are not normally distributed, so it is difficult to calculate approximate confidence intervals. However, the log of the odds ratio is approximately normally distributed. So, you can convert the odds ratio to a log odds ratio, calculate 95% CIs for the log odds ratio using a normal approximation, and then convert the log odds ratio's confidence limits back to the original scale using the inverse log function. The calculation can also be done in a spreadsheet. The natural log of the odds ratio is log(2.8), or 1.03. An approximate formula for the standard error of this log odds ratio is:

$$\text{Standard Error of the Log Odds Ratio} = \sqrt{\frac{1}{a} + \frac{1}{b} + \frac{1}{c} + \frac{1}{d}}$$

In this case, it is:

$$\text{Standard Error of the Log Odds Ratio} = \sqrt{\frac{1}{348} + \frac{1}{1692} + \frac{1}{72} + \frac{1}{978}} = 0.136$$

As usual, the confidence limits are the point estimate (remember that this is the log odds ratio) plus or minus an appropriate z value multiplied by the standard error. If the goal is a 95% CI, the appropriate z value is 1.96. So the confidence limits in this case are 1.03 plus or minus 1.96×0.136, which is 0.761 and 1.29. To convert the confidence interval back to the regular scale, the inverse log of these limits should be calculated, which leads to a 95% CI of 2.14–3.64.

Questions

1. List 4 advantages and 4 disadvantages of cross-sectional studies.

2. Do you agree with the following statement? "It is impossible to make causal inference from cross-sectional data." Why or why not?

3. Using the data from Table 23:
   a. What is the prevalence of impulse-control disorders in this population?
   b. Calculate an approximate 95% CI for this proportion.

4. Using the data from Table 23, calculate a prevalence difference for the use of a dopamine agonist.

5. Using the data from Table 23:
   a. Calculate the log odds of having an impulse-control disorder for the exposed and nonexposed subjects.
   b. With the help of an indicator variable assuming values of 0 for the nonexposed group and 1 for the exposed group, formulate an equation of the linear form $y = \alpha + \beta X_e$ that can represent the 2 log odds of impulse-control disorder.
   c. Calculate the inverse log of your β coefficient from part b of this question. What does this represent?

6. The odds ratio can be used as an indicator of the accuracy of a diagnostic test. When used in this way, the odds ratio is called a *diagnostic odds ratio*.[169] Using the data from Table 11 (see page 94), calculate the diagnostic odds ratio.

7. A survey of vitamin D levels in a population living near James Bay collected data using questionnaires and collected blood to measure vitamin D status. The study found that vitamin D deficiency had a higher prevalence in the winter than in the summer.[168] So, in this study, the results varied depending on the timing (e.g., season) of data collection.

   a. Since some of the data were collected in the spring and some in the summer, is it correct to classify this as a cross-sectional study?

   b. A disadvantage of cross-sectional studies is that they can be sensitive to time-dependent frequency changes, which can lead to different estimates depending on the time of year of data collection. Do you think that this general disadvantage of cross-sectional studies is a disadvantage of the Riverin et al study?

8. Point prevalence is the proportion of a population that has a disease at a point in time; the ratio of prevalence in exposed and nonexposed groups is a prevalence ratio (a measure of association). An elevated ratio suggests a higher prevalence in people exposed to the risk factor. However, causal inference is not usually ascribed to cross-sectional estimates. List 2 important reasons why a prevalence ratio should not be used to make causal inferences.

9. If it is generally true that causal inference cannot be made from cross-sectional data, is it fair to say that cross-sectional studies are inherently descriptive in nature?

10. Statistics Canada conducts large cross-sectional household health surveys every year—for example, the Canadian Community Health Survey. However, cross-sectional studies are usually not capable of supporting causal inference. Do you think that Statistics Canada should conduct more longitudinal and fewer cross-sectional studies?

Case-control studies

OBJECTIVES

- Define case-control studies.
- Explain how to interpret measures of association calculated from case-control data.
- Describe recall bias.
- Describe the rare disease assumption.
- Distinguish between induction and latency periods for disease, and describe the dynamic of component causes of disease.
- Define primary, secondary, and tertiary prevention.
- List strengths and weaknesses of case-control studies.

What is a case-control study?

Case-control studies usually have analytic goals: they usually aim to evaluate hypotheses about disease etiology (what causes disease). Some case-control studies have descriptive aims: to generate hypotheses rather than testing them.

Case-control studies differ from cross-sectional studies in their selection of research participants. In a case-control study, participants are selected based on their disease status. This is a radical departure from the typical cross-sectional study, which aims for simple random samples (where each person in the population has an equal probability of selection) or other types of probability samples (where each person has a known probability of selection). Case-control studies really have 2 processes of selection, because they select 2 groups: a group of cases and a group of controls.

Since selection is based on disease status, these studies cannot estimate the frequency of disease. Instead, they focus on estimating associations between risk factors and disease.

Key point: Case-control studies aim to estimate associations between risk factors and disease, and are therefore usually analytical in their orientation.

Design of case-control studies

Case-control studies involve identifying a set of cases (people who have a disease under investigation) and a set of controls (people who do not). Their goal is to assess exposure in both groups, and so disease etiology.

Assessment of exposure in case-control studies is, by necessity, retrospective, because people in the "case" group already have the disease under investigation. This means that case-control studies literally look back in time. They select cases and controls in the "here and now," and then assess past exposure (retrospectively) in each group.

Some investigators used to call case-control studies *retrospective studies*, but this term is now considered obsolete. Although case-control studies are almost always retrospective, other study designs also look back in time.

Figure 10 presents a schematic of the case-control study design.

FIGURE 10. SCHEMATIC OF THE CASE-CONTROL STUDY DESIGN

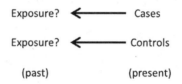

Key point: Case-control studies have 2 key characteristics: they select participants based on disease status (cases and controls), and they assess exposure retrospectively.

Association in case-control studies

A 2 × 2 contingency table, like Table 24, is a good starting point for understanding how case-control studies can estimate risk-factor associations. This table has some familiar features and a few new wrinkles.

The use of lowercase letters shows that this table represents sample data. Because the cases and controls are differentiated based on their disease status, the column headings now reflect this terminology: they refer to cases and controls, rather than disease and nondisease. Also, because the design of the study affects the proportion of participants selected as cases and controls, the table has a row for the total in each group.

TABLE 24. 2 × 2 TABLE FOR DATA FROM A CASE-CONTROL STUDY

	Cases	Controls
Exposed	a	b
Nonexposed	c	d
Total	n_{cases}	$n_{controls}$

Think back to the features of cross-sectional studies based on simple random samples: because the selection probabilities are equal for each member of the population sampled, the expected values falling into each contingency cell (a, b, c, d) reflect those same contingencies in the population. At least this is true in the absence of study-design defects involving participation and classification. In case-control studies, the situation is different: the investigator decides how many cases and how many controls will be in the study. For this reason, unlike cross-sectional studies based on simple random samples, case-control studies have no expectation that the proportion of cases provides an estimate of the population prevalence:

$$e\left(\text{Prevalence}\right) \neq \frac{a+c}{a+b+c+d}$$

In a cross-sectional study, if the selection probabilities are higher for those with a disease, it follows that prevalence will be overestimated due to selection bias. If the selection probabilities for those with a disease are lower than for those without a disease, a prevalence estimate will underestimate the population prevalence.

In a case-control study, the unequal selection probabilities are not a study-design defect leading to bias, but a deliberate study-design feature. The selection probability for cases is always much higher than for controls, but this does not preclude estimating the association. These studies are designed to produce valid estimates of disease-exposure associations, not estimates of prevalence.

> *Key point:* In a case-control study, the selection probabilities for cases are typically much higher than those of controls.

THE IMPACT OF DIFFERENT SELECTION PROBABILITIES FOR CASES AND CONTROLS

In fact, far from representing a study-design defect, the ability to have different selection probabilities for cases and controls is a major advantage of the case-control design and a key reason for its enduring popularity. It allows investigators to selectively recruit cases, even of rare diseases, into a study.

This possibility can be exploited to an extreme degree in case-control studies. Imagine a rare disease for which all of the cases in a health region or province are treated at a single clinic. In this situation, you could conduct a case-control study with a selection probability for cases of 1.0 (100%), meaning that the study would include every single case. However, it would be very inefficient to attempt to have the same selection probability for controls. The value of the case-control design is its ability to use a subset of potentially eligible controls in the population as a referent against which to compare the cases.

The selection of cases is only a part of subject selection in case-control studies. It is usually the easier part. The most difficult challenges involve the selection of controls. The selection of controls must occur in a way that supports valid estimation. The rationale of this study design is that differences in exposure between cases and controls should reflect etiology of the disease, so selection must not depend on exposure in any way that differs between the cases and controls. Otherwise, differences observed may partially or wholly represent methods of selection rather than a disease-exposure association. Here's an example of a tricky problem in control selection. Suppose that a case-control study of a rare disease selects its cases from a specialized clinic. Various exposures might have affected the probability of a case attending that clinic. For example, people with other illnesses, or with worrisome lifestyle characteristics such as smoking or alcohol consumption, may have a higher likelihood of being referred to such a clinic. If exposures of interest to a case-control study have an influence on the selection of cases, a control group with exactly the same influence of exposure on selection would need to be found.

To understand the impact of different selection probabilities on estimating exposure-disease associations in case-control studies, let's revisit the familiar 2 × 2 table for sample-based data, as presented in Table 24. Because the 2 × 2 data no longer reflect the prevalence of disease, a prevalence ratio or prevalence difference is no longer a suitable measure of association. The best measure of association is the odds ratio. Another look at the formula for an odds ratio helps to explain why:

$$\text{Odds Ratio} = \frac{\dfrac{a}{c}}{\dfrac{b}{d}} = \frac{ad}{bc}$$

Higher selection probabilities for cases (a and c) and lower selection probabilities for controls (b and d) will not necessarily introduce bias into the estimated odds ratio, because the odds ratio is not dependent on the counts in the different cells. Instead, the odds ratio depends on the odds of exposure in cases relative to controls. For this reason, even if the selection probabilities for cases and controls are very different (they always are), a case-control study can still produce valid estimates of the underlying population odds ratio.

> *Key point:* If properly conducted, case-control studies can provide valid estimates of the odds ratio for an epidemiologic association.

The efficiency of case-control studies

You may reasonably ask: So what? After all, a simple random sample can also produce unbiased estimates of the odds ratio. Indeed, a simple random sample seems more straightforward, since the contingency table for the sample will then directly represent the population contingencies.

The value of the case-control study, however, lies in its efficiency. Efficiency is the extent of precision (width of the confidence intervals) that a given investment of resources in a study can obtain. In a case-control study, you can obtain cases from places such as cancer registries or health care settings. This is extremely efficient compared to simple random sampling, especially for rare diseases. A simple random sample would result in a small number of cases (especially for a rare disease)—so even if the sample size were very large, it would likely generate imprecise estimates. Essentially, the case-control design allows for the more efficient use of a smaller subset of population members than a simple random sample, leading to gains in efficiency.

> *Key point:* The main advantage of the case-control design is its efficiency. The design is efficient because selection of cases can be accomplished flexibly and the control group is usually only a small subset of the analogous group in the general population.

The organization of the Canadian health system can add to the efficiency of case-control studies. The Canadian health system operates largely on a single-payer model, so it often pursues population-based clinical services to reduce duplication of services. If the population served is geographically defined (e.g., a health region or province), it is referred to as a *catchment area* for that clinical service. Catchment areas are ideal for conducting case-control studies. If a clinic serves all members of the catchment area population with a specific disease, selection cannot depend on exposure in the cases. Similarly, any noncase (potential control) in the catchment area would have been a case had they developed the disease, regardless of exposure. Other types of health system organization can also interface very well with the case-control design. For example, many case-control studies use hospital-based cases: some select all patients presenting to a particular hospital for a particular disease during a defined period.

Examples of case-control studies

Hackam et al[170] conducted a case-control study in Ontario to assess the potentially protective role of angiotensin-converting enzyme inhibitors (ACE inhibitors) in preventing rupture of aortic aneurisms. This study used linked administrative data to identify patients admitted to hospital with ruptured aneurisms. This was the case group. Patients admitted to hospital with unruptured aneurisms were the control group. The investigators observed a significant protective effect of ACE inhibitors: the odds ratio was 0.82, with a 95% CI of 0.74–0.90. The odds ratio, as with other ratio-based measures of association, has a null value of 1.0: values less than 1.0 are interpreted as being protective. In the study by Hackam et al, the upper limit of the confidence interval does not reach this null value, which is the basis for the investigators' assertion that ACE inhibitors have a significant effect. In situations where a 95% CI for a measure of association does not include the null value, the result will be significant at the 5% level of confidence. The confidence limits clarify that the protective effect may be as strong as odds ratio = 0.74, or as weak as odds ratio = 0.90.

Pahwa et al sought to evaluate the role of pesticide exposures in causing multiple myeloma, a cancer of plasma cells (antibody-producing white blood cells).[171] This type of cancer has been reported as more common in agricultural workers. As a source of cases, the researchers used cancer registries in 5 provinces (Ontario, Manitoba, Saskatchewan, Alberta, and British Columbia) and hospital-based ascertainment in a sixth (Quebec) to identify men with a first diagnosis of multiple myeloma ($n = 342$). In these same provinces, they used administrative databases (health insurance records, telephone lists, or voter lists), to which they applied age constraints, in order to identify 1506 controls matched for age and province of residence. Exposure data were collected using postal questionnaires and telephone interviews. Cases and controls were similar in their overall exposure to pesticides, but when specific chemical types of pesticide exposure were examined, an elevated odds ratio was seen for carbamate insecticides and captan fungicides.

Pan et al[172] conducted a case-control study to assess the effect of lifestyle-related risk factors for salivary gland cancer. This is an uncommon cancer, affecting about 500 people in Canada each year, making a case-control study the logical choice for study design. The study was part of a larger initiative called the Canadian National Enhanced Cancer Surveillance System, based on collaboration between Health Canada and cancer registries in 8 of the 10 provinces. A control group was selected from the general population with frequency matching for age, sex, and province. The analysis included 132 incident cases and 3076 controls. A goal of the study was to examine the role of processed meat consumption as a possible risk factor. This variable was categorized at 3 levels: < 1.4 servings per week ("group 1"), 1.4 to < 4 servings per week ("group 2"), and ≥ 4 servings per week ("group 3"). These 3 levels of exposure create a more complex situation than a binary exposure: in this situation, the lowest level of exposure (group 1) is treated as the "nonexposed" state and 2 odds ratios are calculated, comparing each of the higher levels of exposure (groups 2 and 3) to the lowest level (group 1). This is the best approach for epidemiologic analyses dealing with nonbinary exposure data. The odds ratios—adjusted for age, sex, province, and total energy intake— were 1.02 for the group-2-to-group-1 comparison, and 1.62 for the group-3-to-group-1 comparison. The 95% confidence interval for the ≥ 4 servings group (1.02–2.58) did not cross the null value, suggesting that a significantly elevated risk was associated with this exposure.

Selection bias in case-control studies

The efficiencies of the case-control design come at the cost of 2 main vulnerabilities: selection bias and misclassification bias.

Selection bias is not necessarily a point of vulnerability for every case-control study. In general, however, the case-control design is vulnerable to selection bias.

The concept of selection bias is more complicated for case-control studies than for simple parameters such as prevalence.

For simple parameters, there is a single outcome, usually a disease. If the presence of the disease affects the probability of selection, bias results. In other words, if the selection probability for those with the disease differs from the selection probability for those without the disease, this defect produces bias. This is a fairly simple rule to follow.

More complex rules are needed to assess whether selection bias has affected the estimated odds ratio in a case-control study. To grasp these complex rules, it is best to view the odds ratio as an actual ratio of odds and not as a cross product. In other words, it is best to think of the odds ratio as this:

$$\text{Odds Ratio} = \frac{\dfrac{a}{c}}{\dfrac{b}{d}}$$

Rather than this:

$$\text{Odds Ratio} = \frac{ad}{bc}$$

Also, it's useful to approach the more complex rules in terms of the simple rule—as the simple rule applied twice, once for the numerator and once for the denominator. This involves thinking about a case-control study as 2 studies. One "study" seeks to estimate the odds of exposure in cases and the other "study" seeks to estimate the odds of exposure in controls. This leads to some additional rules and insights. If the numerator of the odds ratio is too big, the odds ratio will be overestimated. If the denominator is too big, the odds ratio will be underestimated. And there is 1 other possibility: if the odds of exposure are elevated, or diminished, but to the same extent in the cases and controls, then the numerator and denominator are altered to the same extent and the ratio of the odds of exposure in cases and controls (the odds ratio) will not be biased.

In principle, if these 2 odds represent the odds of exposure in the underlying populations of cases and controls, then the expected value of the estimated odds ratio will be the true population value. This is the proof in principle that the case-control design can work. The expectation (which should be understood as an intuitive expectation, not as a more strictly defined statistical expectation) is:

$$\text{e}(\text{Odds Ratio}) = \frac{e\left(\dfrac{a}{c}\right)}{e\left(\dfrac{b}{d}\right)} = \frac{\dfrac{A}{C}}{\dfrac{B}{D}} = \frac{AD}{BC}$$

Imagine, for example, a hospital-based case-control study investigating association between asthma and smoking. The case group is special in certain respects because its subjects are selected from a hospital. There are many health-related behaviours and characteristics that could increase the chance of hospitalization and hence the probability of selection of cases. For example, people with asthma are more likely to be admitted to hospital if they smoke. The odds of smoking for cases of asthma will be higher if those cases are selected from a hospital. Let's imagine that hospital-based selection doubles the probability of exposure to smoking. If the control group were selected in such a way that its subjects also had similarly elevated odds of exposure (perhaps they are also selected from the same hospital and have other conditions for which smoking doubles their chances of admission), selection bias would not occur. Even though the odds of exposure are twice as high in the cases and controls—indeed, because they are twice as high in both the cases and controls—bias will not occur:

$$\text{e}(\text{Odds Ratio}) = \frac{e\left(\dfrac{a}{c}\right)}{e\left(\dfrac{b}{d}\right)} = \frac{2\times\left(\dfrac{A}{C}\right)}{2\times\left(\dfrac{B}{D}\right)} = \frac{AD}{BC}$$

This is a challenging concept to grasp, but it does lead to a general rule about how a case-control study's estimated odds ratio can avoid selection bias. The rule can be stated as follows: the probability of selection for cases and controls should not depend on exposure in any way that differs between the 2 groups.

This rule can also anticipate the direction of possible bias. For example, if the procedure used to select cases overrepresents exposure, the selection of controls must overrepresent exposure to the same extent. If exposure has an impact on the selection of cases and not on the selection of controls—or not as much—the odds ratio will be biased. In this case, the direction of bias would be positive: the estimated odds ratio would systematically overestimate the population value. As usual, this selection bias comes from a defect in the design of the individual study: increasing the sample size would not fix it. This is systematic error, not random error. The defect is not that the probability of selection depends on exposure, but that it does so in a way that differs between cases and controls. Of course, if the selection of cases and controls did not depend at all on exposure (another way to say this: if the process of selection were independent of exposure), there would be no bias. This is a special instance of the rule stated above: the probability of selection does not depend on exposure in this scenario in a way that differs between cases and controls.

Key point: Selection bias results if selection of cases and controls depends on exposure in some way that is not equivalent between the 2 groups.

Data sources and selection bias in case-control studies

It is easiest to be confident that selection bias has not occurred if the selection of cases and controls does not depend in any way on exposure. If this is the case, it is more obvious that the impact of exposure on selection does not differ between cases and controls.

In Canada, this is sometimes possible due to the existence of population-based data. For example, Canadian cancer registries register all cases of cancer. Registration does not depend on exposure in any way. Case-control studies that use these cancer registries as a source of cases typically use a selection procedure for controls that also does not depend at all on exposure, such as sampling the general population via random digit dialing. For example, Friedenreich et al[173] followed this procedure in their study of alcohol consumption and endometrial cancer risk.

If case-control studies use administrative data to select cases and controls, it is important that coding of disease status (and hence the probability of selection of cases) not depend on exposure status, at least not in a way that differs between cases and controls. A person recorded as having a disease in physician-billing data or hospital-discharge data has seen a physician or been admitted to hospital. Exposure could potentially affect selection among such cases. The selection of the control group would need to include exactly the same impact of exposure.

Several pivotal case-control studies have used administrative data. An example is a case-control study by Rothwell et al,[174] which used Ontario hospitalization records to identify cases of vertebrobasilar dissection or occlusion, and selected controls from the Ontario Registered Persons Database. This database contains a list of everyone covered by the provincial health care insurance plan, which is essentially the entire population. These investigators were interested in whether chiropractic neck manipulation might increase the risk of stroke due to dissection or occlusion of the vertebral arteries. They used administrative data to identify whether cervical visits for chiropractic services had occurred. They reported a fivefold elevation in the odds of this type of stroke when cervical manipulation had occurred in the prior week.

De Gage et al[175] used administrative data from Quebec to examine a possible association between benzodiazepine use and Alzheimer disease (benzodiazepines are used as anticonvulsants and muscle relaxants, and for reducing anxiety and promoting sleep). Their study included 1796 incident cases of Alzheimer disease and 7184 matched controls identified in the database of Quebec's Régie de l'assurance maladie du Québec (RAMQ). The odds ratio for every exposure to benzodiazepines (after adjustment for a set of potentially confounding variables) was 1.51 (95% CI 1.36–1.69), suggesting a possible causal role for these medications. A special feature of this study was its use of incidence density sampling for the controls. This procedure is one the best ways to select controls in a case-control study. It selects controls from among those at risk at the time that each case is diagnosed.

BERKSON'S BIAS

Selection bias that arises from the use of hospitalized cases in a case-control study has a special name: *Berkson's bias*. Berkson published a paper about this form of bias in 1946.[176]

When hospitalized cases are used, it is often difficult to identify an appropriate control group. The controls should be selected such that they would have been cases had they developed the disease. They could, for example, be selected from the catchment area of the hospital from which the cases were recruited, or from among patients admitted to the same hospital for another reason. This other reason would need to be another disease that is not related to the risk factor in question—a tricky distinction. Some risk factors influence decisions to admit patients with certain diseases to hospital, increasing the odds of exposure among hospitalized cases with those diseases, but not necessarily doing the same thing for controls. If these challenges are not navigated successfully, Berkson's bias will occur.

Misclassification bias in case-control studies

Misclassification bias, like selection bias, is more complicated for odds ratios from case-control studies than for simple parameters such as prevalence.

In simple parameters, insensitive measures of disease status result in frequencies biased downwards: erroneous negative classification of people with a disease moves these people from the numerator to the denominator of the frequency or odds being estimated. Nonspecific measures of disease status result in frequencies biased upwards: false-positive errors result in misclassification from the denominator to the numerator of the frequency or odds, which inflates the estimate compared to the true population parameter.

Where an odds ratio is concerned, the situation is more complex because it involves consideration of 2 elements: the numerator of the odds ratio and the denominator. Again, it is helpful to consider the odds ratio in its raw form as a ratio of 2 odds, rather than in its cross-product form:

$$\text{Odds Ratio} = \frac{\dfrac{a}{c}}{\dfrac{b}{d}}$$

This makes it easier to think of the odds ratio in the same terms as a frequency or odds-based measure—but now with 2 odds of exposure, 1 in the numerator and 1 in the denominator.

If the numerator of the odds ratio is too large relative to the denominator, a positive bias results. This would occur if the specificity of the measure of exposure status were lower in cases than controls: a would be too large (it would be inflated by false-positive exposure assessments that should have been included in c) and, all else being equal, this would bias the odds ratio upwards. By contrast, if the numerator of the odds ratio is too small, a negative bias results. This happens if the sensitivity of the measure of exposure in cases is low: a becomes be too small relative to c, because false-negative classification moves people who should be included in a to c.

Misclassification of exposure can also affect the denominator of an odds ratio estimate. If a measure of exposure is nonspecific among controls, then the number of exposed controls will be inflated by false positives, the denominator of the odds ratio will enlarge, and the expected value of the estimated odds ratio will diminish. If measurement of exposure in controls is insensitive, the odds of exposure in the controls will be underestimated, making the denominator of the odds ratio too small, and the odds ratio inflated.

Key point: By considering the effects of misclassification on estimates in the numerator and denominator of an odds ratio separately, the direction of the resulting bias can be anticipated. If the numerator is inflated, the estimate of the odds ratio will be too high. If the denominator is inflated, the estimate of the odds ratio will be too low.

Differential and nondifferential misclassification bias

Our discussion of misclassification bias so far has shown several examples of what is called *differential misclassification bias*, where errors in classification occur at a different rate in the cases and controls. The first example was a lack of specificity for classification of exposure that occurs only among the cases. This would inflate the estimated odds ratio. The second example was a lack of sensitivity among the cases, which would result in a negative bias.

There are 2 other possible mechanisms of differential misclassification bias. A lack of specificity in the classification of exposure that occurs predominantly among controls would bias the odds ratio downwards (negative bias). A lack of sensitivity for exposure that occurs exclusively among controls would lead to overestimation of the odds ratio (positive bias).

Nondifferential misclassification bias occurs when classification is inaccurate, but equally so for cases and controls. This type of bias cannot be characterized as positive or negative. Instead, it displays a different behaviour: bias towards the null value. Remember that the null value for an odds ratio is 1. Therefore if the exposure is a risk factor, the association will appear smaller than it really is. If the exposure is a protective factor, the odds ratio will be larger than it should be (closer to 1).

RECALL BIAS

Case-control studies are vulnerable to recall bias, a kind of differential misclassification. This is because they assess exposure retrospectively.

Retrospective assessment of exposure does not always depend on the memory of subjects (e.g., the study of ACE inhibitors assessed exposure using administrative record linkage[170]). But when it does depend on the memory of subjects, there is a concern that disease status will affect recall of exposure. The usual concern is that people who are sick are motivated to think harder about reasons for their illness. So, their recall of exposure may be more sensitive than that of controls.

Recall bias creates a tendency for exposed controls to more often be misclassified as false negatives (for exposure), which diminishes the odds of exposure in controls relative to cases and leads to a positive bias (overestimation) of the odds ratio.

Although this type of bias has a name, it doesn't really need a special label. Recall bias can be described as a form of differential misclassification in relation to sensitivity for exposure classification in cases and controls.

Other aspects of case-control studies

Odds of disease and exposure

In the case-control design, the odds ratio—which contrasts the frequency of exposure in cases and controls—seems to transpose the basic idea of contrasting the frequency of disease in exposed and nonexposed groups. Fortunately, this transposition is not problematic. The reason is a matter of arithmetic related to the properties of this parameter.

Think back to Table 24—the standard 2 × 2 table from a case-control study. If you base the calculation of the odds ratio on the odds of disease in the exposed and nonexposed groups—rather than comparing the odds of exposure in cases and controls—the equation would be as follows:

$$\text{Odds Ratio} = \frac{\dfrac{a}{b}}{\dfrac{c}{d}}$$

This odds ratio reduces to the following familiar cross-product formula:

$$\text{Odds Ratio} = \frac{\dfrac{a}{b}}{\dfrac{c}{d}} = \frac{ad}{bc}$$

Fortunately, the odds ratio calculated from case-control data is a valid means of estimating the association between a risk factor and a disease outcome. The Ontario study about ACE inhibitors discussed earlier in this chapter, for example, showed lower odds of exposure to these inhibitors in people with ruptured aneurisms, which implies that ACE inhibitors lower the risk of ruptured aneurisms.

Incidence and prevalence effects

So far, we have talked about cases and controls with a labelling convention based on disease-exposure contingencies. However, all cases of disease are not the same.

A case of disease can be a prevalent case—a person having the disease at a point in time. Alternatively, a case can be an incident case—a newly developed case. This distinction is absolutely critical for interpreting the odds ratios that arise from case-control studies. If a case-control study uses incident cases, the odds ratio will estimate the ratio of incidence (expressed as an odds rather than the usual proportion) in the population, and the resulting estimate will be an estimate of the incidence odds ratio in the population. By contrast, if a study uses prevalent cases, it will estimate the prevalence odds ratio.

Why is this distinction important? Recall that prevalence reflects the end result of several underlying dynamics. Partially, it reflects the risk of a person developing a disease (incidence) and partially it reflects the duration of illness among those developing the disease. Recall also that the purpose of using ratio-based measures is to create a single parameter that embodies a comparison between exposed and nonexposed groups. So, a prevalence odds ratio reflects a comparison of prevalence in exposed and nonexposed people.

Prevalence odds ratios do not directly reflect etiology. Rather, they make a statement about how common a disease is in people with and without exposure. It is an error to interpret these parameters as if they conveyed information about risk factors. For example, a prevalence odds ratio of 2 does not mean that the risk factor in question doubles the risk of disease: it only means that the odds of disease are twice as high in those with the exposure as in those without the exposure. The prevalence odds ratio reflects both the effect of exposure on risk and duration. The implications of this distinction are not trivial. If an exposure is a determinant, this will affect the prevalence odds ratio. If the exposure makes people more likely to die from a disease, it will make the prevalence odds ratio smaller, not larger, because death shortens the duration of disease. If the exposure makes an episode of illness last longer, for example by prolonging survival, it will make the prevalence odds ratio larger even if it has no impact on risk.

If incident cases are used in a case-control study, the resulting incidence odds ratio will reflect an effect of the exposure on the incidence (risk) of the disease.

Key point: The use of incident versus prevalent cases in case-control studies is key to interpreting the resulting odds ratio, even if the formula looks the same in both cases.

TEMPORALITY, INCIDENCE, AND PREVALENCE

Case-control studies can have challenges with temporality similar to cross-sectional studies. As noted in chapter 10 (see page 147), cross-sectional studies are generally precluded from assessing etiology because they cannot clarify the temporal association between disease and exposure. A case-control study that uses incident cases is better able to assess etiology than a cross-sectional study, but this is not true for a case-control study that uses prevalent cases.

In case-control studies that use prevalent cases, questions about temporality can arise and draw into question the cause-effect relationships that the study is attempting to address.

The rare disease assumption

Even though an odds ratio from a case-control study can estimate the odds ratio in a population, debates sometimes arise about whether it can estimate the ratio of 2 frequencies in a population. The key question is: When is an odds ratio a good estimate of the equivalent ratio-based measure that is based on proportions rather than odds? Put into other words, this is the question of whether a prevalence odds ratio can be interpreted as a prevalence ratio, and whether an incidence odds ratio can be interpreted as a risk ratio.

The answer to this question hinges on whether the disease in question is rare. Let's revisit Table 5 (see page 20), the 1 × 2 table that labels those with a disease as a and those without the disease as b. The odds of disease are very similar to the proportion having the disease when a is small, because the denominator of the odds is b and the denominator of the proportion is $a + b$. These 2 denominators are very similar when a is tiny.

To further illustrate: imagine a sample of $n = 100$ where the proportion with the disease is 1/4 (25%). Here, the odds and the proportion are substantially different: odds = 1/3 (0.333) and proportion = 1/4 (0.25). If the proportion having the disease is 1/100 (1%), however, then the odds are 0.0101, which is almost identical to 1% or 0.01.

This tendency of odds ratios to resemble ratios of 2 proportions only when a disease is rare has a name: the *rare disease assumption*. The term is unfortunate because it seems to suggest that the validity of the odds ratio is dependent on an assumption that a disease is rare. This is not true at all. In epidemiology, valid estimates of a parameter are estimates that do not systematically deviate from the underlying population value. An odds ratio is valid if its distribution does not systematically deviate from the underlying population odds ratio. The rare disease assumption merely points out that an odds-based parameter will only be a close approximation of a related proportion-based parameter if the disease is rare.

Key point: The validity of an odds ratio does not depend on the assumption that a disease is rare.

Induction and latency periods

A case-control study can investigate exposures to risk factors that occur many years before the emergence of the diseases caused by those exposures. This period between exposure to a risk factor and emergence of a disease process (even if the disease is not yet evident) is called the *induction period*. Infectious diseases can have short induction periods: diseases often follow rapidly after exposure to infectious agents. Chronic diseases can have very long induction periods.

A latency period is the time between the onset of a disease and its emergence as a clinically evident entity. Some diseases may exist for years in a latent, or hidden, phase and only become clinically apparent in an advanced stage.

Diseases with long induction or latency periods can pose challenges for epidemiological research. If researchers investigating such a disease begin with, say, a random sample and then follow the participants in the sample prospectively to see who develops the disease, they might need to follow the participants for many years waiting for cases to accrue or become apparent. A case-control study, though, can start with people who are already known to have the disease and enquire retrospectively about their exposures. Case control studies are therefore much more efficient than prospective studies for diseases that have long induction and latency periods.

INDUCTION PERIODS AND COMPONENT CAUSES OF DISEASE

Diseases do not usually have a single cause: exposure to a single risk factor is not typically enough in itself to trigger a pathophysiologic disease mechanism. Instead, additional effects from other exposures are usually necessary.

These dynamics have been articulated in a model that posits the existence of multiple component causes for most diseases. This model was developed by Rothman and is therefore often called the *Rothman model*, but is also named (by Rothman) the *causal pie model* of disease etiology.[177] Another name is the *sufficient-component cause model.*

In brief, this model posits that the cause of a disease is a specific combination of component causes. Each component cause is like a piece of a pie: when the pieces fit together into a causal mechanism—a complete "pie"—the disease has its onset.

Figure 11 shows an example of 2 causal mechanisms, depicted as causal pies. The first sufficient-cause mechanism, on the left, shows 4 component causes combining to cause the disease. The mechanism on the right shows a sufficient-cause mechanism composed of 2 component causes, D and E. Note that component cause D is present in each of the causal mechanisms. Each of A, B, C, D, and E are component causes, but D is a necessary component cause. A public health action that could eliminate the effects of exposure D could prevent all cases of the disease. An action that eliminated the effects of A would prevent the cases arising from the first, but not the second, mechanism.

FIGURE 11. SIX COMPONENT CAUSES FORMING 2 CAUSAL MECHANISMS

Through the lens of this model, induction periods occur because the completion of a causal mechanism may involve the collection of component causes through time. It is best to think of an induction period as the time between (1) exposure to a specific risk factor under study and (2) exposure to all component causes related to causal mechanisms that include that specific factor (i.e., the point when a sufficient cause has occurred).

PRIMARY, SECONDARY, AND TERTIARY PREVENTION

Primary, secondary, and tertiary prevention are related to induction and latency.

Primary prevention comprises measures to prevent the occurrence of disease. It is a key application of epidemiological research. In the language of the causal pie model, it involves eliminating exposure to component causes (risk factors) for disease, as identified by analytical epidemiological research. By removing a component cause that is a part of 1 or more etiological mechanisms, the onset of disease through those mechanisms is prevented. Primary prevention operates before the onset of disease. For example, reducing the frequency of smoking is primary prevention: it removes a component cause of cardiovascular disease and many types of cancer,[178] and so reduces the incidence of these diseases. Another example of primary prevention is vaccination for human papilloma virus (HPV). HPV is a component cause, and a necessary cause, of certain cancers,[179] meaning that all known causal mechanisms involve the infection. By preventing infection (a component cause) the vaccine prevents the completion of most, or perhaps even all, causal mechanisms leading to those cancers.

Secondary prevention, also known as screening, is based on early detection of established disease. Early detection allows treatment to begin earlier, during the latency phase, before the disease would normally come to clinical attention. In certain instances, this leads to dramatically better outcomes. For example, in congenital hypothyroidism, newborn babies are unable to produce thyroid hormone. Thyroid hormone is essential for development, so this condition leads to serious problems. By the time the condition becomes apparent clinically—through delayed development—irreversible damage has been done. To address this problem, all newborns in Canada are screened for congenital hypothyroidism at birth. Through early intervention, the negative effects can easily be prevented through supplementation treatment.

Tertiary prevention comprises interventions after the overt manifestations of disease have occurred. The goal is to diminish the impact of disease through measures such as treatment or rehabilitation.

These concepts are illustrated in Figure 12. In the diagram, there are 3 component causes, labelled *A*, *B*, and *C*. Exposure to *C* completes the causal mechanism and coincides with disease initiation. The induction period for component cause *A* is the period of time between exposure to *A* and disease initiation. After that, there is a period of time when the disease is present, but not yet apparent clinically (the latency phase). This is followed by a manifest clinical phase when the disease produces signs, symptoms, and functional impairments that make it clinically apparent.

FIGURE 12. INDUCTION AND LATENCY

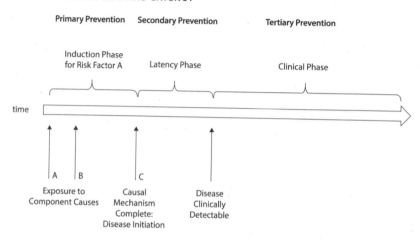

Key point: The induction period occurs before disease onset. The latency period occurs after disease onset, but before the disease has become clinically evident.

Primordial (or primal) prevention

Some epidemiologists like to think of 4 levels of prevention rather than 3. They add primordial (or primal) prevention to the 3 categories listed above. Whereas primary prevention involves reducing exposure to risk factors in order to prevent disease, primordial prevention seeks to prevent the occurrence of the risk factors themselves. Primordial prevention involves changing the social, economic, and environmental conditions in which risk factors emerge. These conditions comprise the social determinants of health.[180] Social determinants of health relevant to Canada include:[181] disability, early child development, education, employment and working conditions, food insecurity, gender, geography, globalization, health services, housing, immigration, income and income distribution, Indigenous ancestry, race, social exclusion, social safety net, and unemployment and job security.

Strengths and weaknesses of case-control studies

Strengths

Efficiency: Case-control studies are generally viewed as an efficient, and therefore reasonably inexpensive, approach to studying an epidemiological association. Since the orientation of case-control studies is retrospective, the studies can be conducted fairly quickly. Long periods of follow-up are not required, as they are for some other study designs.

Fit with rare diseases: For rare diseases, the efficiency and opportunity (especially the ability to use clinical subjects) provided by the case-control design often make it the most feasible option. However, as with cross-sectional studies, case-controls studies are not necessarily efficient when the exposure is very rare. Even the ability to accrue a large number of cases will not result in precise estimates of association if the number of exposed participants is small.

Fit with long induction and latency periods: In a longitudinal study, induction and latency periods can create long delays and require years of follow-up, which is often impractical. A case-control study, due to its retrospective assessment of exposure, can accommodate long delays.

Ability to examine multiple exposures: With appropriate selection of cases and controls, multiple potential determinants can be examined in a case-control study.

Weaknesses

Vulnerability to selection and misclassification bias: The case-control design is vulnerable to selection bias. To ensure that selection bias does not occur, it is necessary to ensure that any effect of exposure on selection is exactly the same for cases and controls. Yet, cases and controls differ on an important characteristic—whether they have a disease or not. This can affect many aspects of behaviour and function. These, in turn, may relate to both exposure and selection, leading to bias. As a result, it is often difficult to be certain that a case-control study is not biased due to selection.

The case-control design is also vulnerable to misclassification bias—in particular, when these studies rely on the memory of subjects to assess exposure. People with disease (cases) may be more likely to recall exposure than people without disease (controls).

Key point: Case-control studies are vulnerable to recall and selection bias.

Inefficiency for rare exposures: Case-control studies are inefficient for rare exposures.

Limits on estimation: Case-control studies are limited to estimating the odds ratio, which is a measure of association. They cannot estimate actual risks since they cannot estimate incidence proportions or incidence rates.

Can only examine one disease at a time: Since these studies are based on the selection of a case group, a case-control study can only examine risk factors for a single disease at a time.

Thinking deeper

Selection bias and selection odds ratios

One of the most challenging tasks in critical appraisal is the prospect of judging whether an estimate has been systematically distorted by selection bias. The task is easier in descriptive studies, where the parameter being estimated is a frequency or odds. It is always more complex in analytical studies, where the intention is to estimate a complex parameter such as an odds ratio.

So far, we have approached this task by looking at the odds ratio as a true ratio of odds (and setting aside the familiar cross-product equation for calculating this parameter). This breaks the task into 2 parts—since the odds ratio, when considered this way, has a more understandable numerator and denominator—and allows you to connect the assessment of selection bias for this complex parameter to the simpler rules that govern selection bias for odds in general. By considering the effect of selection on the 2 parts individually (the numerator and denominator of the odds ratio), you can begin to approach the problem of whether bias would occur and, if so, in what direction it would tend to go.

Kleinbaum et al[182] many years ago described another approach based on selection probabilities. We introduced the idea of selection probability in chapter 8 (see page 94). There, in a discussion of selection bias in prevalence studies, we identified 2 selection probabilities as important: the selection probability for those with the disease and the selection probability for those without.

In a case-control study, there are 4 relevant selection probabilities, which Kleinbaum et al labelled with the Greek letters α, β, γ and δ. These probabilities can be defined as follows (as usual, uppercase letters signify population data and lowercase letters signify sample-based data):

$$\alpha = \frac{a}{A}$$

$$\beta = \frac{b}{B}$$

$$\gamma = \frac{c}{C}$$

$$\delta = \frac{d}{D}$$

From this set of 4 selection probabilities, you can produce a parameter that Kleinbaum et al called the *selection odds ratio*:

$$\text{Selection Odds Ratio} = \frac{\alpha\delta}{\beta\gamma}$$

This is an imaginary construction in the sense that it would rarely, if ever, actually be calculated. If A, B, C, and D were actually known, there would be little interest in sample-based estimates—the estimates would serve no inferential purpose.

The construction, however, provides an additional framework for evaluating the impact of selection bias in a case-control study. A strong feature of this parameter is that it forces a critical reader to examine a study's design carefully and to think systematically about the probability of selection in each of the 4 relevant contingencies. This, in itself, is a valuable start on thinking through a complex issue such as selection bias.

In addition, the selection odds ratio can help sort out the direction of bias. For example, suppose there is concern that an exposure might favour selection among cases but not controls. This would increase the selection probability for exposed cases relative to other selection probabilities. The equation below clarifies that this methodological flaw would tend to produce a positive bias, because it would inflate the numerator of the selection odds ratio:

$$\text{Selection Odds Ratio} = \frac{(\alpha\uparrow)\delta}{\beta\gamma}$$

If the selection of controls resulted in a similar higher probability of selection due to exposure—in other words, if exposure influenced selection of cases and controls to the same degree—then β would be increased to a similar extent as α, eliminating the bias:

$$\text{Selection Odds Ratio} = \frac{(\alpha\uparrow)\delta}{(\beta\uparrow)\gamma}$$

Some students of epidemiology find this type of schematic useful as a tool for critical appraisal.

Questions

1. List 4 advantages and 4 disadvantages of case-control studies.

2. In infectious disease epidemiology, the period between exposure to an infectious agent and the emergence of signs and symptoms of infectious disease is called the incubation period. For example, the initial report on the Wuhan outbreak of COVID-19 disease reported a mean incubation period of 5.2 days.[183] Is the incubation period best regarded as an induction or latency period?

3. The table below presents data from the Hackam et al[170] study of ACE inhibitors in preventing rupture of aortic aneurisms. This is the crude 2 × 2 table from the study.

	Cases	Controls
Exposed	665	2761
Nonexposed	2714	9186
Total	3379	11947

   a. Calculate an odds ratio from this 2 × 2 table data.

   b. Calculate the extent to which the odds of exposure are decreased in the case (ruptured aneurism) group compared to the controls.

4. In plain language, what is your interpretation of the odds ratio calculated in question 3? Do you feel that the odds ratio may be invalidated by the rare disease assumption?

5. Depression is a common health issue in primary care. It is often not detected in clinical practice. Some experts have recommended "screening" to deal with this problem. "Screening" involves the distribution of rating scales to primary-care patients and offering a clinical assessment to people who screen above a threshold score. Would you classify depression screening as primary, secondary, or tertiary prevention?

6. What is wrong with the following statement? "The selection probabilities in a case-control study depend on disease status, therefore these studies are always biased."

7. Do you agree with the following statement? "Because of the rare disease assumption, odds ratios from case-control studies of common diseases are not valid."

8. What is the best type of public health intervention: primary, secondary, or tertiary prevention?

9. List key characteristics that identify a disease for which screening is likely to be an effective intervention.

10. Explain why the inverse logarithm of ß coefficients in a logistic regression model is an odds ratio.

Differential and nondifferential misclassification bias in analytical studies

---

OBJECTIVES

- Distinguish differential and nondifferential misclassification bias.
- Explain the effect of differential and nondifferential misclassification bias on the interpretation of epidemiological parameters.
- Describe blinded outcome assessment.

Differential and nondifferential misclassification bias in context

Epidemiology has many study designs, but the 3 major types of study are cross-sectional studies, case-control studies, and prospective cohort studies.

The design of case-control studies and prospective cohort studies give them explicitly analytic goals (which they may or may not achieve). All studies that estimate associations—descriptive and analytic—are vulnerable to differential and nondifferential misclassification bias.

Chapter 11 discussed case-control studies, and introduced the concepts of differential and nondifferential misclassification bias. Chapter 13, on prospective cohort studies, will revisit them.

This chapter discusses these types of bias in more detail because of their key importance in analytical studies.

Bias in review

The types of bias discussed in this chapter have the same characteristics as all types of bias. Here's a review of the key characteristics:

Bias comes from study-design defects. If the classification of study variables is perfect, there can be no misclassification bias. If perfect participation is achieved, there can be no selection bias.

Bias cannot be corrected by increasing the sample size. The occurrence of a study-design defect means that a study is estimating something other than its intended target of estimation. Increasing the sample size will merely result in narrower confidence intervals around an erroneous estimate, providing a false sense of precision.

Bias can be prevented, but not often corrected. Investigators can avoid bias by careful thinking at the stage of study design. Once bias has occurred, it cannot usually be corrected after the fact.

BIAS IS NOT AFFECTED BY SAMPLE SIZE

The second key characteristic listed above deserves additional emphasis. Consider a case control study with 1000 cases and 1000 controls. The odds of exposure in cases within the population is 0.2 and the odds of exposure in the controls is 0.1. This means that the true odds ratio is 2. Assume that no measurement error occurs. Due to random error, the estimated odds ratio in a particular study of this size will not always be exactly 2. If this study were conducted 1000 times, the distribution of estimated odd ratios would be similar to that shown in Figure 13, where, although random variation occurs, the estimates cluster around the true value of 2, indicating no systematic distortion of the results. By contrast, if the sensitivity of measurement of exposure is only 80% in the controls (assume the cases include no errors of measurement), as might occur due to recall bias, approximately 20% of the exposure-positive controls will be misclassified as nonexposed. The distribution of 1000 estimates of the resulting, biased, odds ratio is presented in Figure 14, where, although random variability continues to occur, the distribution of values no longer centres on the true odds ratio in the population. The estimate of the population parameter has been systematically distorted in the direction of overestimating the true odds ratio. Figures 15 and 16 show the same bias in case-control studies with much larger sample sizes (10 000 cases and controls). Random variation diminishes due to the increased sample size, but the systematic distortion of nondifferential misclassification bias persists.

Differential misclassification bias

Let's review how differential misclassification can affect case-control studies.

The retrospective measurement of exposure status in case-control studies often relies on recall. This may result in recall bias. People with a disease (cases) are more likely to recollect exposures. This means that questions and instruments seeking to elicit exposure history are likely more sensitive in

FIGURE 13. FREQUENCY DISTRIBUTION OF ESTIMATED ODDS RATIOS IN
1000 SIMULATED CASE-CONTROL STUDIES

For each, n = 1000 cases and n = 1000 controls; population odds ratio = 2

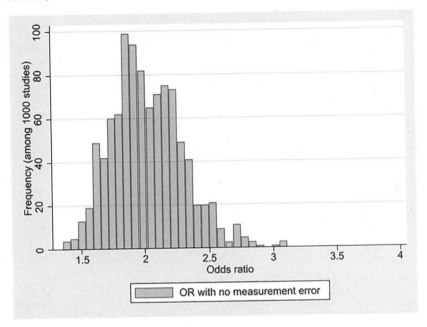

FIGURE 14. FREQUENCY DISTRIBUTION OF ESTIMATED ODDS RATIOS WITH
MEASUREMENT ERROR IN 1000 SIMULATED CASE-CONTROL STUDIES

For each, n = 1000 cases and n = 1000 controls; population odds ratio = 2

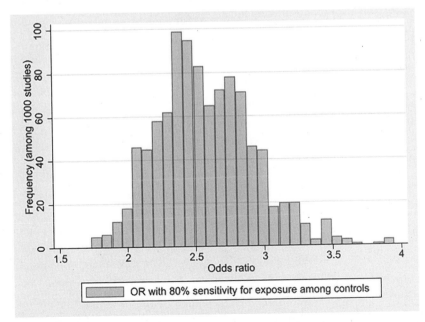

FIGURE 15. FREQUENCY DISTRIBUTION OF ESTIMATED ODDS RATIOS IN
1000 SIMULATED CASE-CONTROL STUDIES

For each, n = 10 000 cases and n = 10 000 controls; population odds ratio = 2

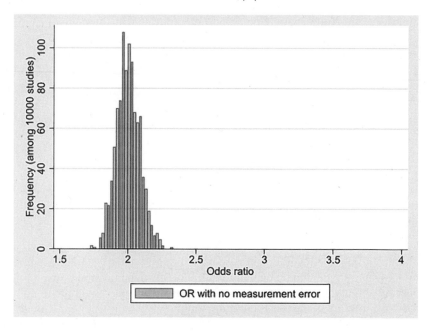

FIGURE 16. FREQUENCY DISTRIBUTION OF ESTIMATED ODDS RATIOS WITH
MEASUREMENT ERROR IN 1000 SIMULATED CASE-CONTROL STUDIES

For each, n = 10 000 cases and n = 10 000 controls, population odds ratio = 2

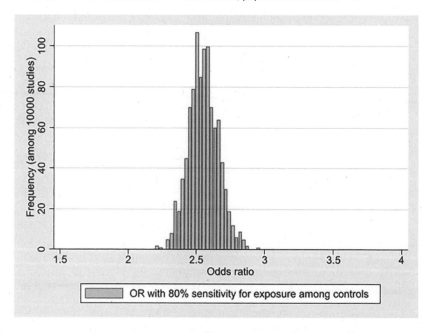

cases than in controls, so that misclassification of exposure happens in a way that differs depending on case or control (disease) status.

Here's another way of thinking about recall bias, using the classic 2 × 2 contingency table of exposure versus disease. You could say that, in recall bias, misclassification happens across the "exposure" axis of the table and depends on the "disease" axis.

Recall bias is only one example of differential misclassification bias. The 2 × 2 contingency table helps us imagine another example, where misclassification happens across the "disease" axis and depends on the "exposure" axis.

In general, misclassification is differential if the misclassification of exposure or disease depends on the other axis.

Magnitude and direction of differential misclassification bias

There are no simple rules for understanding the behaviour of differential misclassification bias. You have to think through the expected impact of the misclassification (see page 161).

In the case of recall bias in a case-control study, since the classification of exposure in the controls lacks sensitivity, the odds of exposure in the controls will tend to be underestimated. This makes the denominator of the odds ratio smaller and consequently the value of the odds ratio larger. This particular mechanism of bias is likely to inflate the observed value of the odds ratio.

Key point: When misclassification is differential, there are no simple rules about the direction or magnitude of bias. Each case needs to be thought through individually.

Nondifferential misclassification bias

Misclassification in general happens because the procedure for classifying exposure or disease has a sensitivity or specificity—or both—of less than 1.

In differential misclassification bias, misclassification occurs and its occurrence depends on the other axis of the contingency table.

In nondifferential misclassification bias, misclassification occurs and its occurrence does not depend on the other axis of the contingency table.

Let's think about this in the context of case-control studies, where most of the concern surrounds the classification of exposure. Nondifferential misclassification bias would mean the frequency with which classification errors occur does not differ depending on case-versus-control status.

This type of misclassification occurs commonly. In a case-control study that measures exposure using a procedure that does not depend on recall, there may be no reason to believe that the errors in classification would depend on outcome (i.e., disease or no disease). In Canada, many case-control studies use record linkage to administrative data to avoid a reliance on recall. However, this is only feasible when the exposure of interest is an event recorded in administrative data.

Magnitude and direction of nondifferential misclassification bias

The direction of bias introduced by nondifferential misclassification errors is almost always towards the null value of the parameter being estimated.

All of the complex parameters that are intended to embody an association between risk factors and disease have null values. In a case-control study, where the measure of association must be an odds ratio, the null value is 1 because this value implies an absence of effect of the exposure. This means that for a protective association (where the odds ratio is less than 1), the estimated odds ratio will be systematically higher than the true population value. It will appear less protective than it actually is. When a risk factor elevates the risk of disease, the odds ratio is greater than 1, but nondifferential misclassification bias will bring the estimate closer to the null value of 1. (Note that difference-based measures have a null value of 0.)

Nondifferential misclassification bias is unique: other sorts of bias affect estimates by making them too large or too small, and cannot generally be identified as going in any specific direction with respect to a null value. Nondifferential misclassification bias does not inflate or suppress estimates of effects, but rather dilutes the actual effect. The direction is predictable in this sense.

Key point: The effect of nondifferential misclassification is bias towards the null value.

Addressing misclassification bias in critical appraisal

During critical appraisal of a study, it is essential to examine how the study measured disease and exposure variables.

Assessing the quality of measurement strategies

Critical appraisal should include consideration of the quality of a study's measurement strategies. The selection of high-quality measurement strategies is key to avoiding misclassification. Many studies, however, rely on poorly validated scales and measures. They may also fail to employ proper procedures, such as training study staff in the use of measurement instruments.

Blinding: a way to avoid misclassification bias

Critical appraisal also requires careful assessment for differential misclassification bias: Would misclassification of disease occur at a different frequency depending on exposure, or would misclassification of exposure occur at a different frequency depending on disease? In studies that use raters to determine disease or exposure status—for example, through interviews or clinical examinations—the raters can be a source of differential misclassification bias. These studies often use a procedure called *blinding* (also known as masking) to avoid differential misclassification. Blinding ensures that raters do not know the disease or exposure status of study subjects. If raters did know, this knowledge could influence their classification. For example, if a rater in a case-control study knew a subject was a case (had a disease), the rater might (perhaps subconsciously) probe more deeply for evidence of exposure.

Interpreting nondifferential misclassification bias

Critical appraisal must finally consider the impact of possible nondifferential misclassification bias. A study that fails to find an exposure-disease association should not be taken seriously if considerable nondifferential misclassification bias may have occurred. This methodological flaw could explain the study's negative result. By contrast, in a study that finds an association, nondifferential misclassification bias would mean that the effect reported is probably stronger than it appears.

Key point: The implications of nondifferential misclassification bias are related to its expected direction (towards the null). A weak (or no-effect) result may not be a credible finding in a study that is biased towards the null, but a strong effect may be even more impressive in the face of such bias.

Thinking deeper

Exploring the mechanisms of differential and nondifferential misclassification bias

Let's do some simple calculations based on hypothetical 2 × 2 tables to more fully understand differential and nondifferential misclassification bias.

Consider a case-control study where a measure of exposure is insensitive. Further imagine that this lack of sensitivity is nondifferential—in other words, the probability of false-negative classification is the same in cases and controls. In this situation, you would expect underestimation in both the numerator (the odds of exposure in the cases) and the denominator (odds of exposure in the controls). You might also expect these underestimations to cancel out—however, they don't. If the odds of exposure are actually higher in the cases, the extent of misclassification will also be greater in the cases, making them (relatively speaking) more like the controls. In any situation in which there is a positive association (odds ratio > 1), nondifferential misclassification results in bias of the estimated odds ratio towards the null value.

Table 25 presents the first hypothetical contingency table. In Table 25, the odds ratio is 1.

TABLE 25. 2 × 2 TABLE FOR DATA FROM A CASE-CONTROL STUDY: NO EFFECT OF EXPOSURE, NO MEASUREMENT ERRORS

	Cases	Controls
Exposed	100	100
Nonexposed	100	100
Total	200	200

Now, imagine that the method of classification of exposure had a sensitivity of only 0.50, or 50%. You would expect, on average, half of those who really are exposed to be misclassified into the nonexposed group. The expected 2 × 2 table will now look like Table 26—which, however, again has an odds ratio of 1.

TABLE 26. 2 × 2 TABLE FOR DATA FROM A CASE-CONTROL STUDY: NO EFFECT OF EXPOSURE, 50% SENSITIVITY FOR EXPOSURE

	Cases	Controls
Exposed	50	50
Nonexposed	150	150
Total	200	200

Because nondifferential misclassification of this type is always towards the null, it is not surprising that nondifferential misclassification in a situation of no effect does not cause bias.

When there is an effect, however, the situation is different. Table 27 shows a case-control study with a positive exposure-disease association and an odds ratio of 3. Table 28 shows the expected 2 × 2 table in the same case-control study with a positive exposure-disease association and a 50% sensitivity for exposure.

TABLE 27. 2 × 2 TABLE FOR DATA FROM A CASE-CONTROL STUDY: POSITIVE ASSOCIATION OF EXPOSURE WITH DISEASE

	Cases	Controls
Exposed	150	100
Nonexposed	50	100
Total	200	200

TABLE 28. 2 × 2 TABLE FOR DATA FROM A CASE-CONTROL STUDY: POSITIVE ASSOCIATION OF EXPOSURE WITH DISEASE, 50% SENSITIVITY FOR EXPOSURE

	Cases	Controls
Exposed	75	50
Nonexposed	125	150
Total	200	200

In Table 28, the odds ratio is 1.8. The nondifferential misclassification of exposure in this case-control study has resulted in a major dilution of the observed association. Seventy-five of the cases ended up being misclassified compared to only 50 in the control group.

Questions

1. Weintraub et al[167] used various scales to identify impulse-control disorders in their case-control study evaluating the association of these disorders with dopamine-agonist treatment in people with Parkinson disease. One of these was the Minnesota Impulsive Disorders Interview, which was used to assess compulsive buying and sexual behaviour. Such interviews can be embarrassing for respondents to complete, so they may try to withhold their reporting of certain behaviours.

   a. What sort of misclassification errors could embarrassment cause?

   b. What kind of bias would you expect from these errors?

   c. What direction of bias do you anticipate?

2. Case-control studies are considered vulnerable to recall bias.

   a. What subtype of misclassification bias underlies the phenomenon of recall bias?

   b. In what direction does the error associated with recall bias usually go?

   c. Can you think of a disease in which recall bias might make an association appear weaker than it actually is?

3. Hackam et al[170] relied exclusively on administrative data to assess exposure and disease in their study of the association between ACE inhibitors and rupture of aortic aneurisms. Since they did not need to rely on recall, can their study be considered perfectly safe from misclassification bias?

4. Friedenreich et al[184] conducted a case-control study to evaluate associations between metabolic syndrome (a group of risk factors for diabetes and cardiovascular disease such as large waist size, elevated triglycerides, abnormal lipid profiles, high blood pressure, and elevated blood glucose) and endometrial cancer. The cases were selected from a cancer registry and controls were selected from the general population using random digit dialing to identify people that had not been diagnosed with cancer. Assessment of the metabolic syndrome involved detailed and carefully conducted in-person interviews, anthropometric measurements, and 8-hour-fasting blood draws.

   a. Do you view this study as vulnerable to misclassification bias?

   b. Although the study excluded controls that had been diagnosed with cancer, some controls may have had cancer that was not yet detected. This would result in misclassification of disease status. What are the implications for bias?

5. Villeneuve et al[185] conducted a case-control study to examine the association between lung cancer and long-term exposure to ambient volatile organic compounds and nitrogen dioxide. Cases were recruited from 4 Toronto hospitals. Two sets of controls were selected: a population-based set and a set from a family-medicine clinic. Long-term exposure to ambient pollution is difficult to measure and these investigators needed to rely on models developed during monitoring campaigns to classify exposure. They reported moderate

associations (e.g., an odds ratio of 1.59 for increased nitrogen dioxide exposure) in the analyses using population controls. What impact should the possibility of exposure misclassification have on interpretation of the results?

6. Which is worse: differential or nondifferential misclassification bias?

7. List several strategies to minimize differential misclassification bias in case-control studies.

8. In Canada, research often uses health system administrative data. These are data routinely collected during administration of the health system. For example, physicians must submit diagnostic codes to a provincial health insurance program when they seek payment for services such as consultations and procedures. When a person is discharged from hospital, a discharge abstract is created that records diagnoses. To use these data for research, it is necessary to create algorithms called *case definitions*. For example, Crighton et al[186] used the following case definition to identify chronic obstructive pulmonary disease: being 35 or older, and having 1 hospitalization and/or 1 ambulatory care claim recording an ICD-9 code for chronic obstructive pulmonary disease. Komenda et al[187] used gold standard clinical information from the Manitoba Renal Program database to evaluate several case definitions for end-stage renal disease. They found that 2 claims for outpatient dialysis (an example of a case definition defined by administrative data) was 74.6% sensitive and 94.4% specific for end-stage renal disease. Ideally, case definitions should be validated against a gold standard criterion, such as a detailed review of medical records or a detailed clinical definition. However, case definition algorithms are sometimes validated merely by confirming that they produce age- and sex-specific prevalence patterns consistent with expectations for that disease. Can you think of any pitfalls related to the use of such "validated" case definitions in analytic research? Could a case definition that produces valid prevalence or incidence estimates lead to invalid risk ratios or odds ratios?

9. Recall bias is a classical form of differential misclassification bias in case-control studies. What is the direction of such bias? Will it tend to over- or underestimate the odds ratio?

10. Recall bias is a big concern in case-control studies. Is it also a concern for cross-sectional studies seeking to estimate prevalence odds ratios in a population?

Prospective cohort studies

OBJECTIVES

- Define prospective cohort studies.
- Describe measures of association in prospective cohort studies: risk ratios, incidence rate ratios, and hazard ratios.
- Explain how to interpret measures of association calculated from prospective cohort data.
- List strengths and weaknesses of prospective cohort studies.

What is a cohort study?

Cohort is an ancient Roman military term, but it has come to mean any group with a shared characteristic. In epidemiology, cohort studies assemble groups of subjects, often based on an exposure, and then compare outcomes in relation to this exposure over time.

There are 2 types of cohort-study designs: prospective and retrospective. These differ in temporal direction: a prospective cohort study looks forward in time (from the present to the future) and a retrospective study looks back in time (from the present to the past).

Temporal direction, logical direction, and study-design classification

Cohort studies can differ in temporal direction, but they always have the same logical direction of inquiry. A study's logical direction of inquiry involves how it explores cause and effect. The logical direction in case-control studies is backward: these studies start with an effect (cases have the disease) and then look for a cause (exposures). By contrast, cohort studies have a forward logical direction: they start with a possible cause (exposure) and then look for effects (disease).

Temporal direction and logical direction are very useful concepts for classifying study designs. Figure 17 presents a classification of study designs according to these key characteristics.

FIGURE 17. TEMPORAL AND LOGICAL DIRECTION OF DIFFERENT STUDY DESIGNS

	Logical direction: cause to effect (forward)	Logical direction: effect to cause (backward)
Temporal direction: retrospective	Retrospective cohort study	Case-control study
Temporal direction: prospective	Prospective cohort study	--

Even though cross-sectional studies do not appear in Figure 17, the concepts of temporal and logical direction are also useful for distinguishing cross-sectional studies from case-control and cohort studies. Since cross-sectional studies begin with a sample intended to represent a population at a point in time, they do not have direction to their logical inquiry. Since they are intended to provide a snapshot at a point in time, they are neither prospective nor retrospective in their temporal direction. This means cross-sectional studies have neither temporal nor logical direction. (It is important to remember that many cross-sectional studies use questionnaires that ask about past events, such as the age at which a respondent started smoking. This in itself does not make these cross-sectional studies retrospective since the variables are all measured at a single point in time.)

The prospective cohort study is a classic analytical epidemiology study, which is why it forms the focus of this chapter. Assessment of causal relationships is the usual reason for choosing this design, so prospective cohort studies almost always have analytic, rather than descriptive, aims.

Don't forget, though, that the analytic-versus-descriptive nature of a study is a soft distinction. Investigators may have a variety of motivations for their research. With prospective cohort studies, they likely have analytical motivations, but they may also have descriptive aims—for example, they may want to generate new hypotheses or describe noncausal associations between some variables. The distinction between analytic and descriptive aims—because soft—is a weak criterion for study-design classification. The characteristics of temporal direction and logical direction—because more tangible—are more useful for study-design classification.

Key point: Temporal direction and logical direction are tangible study-design characteristics that are very useful for study-design classification.

Design of prospective cohort studies

The prospective cohort study design clarifies the temporal relationship between exposure and disease—an important advantage. This type of study can assess risk. Prospective cohort studies can either be based on large multipurpose cohorts, or they may specifically select exposed and nonexposed participants.

To assess risk, it is necessary that the population under study not have the condition under investigation at the start of the observation period. This means that a prospective cohort study needs to eliminate people who already have the disease (or other outcomes) at a baseline time point before commencing follow-up.

Figure 18 presents a schematic of a typical prospective cohort study, as carried out using a data set from a large multipurpose cohort. First, prevalent cases are excluded (although they remain members of the underlying multipurpose cohort). Next, the "at risk" cohort is divided into exposed and nonexposed groups, and is followed prospectively to determine the incidence of disease based on exposure.

FIGURE 18. SCHEMATIC OF A TYPICAL PROSPECTIVE COHORT STUDY DESIGN: EXISTING MULTIPURPOSE COHORT

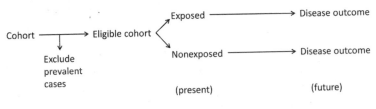

In a study seeking to examine the effects of a single exposure, exposed and nonexposed cohorts may be selected from an underlying source population.

In this case, for reasons of efficiency, the selection probabilities for the exposed subjects would generally be much higher than for the nonexposed. However, the key aspects of the study design—its forward temporal direction and logical direction—remain the same (see Figure 19).

FIGURE 19. SCHEMATIC OF A PROSPECTIVE COHORT STUDY: SELECTION OF EXPOSED AND NONEXPOSED COHORTS

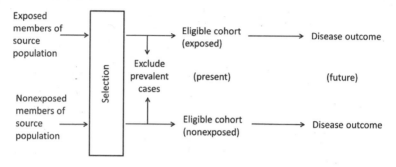

Examples of prospective cohort studies

Prospective cohort studies are expensive to conduct because they usually "follow" cohorts for long periods. So, they need to hire and pay staff for long periods, and they need to maintain contact with study participants for long periods, which is expensive and difficult.

Such large investments of resources need the justification of important goals. As a result, prospective cohort studies typically tackle major analytic questions and often several questions. Multipurpose cohort studies are large-scale projects that address many possible outcomes of many possible exposures.

Prominent examples of multipurpose prospective cohort studies in Canada include the National Population Health Survey (NPHS), and the National Longitudinal Study on Children and Youth (NLSCY). These were large-scale projects that collected baseline data from carefully selected cohorts and then followed the cohorts over time. This allowed for economies of scale and better quality control. Statistics Canada conducted the NPHS and NLSCY. This agency has an established network of interviewers, highly trained personnel, advanced operational systems, and expertise in topics such as sampling and avoidance of attrition. It makes sense that it should play a central role in such national initiatives. Unfortunately, the NPHS and NLSCY were terminated in 2010.

A new and ambitious prospective cohort study of health and aging called the Canadian Longitudinal Study on Aging (CLSA) is currently underway.[188] There is also a large prospective cohort study focusing on cancer etiology called the Canadian Partnership for Tomorrow Project.[189]

In an interesting development, Statistics Canada has begun linking data collected in their surveys to other data sources, such as the Canadian national mortality database and versions of the Discharge Abstracts Database and National Ambulatory Care Reporting System database. Data linkages are either deterministic or probabilistic. Deterministic linkage depends on a variable that is common in 2 data sources, allowing the sources to be merged. Probabilistic linkage uses a set of variables from each data source that, although perhaps not uniquely identifying, together allow records to be connected with a high degree of probability. In linking their surveys, Statistics Canada used probabilistic record linkage.[190] An example is an investigation of the association between major depression (as measured by diagnostic interviews in national surveys) with subsequent mortality data (as determined using linkage to national mortality data).[191] This study found significantly higher mortality in those with major depression. The age-adjusted mortality in the depressed cohort was 60% higher than in the nondepressed cohort.

Some of the most important multipurpose prospective cohort studies have been conducted in the United States. These include the Nurse's Health Study, now in its third iteration,[192] and the National Health and Nutrition Examination Survey (NHANES).[193]

Key point: Major multipurpose prospective cohort studies are large initiatives that lead to analysis of associations between multiple exposures and multiple outcomes.

Assessing associations in a prospective cohort study using ratio-based measures

Prospective cohort studies exclude cases of disease at a baseline point in time, which makes it possible to assess risk for disease in both the exposed and nonexposed groups.

The parameter that quantifies risk may be a risk ratio (incidence proportion ratio), incidence rate ratio, or a hazard ratio.

RISK RATIOS

Where the incidence proportion is concerned, this leads to the familiar 2 × 2 contingency table of exposure versus disease presented in Table 29. Note, however, that this table only looks familiar: it is very different from a contingency table for a cross-sectional or case-control study. In a prospective cohort study, it includes only study subjects at risk of the disease at baseline. The classification of these subjects as having or not having disease depends on whether they develop the disease during the period of observation of the study. This differs from studies that focus on a point in time (cross-sectional studies) and studies that select participants based on disease status (case-control studies).

Key point: The 2 × 2 contingency table for a prospective cohort study looks similar to that of other types of study, but its meaning is different.

TABLE 29. 2 × 2 TABLE FOR A TYPICAL PROSPECTIVE COHORT STUDY

	Incident disease	No incident disease	Total
Exposed	a	b	$n_{exposed}$
Nonexposed	c	d	$n_{nonexposed}$

As always, there is value in using a single parameter to quantify association between exposure and disease. In cross-sectional studies, the prevalence ratio and prevalence odds ratio function as single quantifying parameters. In case-control studies, the odds ratio does this.

In prospective cohort studies, the odds ratio can work to quantify association—you could derive it from Table 29. Note that this odds ratio is, more specifically, an incidence odds ratio.

Prospective cohort studies can also report an estimated association in the form of a risk ratio, which is the ratio of the 2 incidence proportions:

$$\text{Risk Ratio} = \frac{\dfrac{a}{a+b}}{\dfrac{c}{c+d}}$$

The risk ratio could also, and perhaps preferably, be referred to as the *incidence proportion ratio*. This term is not used very often, perhaps because it is awkward to say. The risk ratio is also sometimes also called *relative risk*.

Key point: Superficially similar parameters comprising ratios of proportions have multiple names.

INCIDENT RATE RATIOS

If a prospective cohort study uses a defined risk interval—for example, 16 years (the duration of the NPHS)—not everyone at risk in the cohort at baseline is actually at risk for the whole 16-year period. A study participant who dies after 8 years, for example, is not at risk of disease during the subsequent 8 years.

When there is appreciable movement in or out of the at-risk cohort, the risk ratio is not the ideal parameter to quantify association. It would be better to use a parameter that can account for movement. Rather than calculating the incidence proportion in the exposed and nonexposed groups—as in a risk ratio—it would be preferable to calculate the incidence rate, with its person-time denominator. The person-time denominator of the incidence rate can account for the reality that not every cohort member is followed for exactly the same amount of time.

A ratio of the 2 incidence rates is the incidence rate ratio:

$$\text{Incidence Rate Ratio} = \frac{\text{Incidence Rate}_{\text{exposed}}}{\text{Incidence Rate}_{\text{nonexposed}}}$$

Because cohort studies can use incident rates, the cohorts do not need to be assembled at a single point in time (although they can be, in which case they are called *fixed cohorts*). Some studies use what are called *dynamic cohorts*, meaning that participants can be added or removed from the cohort over time. Since each participant contributes person-time only when they are in the cohort, it is possible to calculate incidence rates and incident rate ratios from a dynamic cohort.

HAZARD RATIOS

Mortality rate ratio is a more specific term for an incidence rate ratio that compares 2 mortality rates. Relative mortality can also be estimated using hazard ratios.

Hazard ratios are associated with survival analysis, a technique that is commonly used in the analysis of data from prospective cohort studies, even when mortality is not the outcome of interest. A hazard rate is the rate of an outcome at a point in time conditional on the outcome not having occurred to that point in time. A hazard ratio is the ratio of 2 hazard rates: that for the exposed divided by that for the nonexposed.

Survival analysis is a sophisticated way of addressing the issues that arise when at-risk subjects leave the at-risk cohort, either because they develop the outcome or for some other reason. Survival analysis addresses this issue by censoring (removing participants from the at-risk cohort) in the calculation of hazard ratios. This approach can be extended to more elaborate models, such as proportional hazards models, capable of addressing complex methodological problems.

The techniques used in survival analysis are complex, but hazard ratios can be interpreted very much like other relative measures of effect and can be treated as such during critical appraisal.

Key point: Comparisons of incidence in prospective cohort studies can be accomplished using several parameters. Basic techniques use ratios of risks. More advanced techniques use ratios of incidence rates or hazard rates.

Assessing associations in prospective cohort studies using difference-based measures

Ratio-based measures are useful because they produce a single value that embodies a comparison of incidence between exposure groups. These measures include prevalence ratios, odds ratios, incidence proportion ratios, incidence rate ratios, and hazard ratios.

Another way to distill a single value from 2 values is to calculate a difference. In a prospective cohort study, this could involve calculating an incidence proportion difference—usually called a *risk difference*—or an incidence rate difference.

Ratio-based measures have an expected value in the event that the exposure has no impact on risk: the null value of 1. Difference-based measures also have a null value: the null value of 0.

Most prospective cohort studies use ratio-based measures of association, but there is nothing wrong with using difference-based measures. Indeed, a study has reported that clinicians understand risk differences better than relative risk when interpreting estimates of treatment effects.[117]

Selection bias in prospective cohort studies

There are many names for different types of bias.[194] *Selection bias* is an overarching term that simplifies terminology by focusing on a common mechanism through which the bias arises. Selection bias comes from study-design defects that affect who does or does not participate in a study. Factors that affect participation include the formal process of sampling, and procedures for obtaining consent, retaining subjects during follow-up, and collecting information from subjects (e.g., if missing data results in exclusion from the calculation of a parameter).

Think back to selection bias in case-control studies (see page 157), which centred on the methods of selecting cases and controls. The key question was whether the selection of cases and controls (based on disease status) depended on exposure in some way that differed between the 2 groups.

The same general considerations apply to the assessment of selection bias in prospective cohort studies, although the story unfolds in a slightly different way.

THE ROLE THAT DISEASE STATUS DOESN'T PLAY

In prospective cohort studies, subjects are selected (or included) in ways that ensure that none of them have the disease at baseline. Also, they are selected (or just divided) into exposed and nonexposed groups. Since the disease is not present at the time of selection, it is not possible for disease status to affect selection (if disease occurs at all, it will occur in the future)—a different situation than in case-control studies. This provides prospective cohort studies with a degree of protection against forms of bias that arise from defective procedures for selecting participants.

ATTRITION

Attrition happens when participants leave a study in ways not planned by the investigators.

People can "drop out" from the sample because they move, are lost to follow-up, withdraw consent, or for many other reasons. Attrition is almost inevitable in real-world research, and may be influenced by disease, or by precursors of disease, or by exposures that affect behaviour. Of particular concern: attrition can depend on factors related to disease in a way that differs depending on exposure. This is the scenario in which selection bias may occur. Some investigators propose the use of weights, calculated as the inverse probability of attrition (called *inverse probability of attrition weights*, or IPAWs) to reduce such bias,[195] but the only certain way to prevent it is to prevent attrition. Selection bias is first and foremost a study-design issue.

Key point: Cohort studies have some protection from selection bias, because disease has not occurred at the time of selection and therefore cannot influence selection. Attrition, however, creates an important vulnerability to selection bias.

MISSING DATA

Missing data is an issue related to attrition.

If there is missing data about the disease outcome, even among respondents who did not withdraw from a study, those respondents are not usually included in the calculation of a study's estimates. This type of bias can be regarded as a defect of participation, because those who do not provide the necessary data cannot be included in the estimate of association and are essentially not participating in its calculation.

Due to this defect involving participation, a study may systematically over- or underestimate the target parameter. If the missing data are unrelated to exposure or disease, and are missing completely at random, bias will not occur. However, if the missing data are related to the disease outcome in a way that differs depending on exposure, selection bias will occur and will follow familiar principles.

Several approaches can be used to analyze data with missing elements: listwise deletion, pairwise deletion, and imputation of missing values.

Listwise deletion involves removing the data of any participant with missing data.

Pairwise deletion involves ignoring observations with missing data on variables included in a particular calculation or procedure, but using other elements of those participants' data in other parts of the analysis. This leads to less data loss than listwise deletion. Both listwise and pairwise deletion can cause bias if the data are not missing completely at random. In addition, because they reduce the number of participants included in an analysis, listwise and pairwise deletion reduce the precision of estimates and the power of statistical tests.

Imputation of missing values involves replacing missing data with substitute values based on an educated guess. In single imputation, the guess simply fills in for the actual data point. Single imputation is problematic because it treats an imputed value as if it were known for certain, although it's really an educated guess. Because of this, statistical analyses of data sets with singly imputed values tend to underestimate the variability in the data, which leads to, for example, confidence intervals that are too narrow. Consequently, the preferred approach to imputation of missing data is multiple imputation. In multiple imputation, multiple data sets are generated with imputed values that can differ within those data sets, reflecting both a best guess about the missing data and also the uncertainty associated with that guess. The imputed data sets are then combined in a way that appropriately represents the uncertainty of the imputed values. Such techniques are beyond the scope of this book and their effectiveness continues to be debated. An important precaution with multiple imputation is this: it is only useful when the missing data can be explained by other variables in the data set, a circumstance confusingly known as "missing at random" (which is distinct from "missing completely at random" and "not missing at random"). If data are "missing completely at random," bias will not occur. If data are "not missing at random," then bias will occur. If data are "missing at random," then multiple imputation can address bias that might otherwise occur. If you are interested in reading more about multiple imputation, an accessible summary is provided by Sterne et al.[196]

Key point: If there are missing values for the study outcome, which can occur in a prospective cohort study even in the absence of attrition, this can introduce systematic error into an estimate of association.

Misclassification bias in prospective cohort studies

Misclassification bias follows similar patterns in prospective cohort studies as in case-control studies. A difference, however, is that it tends to arise from misclassification of disease status rather than exposure status. The mechanism of bias can be differential or nondifferential. In prospective cohort studies, the key distinction is usually whether misclassification of disease status depends on exposure status (differential misclassification of disease status) or not (nondifferential misclassification of disease status). As in case-control studies (see page 161), the behaviour of nondifferential misclassification is predictable. The direction of the bias is towards the null value. For a measure of relative risk, the null value is 1. For a risk difference, the null value is 0. If the misclassification is differential, the bias can go in either direction, depending on the type of inaccuracy in the measures being used.

Key point: The general principles of misclassification bias are the same in prospective cohort studies as in case-control studies. Nondifferential misclassification bias will be in the direction of the null value for a measure of association. The direction of differential misclassification bias depends on the nature of misclassification in a particular study.

In a cohort study, the exposure status of participants can be accurately measured at the time of selection. However, there is likely to be much concern about the subsequent classification of disease status. This is especially true in situations where knowledge of the exposure might affect the accuracy of outcome classification, leading to differential misclassification of outcome.

For example, if there is suspicion among investigators that the exposure in question is a risk factor, this could cause greater attention to detection of the disease in exposed subjects. As a result, the sensitivity of assessment of outcome could be greater in exposed than nonexposed participants. This would make the denominator of the risk ratio too small, increasing the estimate of the risk ratio. The specificity could also be lower in the exposed, making the numerator of the risk ratio too large. Each possibility would result in differential misclassification, because the accuracy of classification of disease is different depending on exposure. The direction of bias in each case would be towards overestimation.

This type of bias—arising from raters having an increased suspicion of disease (and therefore a greater sensitivity and/or lower specificity of assessment of the disease outcome) in exposed subjects—is sometimes called *diagnostic suspicion bias* or *surveillance bias*. Methodologically, blinding is the best safeguard against this type of bias: raters should be unaware of exposure status whenever possible.

Strengths and weaknesses of prospective cohort studies

Strengths

Temporal clarity: The main advantage of prospective cohort studies is their ability to clarify the timing of exposure in relation to disease. This is a major advantage over cross-sectional and case-control studies. Because of the temporal clarity that they can produce, prospective cohort studies are generally more capable of identifying causal effects than case-control or cross-sectional studies. A cause must logically precede an effect, so the ability to confirm temporality is an important advantage of prospective cohort studies. Indeed, this strength of the prospective cohort design is related to its temporal direction, which goes forward in time (from present to future) rather than backward (as in a case-control study or retrospective cohort study) or neither (as in a cross-sectional study).

> *Key point:* An advantage of the prospective cohort study is its forward temporal direction and therefore the clarity that it can provide about the temporal relationship between exposure and disease.

Risk measurement: Data from a prospective cohort study can be used to measure the incidence proportion, incidence rate, or hazard rate in addition to making estimates of association. To illustrate this point, imagine a case-control study that produces an odds ratio of 2. If this is an incidence-based case-control study and if the disease is rare, it may be reasonable to accept this incidence odds ratio as a good approximation of the relative risk. However, the odds ratio would not clarify whether the doubling of risk meant that there was a 2% versus 1% risk, or a 0.002% versus 0.001% risk. So, while case-control and prospective cohort studies can both produce information about associations, prospective cohort studies have the distinct advantage of being able to also examine the actual risks.

> *Key point:* An advantage of the prospective cohort design is its ability to measure risk, something that neither cross-sectional nor case-control studies can do.

Some resilience to selection bias: Prospective cohort studies are often considered less vulnerable to selection bias than case-control studies. However, they are vulnerable to selection bias arising from attrition.

Fit with large numbers of outcomes from single or multiple exposures: Prospective cohort studies can be very efficient for studying a large number of outcomes from a single exposure. Multipurpose cohorts, to the extent that they assess multiple exposures, can be useful for studying multiple risk factors and multiple outcomes.

Weaknesses

Expense: Prospective cohort studies are generally expensive. They often take place over long periods, and require investment in strategies that achieve high rates of response, and careful, accurate measurement.

Lengthy time requirement: In addition to being expensive, they are also time-consuming. In situations where the induction and/or latency periods are very long, prospective cohort studies can be especially time-consuming (and expensive).

Lack of fit for rare outcomes: Prospective cohort studies are not very efficient for studying rare outcomes. When the outcome is rare, even a large cohort may produce only a small number of outcome events, which would diminish the statistical power of the study. The case-control design is a more efficient way to study rare diseases. For rare exposures, however—as opposed to rare diseases (outcomes)—the prospective cohort design has advantages: an exposed cohort can be recruited using high probabilities of selection for the exposed cohort.

Attrition: Prospective cohort studies are vulnerable to attrition because of their long time frame. Attrition can result in selection bias, because it can easily depend on exposure and disease. Of course, the exact reasons for attrition are rarely known, since the "drop outs" are no longer in the study. The only sure way to prevent this type of bias is to ensure a very low rate of attrition from the study.

Key point: Like all study designs, the prospective cohort study design has its strengths and weaknesses. There is no generally superior study design. The best study design must be selected for a particular purpose.

Thinking deeper

A closer look at measures of association

Analytical epidemiology studies almost always include measures of association.

Measures of association distill information from 2 risks or rates down to a single number. Something useful is gained from this: a more accessible quantification of the association. Something is also lost, however: the underlying risks or rates. For this reason, epidemiological data analysis generally includes both the generation and reporting of univariate estimates of parameters (e.g., frequencies) and bivariate parameters (e.g., odds ratios, risk ratios, incidence rate ratios, hazard ratios, and risk differences). In fact, it often goes beyond bivariate estimation to report estimates from multivariable models. Multivariable models quantify exposure-disease associations with various adjustments for the possible effects of other variables. Many epidemiological analyses follow a predictable progression from univariate to bivariate to multivariable procedures. Note the term *multivariable*: some people find the word awkward and prefer to say *multivariate*—but *multivariate* refers to models that have multiple dependent and independent variables. It is preferable to say *multivariable*.

Ratio and difference-based measures of association have null values—another useful characteristic. For a ratio-based measure, the null value is 1. For a difference-based measure, it is 0. Typically, both types of estimates are accompanied by 95% CIs. This makes for a value-added proposition. If the 95% CI does not cross the null value, you can be confident that the association would have been statistically significant had a hypothesis-testing procedure been implemented.

A common mistake among students of epidemiology is to interpret confidence intervals as if they were tests of statistical significance. This is a mistake because it sets aside a more informative approach (confidence intervals) for a less informative approach (statistical tests). The best way to interpret a confidence interval is to consider its width (quantifying the precision of the estimate) together with the location of the upper and lower confidence limits. This provides a lot of information about the estimate, helping to portray the range of possible associations (e.g., from weak to strong, from strong to very strong, etc.).

Here's another mistake associated with interpreting confidence intervals as if they were tests of statistical significance. It is true that the overlap of a confidence interval with a null value is equivalent to a statistical test conducted at that same level of confidence. However, the overlap of 2 confidence intervals has no such implication, despite frequent (erroneous) assertions to the contrary. It is not uncommon for 2 prevalence estimates—for example, 1 for men and 1 for women—to have overlapping confidence intervals and yet be significantly different.

By contrast, nonoverlapping confidence intervals always have statistical significance.

The reason for this inconsistency can be understood by appreciating that the standard error of the difference between 2 proportions is not the sum of the standard errors of the 2 proportions. Recall that the standard error of a prevalence proportion (p) is:

$$\text{Standard Error}(p) = \sqrt{\frac{p \times (1-p)}{n}}$$

But the standard error for the difference between 2 proportions is not just the sum of the 2 standard errors: it is the square root of the sum of the 2 variances (the standard errors squared):

$$\text{Standard Error}(p_1 - p_2) = \sqrt{\text{Standard Error}_1^2 + \text{Standard Error}_2^2}$$

Key point: The overlap of confidence intervals from estimated frequencies does not indicate that the 2 groups are not significantly different.

Questions

1. List 4 advantages and 4 disadvantages of prospective cohort studies.

2. Provide a critique for the assertion that prospective cohort studies are the "best" study design for making causal inference.

3. In the Canadian Multicentre Osteoporosis Study (CaMos),[197] a randomly sampled cohort that included 9423 participants was followed for 10 years and assessed twice, at the 5-year and 10-year time points. The CaMos investigators sought to evaluate whether the use of certain antidepressants was associated with an increased risk of fragility fractures. They conducted an analysis of 6 645 subjects who had a baseline bone mineral density measurement. Among these, 4 011 completed all 10 years of follow-up.

   a. The investigators reported that 978 participants experienced at least 1 fragility fracture during follow-up. Calculate the incidence proportion for fragility fractures.

   b. There was an attrition rate of 40%. What characteristics among the study's "drop-outs" would make the parameter you calculated for fragility fractures an overestimation due to selection bias?

   c. The classification of exposure was difficult in the CaMoS study. Antidepressant use was measured at each of the interviews, but a detailed description of exposure over the entire 10 years was not possible. Could this introduce bias? What type of bias do would you suspect?

4. Suppose that you are the principal investigator of a long-term prospective cohort study. You are studying whether an exposure increases the risk of mortality. What would you prefer to employ as a measure of association: an odds ratio, risk ratio, or hazard ratio?

5. Can you think of an advantage of the prospective cohort design for studying recurrent diseases?

6. A 2016 prospective cohort study by Gray et al[198] examined whether cumulative exposure to a group of medications (benzodiazepines) increased the risk of Alzheimer disease. This study used "two rounds of recruitment (1994-96 and 2000-03) followed by continuous enrollment beginning in 2004." Is this a fixed or dynamic cohort?

7. Would it be possible to use the odds ratio as a measure of association in a prospective cohort study?

8. Businesses often keep detailed health and safety records for their employees, so it is often possible to identify a cohort of people with occupational exposures many years in the past. For this reason, occupational health studies often use the retrospective cohort study design. However, it is often not possible in such studies to select a suitable control group. Therefore, the general population may be used as a control group. (a) Could an SMR be used as a measure of

association in this type of retrospective cohort study? (b) Would it be reasonable to say that the healthy worker effect in such studies is a form of selection bias?

9. Explain why misclassification of disease is generally a bigger concern than misclassification of exposure status in cohort studies.

10. The Canadian Multicentre Osteoporosis Study (CaMoS) collected data over a 10-year period from a community cohort of Canadian residents aged 50 and older.[197] Fracture risk was among the many outcomes assessed. After completion of the follow-up, the investigators looked back at the subset of participants who reported taking antidepressants at the baseline assessment 10 years earlier, and used the CaMoS data to estimate the incidence of fractures and to compare this incidence to those not reporting antidepressant use. Is this a retrospective or prospective cohort study?

Confounding and effect modification in analytical studies

OBJECTIVES

- Define extraneous variables, confounding, and effect modification.
- Describe key procedures to control confounding: standardization, restriction, randomization, matching, stratification, and regression models.
- Identify strengths and weaknesses of key procedures to control confounding.
- Define external validity (generalizability).

Confounding and effect modification in context

Chapter 9 looked at confounding in the context of descriptive studies. This chapter looks at confounding in the more complex context of analytical studies.

This chapter also covers effect modification. Effect modification and confounding are related because both come from extraneous variables, but beyond this they are completely different. We have not looked at effect modification before, because it is only an issue in analytical studies, not descriptive studies. This is because only analytical studies assess exposure-disease association. Effect modification involves the influence of extraneous variables on exposure-disease association.

What are extraneous variables?

Extraneous variables are variables that occur outside of the exposure-disease relationship.

The effects of extraneous variables can become intermixed with the effects of exposures, leading to confounded estimates of exposure-disease associations. Confounding is a serious threat to the fundamental assumption of epidemiology: that diseases distribute in relation to their determinants. Analytical studies have to assume that this distribution-by-determinant relationship provides information about the cause of disease—but confounding draws this relationship into question.

Consider, for example, 2 common exposures that are associated: high levels of coffee consumption and smoking. People who drink a lot of coffee are also more likely to smoke. In a study investigating the potential association of coffee consumption and cancer, smoking becomes an extraneous variable that could confound the observed association. Drinking coffee may be associated with a higher risk of cancer, but—etiologically speaking—the association may have nothing to do with coffee consumption itself. It may merely reflect the associated health behaviour (smoking).

Key point: Association does not always mean causation, even if the estimate is free of bias and the temporal relationships are clear.

Confounding in analytical studies

Confounding literally means intermixing. In analytic epidemiology, the issue is whether 2 causal effects have intermixed in a single measure of association. Confounding is not at issue when 2 causes combine to cause a disease—this can certainly happen, but it is not confounding. Confounding is at issue when the intermixing of independent causal effects occurs in a way that makes the interpretation of measures of association difficult.

Key point: Confounding is a methodological flaw that results in the failure of estimated associations to reflect the independent causal effect of exposures.

More technically, confounding is defined as an intermixing of the effect of an exposure with the effect of an independent risk factor for the outcome (disease), leading to an estimated association that no longer reflects the causal impact of the exposure of interest. There are other ways to define confounding, but this definition is a good place to start.

The confounding triangle

A simple schematic can help clarify the problem of confounding: the confounding triangle (see Figure 20). In this triangle, the horizontal arrow from exposure to disease depicts the association of interest (this is the forward type of logical thinking about causation). The question mark indicates that this is a research question. The investigator wants to establish whether an association exists between exposure and disease and, if it does, to quantify the strength of the association. The potential confounder is depicted at the apex of the triangle.

The triangular schematic helps to identify the 3 key characteristics of a confounding variable. First, the potential confounder is a risk factor (hence, the arrow leading to the outcome has no question mark). Second, it is associated with the exposure of interest. Third, it is not a link in a chain of causal events connecting exposure to outcome. In other words, the confounder has effects that are independent of the exposure. Think back to the coffee-cancer example: confounding does not occur because drinking a lot of coffee makes people smoke—it's just that people who drink a lot of coffee are more often smokers. Because the exposure-confounder association is not causal, it is depicted with a dashed line.

FIGURE 20. THE CONFOUNDING TRIANGLE

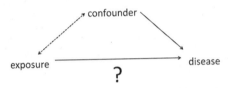

Note that the confounding variable is required to have etiological effects that are independent of the exposure. If the effects of the exposure occurred through a chain of events that included the variable (drinking coffee caused people to smoke and smoking caused them to get cancer), this would be an example of mediation rather than confounding. A mediating variable is a link in a causal chain leading from exposure to outcome. This differs from confounding, which is due to an intermixing of independent effects.

Both upper arms of the triangle need to be present for the association to be confounded. If there is an independent risk factor contributing to the etiology of a disease, this will not cause confounding unless it is also associated with exposure. Similarly, many variables may be strongly associated with exposure, but unless these are also independent risk factors for disease, confounding will not occur.

Confounding is usually identified using some form of adjustment for the potential confounding variable. Actual procedures for such adjustment are discussed later. Most commonly, these adjustments involve stratification on the potential confounding variable or inclusion of the potential confounder in a regression model. When adjustment changes an estimate of effect, confounding is the cause.

Here are some real-life examples of confounding from research about depression. Depression is about twice as common in women as men and is more common in younger than older people. These extraneous variables—sex and age—are important because they are determinants of many health outcomes and likely to be associated with many exposures. They are also not modifiable, so they are classic extraneous variables: their many associations with health outcomes are not very useful for primary prevention, but they can easily distort or modify important associations with modifiable determinants. A study examining association between depression and cataracts (cataracts are an eye problem that affects mostly older people) used data from the Canadian Community Health Survey.[199] It used the prevalence odds ratio as a measure of association, and the unadjusted odds ratio was 0.7 (95% CI 0.6–0.8). This means that the odds of depression seemed to be lower in those with cataracts. However, it might be that the odds are lower simply because people with cataracts tend to be older. After adjusting for age, the odds ratio was 2.5 (95% CI 2.4–2.6), indicating that the association was strongly confounded by age. Another study, examining association between depression and mortality, used longitudinal data from the National Population Health Survey.[199] The unadjusted relative risk of mortality (estimated using a hazard ratio) was 1.0 (95% CI 0.7–1.4), suggesting no association. But older people are much more likely to die than younger people and younger people are much more likely to be depressed. Also, women are more likely to be depressed and typically have lower mortality than men. With adjustment for age and sex, the hazard ratio became 2.0 (95% CI 1.4–2.9), indicating confounding.

A traditional definition of confounding

Building on the confounding triangle depicted in Figure 20, the following is a traditional definition of a confounding variable: a variable that is associated with exposure and is an independent determinant of outcome. Confounding itself can be defined (as suggested by Figure 20) as an intermixing of different causal effects in a single estimate of effect. None of these definitions has used the word *cause*, but they all point towards the importance of confounding for understanding causation. If you are interested in the descriptive question of whether a risk factor or risk indicator is associated with a higher prevalence or incidence of disease, then confounding is not an important issue. Here, a measure of effect is purely a descriptive statement, and a prevalence ratio or difference are merely good ways to provide such descriptive information. But if a measure of effect is intended to show a causal effect of an exposure, then the issue of confounding is of paramount importance.

A different type of confounding triangle

In describing causation, the version of the confounding triangle described above has a limitation: it requires the confounder to be associated with the exposure, but does not say why it is associated. Another way of drawing the triangle addresses this issue and leads to a slightly different definition of confounding. This alternative definition is as follows: a confounding variable is a variable that causes both the exposure and the disease. Figure 21 depicts this version of the triangle. Notice that the causal effects are depicted with single-headed arrows that show the direction of causal effect—for example, the confounder causes the exposure, but the exposure does not cause the confounder. Also, the figure contains no loops: the arrows never create a cycle. These 2 characteristics mean that the Figure 21 shows a directed acyclic graph, or DAG.

Both approaches to drawing the confounding triangle are widely used in epidemiology. The first type of diagram leads to a definition that remains useful in most situations. Consider the example of depression as a risk factor for mortality (see the previous section): age is a potential confounder of the association between depression and mortality. It is easy to think of age as associated with depression and causing mortality, but it is not easy to think of age as a cause of depression. A DAG would need to be more complicated to depict this situation (more information about DAGs is provided later in this chapter). In complicated situations where multiple variables are involved, DAGs can be very helpful for depicting causal mechanisms. In a DAG-based definition, a confounding variable causes both exposure and disease.

FIGURE 21. CAUSAL GRAPH WHERE A CONFOUNDING VARIABLE CAUSES BOTH EXPOSURE AND DISEASE

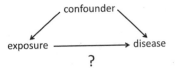

Is confounding a type of bias?

Confounding is not like other forms of bias, even though investigators sometimes use the term *confounding bias*. Bias is a systematic error in estimation of a population parameter such as, for example, an odds ratio. By contrast, confounding has more to do with the interpretation of a parameter than its systematic deviation from a true value. In a study free of defects, with perfect participation and measurement, the odds ratio has an expected value equal to the underlying parameter in the population. It can still be considered unbiased in this sense, even if it represents a mixing (confounding) of independent effects rather than a single causal effect.

In the coffee-cancer example, an elevated risk ratio for coffee consumption may very well centre on the population value for the risk ratio. But the question is: Does that risk ratio reflect an independent effect of coffee consumption or an intermixing of effects of coffee (if any) and smoking?

Key point: Confounding is different than some other types of bias because it does not lead to systematic error in the same way. A confounded estimate can be valid in the sense of not systematically deviating from a targeted population parameter. However, it may nevertheless be misleading if it is intended to represent the causal effect of a single exposure, but actually represents an intermixing of effects of different exposures.

Ways to control confounding: standardization

Chapter 9 covered direct and indirect standardization as procedures to control confounding (see pages XX).

To review: chapter 9 discussed a comparison of mortality in 2 geographic areas, Ontario and Nunavut. This was the concern: that the differences observed in mortality between the populations might merely reflect differences in the distribution of age. Age is a nonmodifiable variable, so it doesn't interest epidemiologists very much, at least not where primary prevention is the goal.

Standardization is a way to ensure that such extraneous variables do not become intermixed with variables of interest. Note that standardization is usually used to adjust rates or frequencies.

Ways to control confounding: other procedures

There are 5 procedures beyond standardization to address confounding. These are typically used in studies estimating parameters such as odds ratios, risk ratios, or risk differences.

The procedures fall into categories depending on when, during a study, you implement them: the design stage, the analysis stage, or both.

DESIGN STAGE CONTROL OF CONFOUNDING: RESTRICTION

Restriction is a procedure for preventing confounding at the design stage. This simply means not allowing people that are exposed to a potential confounder to participate in the study.

Let's take sex as an example of a potential confounder. Sex is a classic example because it is a nonmodifiable extraneous variable. In addition, sex is an independent risk factor for a large number of diseases, and associated with many exposures of interest. So, investigators are often concerned about its potential to introduce confounding.

If a study used restriction to control confounding by sex, it would restrict participation to either men or women.

Think back to the confounding triangle. The concern is that sex—an independent risk factor for many outcomes—may be associated with the exposure of interest. In this case, an apparent effect of exposure could actually be due to sex. However, if the entire sample consists of either men or women, then the effect of sex cannot be intermixed with the effect of any exposure: there is only 1 sex present. Restriction eliminates any association of exposure and the potential confounder (the left-hand side of the triangle), thereby eliminating any possibility of an intermixing of effects.

The main problem with restriction is that it may affect the applicability of the study results to the real world. After all, using sex as an example, the world contains approximately 50% men and 50% women. Study results that derive from men only or women only have questionable applicability to the entire population.

DESIGN STAGE CONTROL OF CONFOUNDING: RANDOMIZATION

In randomization, an investigator randomly assigns an exposure to the study participants and then looks for an effect.

Note that randomization is not the same as random selection of a sample—random selection of a sample is a different procedure and has nothing to do with the control of confounding.

Randomization can only be used in studies where investigators assign an exposure, such as a randomized controlled trial. And it is only possible when assigning an exposure is ethically feasible. It is not feasible to randomly assign study participants to harmful exposures, such as smoking. This would violate the ethical principle of nonmaleficence (see page 115). It is likewise unethical to not expose a research participant to a treatment known to be effective—this would amount to another form of maleficence. Generally speaking, the only exposures allowed for random assignment are treatments of uncertain efficacy. This situation—in which there is reason to hope a treatment may be helpful, but not enough evidence to endorse the treatment as helpful—is called *equipoise*. Equipoise is an ethical requirement for randomized controlled trials.

Why is randomization an effective means of controlling confounding? Refer again to the confounding triangles shown in Figures 20 and 21. Due to the law of large numbers, random assignment helps to ensure that the distribution of confounding variables is approximately equal in exposed and nonexposed groups. This removes the connection between the confounder and the exposure on the left-hand side of the triangle, and precludes the occurrence of confounding. Furthermore, the anticonfounding effect can be expected to work both for known and unknown, measured and unmeasured confounders. The law of large numbers distributes all variables with equal effectiveness. Randomization is the only procedure that can control confounders that are unmeasured or even unknown.

MENDELIAN RANDOMIZATION

Mendelian randomization is a rare but interesting study design in which randomization controls confounding, but where the randomization comes from a natural biological process rather than the actions of an investigator. These studies can be conducted when a variant of a gene strongly determines an exposure and exerts effects on the outcome only through the effects of the exposure. If that exposure is associated with a disease, then it is reasonable to expect that the genetic variant should also be associated with the disease. Genetic variants are typically distributed randomly at the time of conception due to the laws of inheritance—specifically, Mendel's second law. This creates a situation that is similar to a randomized controlled trial: the exposure is essentially randomly allocated at conception. This means that the exposure should not be associated with any other variables that cause the disease, and, consequently, the association is protected from confounding. Also, since conception occurs before disease onset, there is less doubt about whether the exposure is a cause of the disease as opposed to a consequence of the disease.

Mendelian randomization studies have been used to study, for example, whether vitamin D deficiency and obesity may cause multiple sclerosis.[200] In these studies, genetic variants and genetic risk scores known to predict vitamin D levels or obesity were found to be associated with the disease, strongly suggesting a causal role. Mendelian randomization studies remain, however, relatively uncommon. Often, Mendelian randomization cannot be used because there is no suitable genetic variant. Also, it involves assumptions, which are often difficult to evaluate.[201]

DESIGN STAGE CONTROL OF CONFOUNDING: MATCHING

Matching ensures that groups being compared are exact matches in terms of the distribution of confounding variables.

Matching is a type of partial restriction: it does not prevent all subjects exposed to a confounder from participating in a study, but it places some restrictions on who can participate.

Like restriction and randomization, matching targets the left-hand side of the confounding triangle. It eliminates any association between the exposure and the matched confounding variables.

In a prospective cohort study, pair matching involves selecting each member of the nonexposed cohort to have the same value of the confounding variable as a matched member of the exposed cohort. If sex is the target confounder in pair matching, here's what this means: for each exposed male a study selects, it also selects a nonexposed male, and for each exposed female, it also selects a nonexposed female.

In a case-control study, pair matching means that each case with exposure to the potential confounder—we'll use sex again—is matched with a control that has the same exposure to that variable. In other words, each male case would have a matched male control and each female case would have a matched female control.

Pair matching at the design stage has implications for the analysis stage (so, matching is regarded as a procedure that controls confounding both at the design and analysis stage). Normally, each observation in a data set is considered independent of the others and conventional statistics can be used in the analysis. When there has been pair matching, each member of a pair is related to the other member in the sense that they have been selected specifically because they share a characteristic. They are not independent, and special analysis techniques must be used to address this.

The term pair matching is used when study participants are recruited in pairs, but it is also possible to match a case to larger numbers of controls using matching. For example, 3 or 4 controls could be matched to each case. This type of matching still occurs at the level of an individual and is therefore called *individual matching*.

Another approach to matching is frequency matching. Frequency matching ensures that cases and controls have the same frequencies of exposure to potential confounding variables, thereby also eliminating the left-hand side of the confounding triangle. Frequency matching is often easier to do than individual matching because the selection of each individual control doesn't need to be based on the characteristics of an individual case. Also, frequency matching is easier to address in the analysis than pair or individual matching.

Key point: Three study design strategies can be used to address the issue of confounding: restriction, randomization, and matching. The last of these creates a requirement for specialized data-analysis procedures.

ANALYSIS STAGE CONTROL OF CONFOUNDING: STRATIFICATION

The procedures to control confounding during data analysis counteract the intermixing of effects that cause confounding using the same general approach: unmixing them.

Stratification was introduced in chapter 9 in the context of descriptive studies and basic estimates, such as frequencies or rates (see page 123). Stratification is more commonly used in analytical studies as a procedure to detect and adjust for confounding. In analytical studies, it involves stratifying measures of association.

Stratified analysis divides the contingency tables arising from a study into groups (strata). The groups are defined by levels of the confounding variable. In the case of sex, this would mean dividing the data set from a study into sex-specific strata (1 stratum for men and 1 for women) and then examining the effect of exposure separately in each stratum. Since confounding is caused by intermixing, unmixing through stratification will lead to a change in the estimated effect if the unstratified (crude) estimate was distorted by confounding. This is an example of the general principle that confounding is detected by adjusting for the confounder and observing whether this changes the estimated association.

Within strata defined by sex, sex can no longer be a confounder (there can be no association on the left-hand side of the confounding triangle). Therefore, the estimate for each stratum will reflect the effect of exposure and not the effect of exposure mixed with sex.

Stratified analysis leads to a set of adjusted estimates, called *stratum-specific estimates*. Stratum-specific estimates are adjusted for confounding. There is, of course, a drawback to this approach. Since stratum-specific estimates derive from a subset of the sample rather than the whole sample, they are subject to random error to a greater extent. In other words, they tend to be imprecise. Procedures are available to address this problem of imprecision.

ANALYSIS STAGE CONTROL OF CONFOUNDING: REGRESSION MODELLING

Chapter 10 introduced the idea that information about an association could be represented in the form of a linear equation (see pages 144–145). The value of this idea is that regression models based on linear equations have a very important role in the detection of, and adjustment for, confounding.

Regression models produce adjusted estimates. In general, they involve developing a best-fitting linear equation, or a transformed version of such a linear equation. Time-to-event or survival analysis methods are also used for this purpose.

Chapter 10 briefly explored representation of epidemiologic effects in linear models through the derivation of linear equations that basically reproduce the contents of a 2 × 2 table (see pages 144–145). Using statistical software, it is possible to identify an equation of this form that accurately describes more complex data than that of a 2 × 2 table. These more elaborate linear models include not only the exposure of interest, but also potential confounding variables. The estimated effect in such a model (recall that the parameters in these models can be risk differences, log odds ratios, log prevalence ratios, etc.) is adjusted for the effect of the confounders included in the model.

Regression models can separate the independent effects of different variables, and are therefore helpful in identifying and adjusting for confounding effects.

> *Key point:* Procedures to control confounding during data analysis include stratified analysis and regression modelling.

Regression modelling has another use in epidemiological research besides the assessment and control of confounding. Its other use is prediction. In prediction, the goal is to explain as much variability in an outcome as possible. Models focusing on prediction often include variables that are neither confounding nor effect-modifying variables. They may include such variables if inclusion improves the predictive ability of the model. Such decisions may be made based on the statistical significance of model terms or through various goodness-of-fit parameters. The predictive approach to modelling differs from the classical epidemiological approach described in previous sections, an approach that builds from the concepts of stratified analysis and is guided by the need to assess effect modification and confounding.

Strengths and weaknesses of procedures to control confounding

RESTRICTION

Restriction has the advantage of being easily understandable and can, in some instances, be an easy way to allay concerns about confounding. However, it has several disadvantages. The most important disadvantage is the degree of distortion it imposes on population relationships. It makes estimates of association free of the confounding effects of restricted variables, but the frequencies, risks, or rates observed may no longer reflect those of the population. Restriction can also make it more difficult to find study subjects, since they must be determined to be free of the restricted characteristic. Finally, restriction has a negative effect on the generalizability of estimates (for more on generalizability, see page 213).

> *Key point:* Restriction controls confounding, but at a high cost in terms of generalizability.

RANDOMIZATION

Randomization is widely viewed as the best procedure to control confounding due to its unique ability to address both measured and unmeasured confounding variables. Randomization, though, can only be employed in special situations: where equipoise exists. Most randomized controlled trials employ restriction in addition to randomization, and have long lists of inclusion and exclusion criteria to safeguard their internal validity. As in all cases of restriction, this can affect the generalizability of estimates.[202]

A literature of studies seeking to evaluate whether beta-carotene (a precursor of vitamin A) can prevent lung cancer underscores the importance of randomization. As described by Demetrius Albanes,[203] a large number of observational studies in the past suggested that a high intake of beta-carotene reduced the risk of lung cancer by about half. However, when a randomized controlled trial was conducted there was no effect, and the results suggested a possible 16% increase in cancer incidence among those consuming high levels of beta-carotene. The difference may have been due to confounding by the amount of fruits and vegetables consumed. A diet high in fruits and vegetable is associated with higher intake of beta-carotene and is also known to be protective against cancer. Superior control of the consequent confounding in randomized trials of supplemental beta-carotene may have thereby eliminated the apparent protective effect.

Key point: Randomization is the best way to control confounding, but it is often not practical or ethical to use.

MATCHING

Matching has several disadvantages: it distorts population relationships; it can be expensive and inefficient; and in situations where several potential confounders are being matched simultaneously, it can have severe impacts on recruitment into a study.

However, matching can sometimes be easy and inexpensive. And, when the variable at issue is a strong confounder, it can increase efficiency, leading to narrower confidence intervals around a measure of effect than would otherwise occur. Matching can also help control subtle, difficult-to-measure variables—a study can, for example, recruit matched subjects from the same neighbourhood to adjust for effects that can otherwise be difficult to measure (e.g., social standing, living environment). Stratification and modelling, by contrast, can only adjust for quantifiable variables.

Matching, however, should not be viewed as a default procedure for control of confounding: its disadvantages are significant. It is sometimes seen, incorrectly, as a default procedure by investigators who are unfamiliar or uncomfortable with statistical procedures (stratification and modelling).

Key point: Matching can control confounding and sometimes increase efficiency, but these advantages come at the cost of distortion of population estimates. Matching can also lead to operational complexities and extra expense.

STRATIFICATION AND MODELLING

Stratification and modelling are closely related procedures. Stratification is a foundational skill for epidemiologists, but in current research it mostly functions as a preliminary procedure for more advanced analysis using statistical models. When these models are encountered in the literature, they can be very complex and difficult to understand. For example, they may include many variables and it may not be clear which, if any, are actual confounders. The procedures for selecting variables to include in the model are often unclear as well. The motivation for presenting complex models is to report estimates that are simultaneously adjusted for many potential confounders, but this approach comes at the cost of diminished transparency. Stratified analysis is much more clear, but it is usually only possible to stratify on 1 or 2 extraneous variables at a time, so it takes a great deal of space to present stratified analyses for a variety of extraneous variables. The needed space often exceeds the limits of journals that publish studies.

CRITICAL APPRAISAL AND COMMON MODELS TO CONTROL CONFOUNDING

Key models

General familiarity with a small number of modelling approaches is sufficient to critically appraise studies using these tools.

Linear regression models use linear equations to describe data. They predict the mean value of an outcome variable from several predictors included in the model's linear equation. Linear regression models are frequently encountered in the social science literature, where they are usually used to predict the mean value of a continuous variable. A frequency is a type of mean that is calculated from a variable that assumes values of 0 or 1, so it is not surprising that linear regression models are also used in epidemiology. The β coefficients in such models can be interpreted as differences. Depending on the type of frequency data, these may be prevalence differences or risk differences.

Log-transformed models have β coefficients that represent ratios. In logistic regression, the β coefficients are log odds ratios. In models fitting a log frequency rather than a log odds, the coefficients may be log prevalence ratios or log risk ratios, depending on the nature of the underlying data.

Other models produce coefficients that reflect rate ratios and hazard ratios (see page 188). In critical appraisal, the importance of these models is that they contain the exposure of interest as well as other (extraneous) variables.

In each of these approaches to modelling, the method for detecting confounding is the same. The procedure is to examine the parameter quantifying the association without any adjustment, and then to compare this to the estimate after adjustment. If adjustment results in a change of the estimated effect, then confounding has occurred.

An example study

A study by Modgill et al[128] provides an example of models to adjust for confounding. This study used data from the National Population Health Survey to examine the impact of migraine on depression incidence. The investigators used a type of survival analysis called a proportional hazards model and reported an unadjusted (or crude) hazard ratio of 2.1. When sex was included in the proportional hazard model, the hazard ratio (now a sex-adjusted hazard ratio) diminished to 1.9, indicating confounding by sex. Female sex is known to be associated with an elevated incidence of depression and also to be positively associated with migraine. Therefore confounding by sex is expected (see Figure 20). A component of the crude association between migraine and depression reflects that women are more susceptible to migraine and have a higher risk of depression. In the absence of adjustment, therefore, the effect of sex is intermixed with the effect of migraine.

The general approach to confounding is always the same, no matter the details of the mathematical and statistical models a study may employ. A crude estimate is calculated first. Then the estimate is adjusted for the potential confounder (in this case, the adjustment is based on a proportional hazards model and the potential confounder is sex). If the adjustment changes the estimated effect (if the adjusted estimate—a hazard ratio in this case—changes when the potential confounder is included in the model used in making the adjustment), then confounding has been demonstrated. In this study, the effect of migraine, independent of the effect of sex, is represented by the adjusted hazard ratio of 1.9.

Key point: Models detect confounding when they identify a change in the exposure-disease relationship on adjustment for a potential confounding variable.

Using models to control confounding involves challenges such as selecting the best type of model and selecting the variables that should be included in the model. As discussed above, a variable that acts as a confounder, and that is detected as such because its inclusion in the model affects the estimated effect of the exposure, must be included if the model is to provide a valid adjusted estimate. Directed acyclic graphs, mentioned earlier in this chapter (and discussed in more detail later), can also provide guidance for variable selection. Specifically, if a variable falls on 1 or more of several causal paths that link the exposure to the disease, then the variable is a mediator and adjustment for it will lead to an underestimate of effect. This is depicted using a DAG in Chapter 18. In a situation in which a variable mediates all of the effects of exposure, adjustment for that mediator will remove the entire effect of exposure. This problem of incorrectly adjusting for mediating variables, leading to a distorted estimate of the effect of exposure, is called *overadjustment* in the epidemiologic literature. If unnecessary adjustments are made, which in a regression model means that variables that are not confounders or mediators are included in the model, the usual result is a loss of precision. In distinction to overadjustment, this is called *unnecessary adjustment*.[204]

The limits of models

In critical appraisal, it is important to remember that models can only handle variables that were measured, and only report on variables investigators included in the models. It is therefore important to ask not only whether a variable looks like a confounder in the analysis reported in a study, but also whether all of the most important potentially confounding variables were addressed at all.

Table 30 shows a summary of ways to address the issue of confounding, classified according to whether these are implemented at the study-design phase or the data-analysis phase. Note that matching is a study-design procedure, but it requires the use of special data-analysis techniques, and so it affects both study design and analysis.

TABLE 30. 2 × 2 STUDY-PHASE CLASSIFICATION FOR PROCEDURES TO CONTROL CONFOUNDING

	Implemented at the study-design phase	Implemented at the data-analysis phase
Standardization		X
Restriction	X	
Randomization	X	
Matching	X	X
Stratification		X
Regression models		X

CRITICAL APPRAISAL AND GENERALIZABILITY

A study is internally valid if it produces unbiased estimates for its target population.

If it is internally valid, it may also be externally valid: its unbiased estimates might apply to other populations. *Generalizability* is another term for external validity. (If an estimate is not valid, its generalizability is a moot point. There would be no point in trying to apply an invalid estimate to other populations.)

Consider an epidemiological estimate from a US study. If the study has an adequate sample size (is not vulnerable to random error) and no study-design defects (these would introduce systematic error), the study can be viewed as internally valid. The question of whether the study could be considered valid in another country (e.g., Canada) is a question of external validity or generalizability.

Many of the most important national surveys in Canada have used sampling frames that exclude homeless persons, members of the armed forces, residents of aboriginal settlements and remote areas, and residents of institutions. Are estimates arising from these surveys valid for these populations? This is a question of generalizability.

We have explored tools to assess whether bias and confounding have compromised a study's internal validity. Assessing a study's generalizability— its external validity—is different: it is purely a matter of judgement.

Judgements about generalizability that are too restrictive will result in "reinventing the wheel"—unnecessary confirmatory studies in different populations.

Judgements that are too cavalier can lead to actions harmful to public health.

Key point: Internal validity is a necessary but not sufficient condition for external validity.

Effect modification

Confounding is one way in which an extraneous variable can enter into epidemiological analyses. The other way is effect modification.

Effect modification, as the name implies, happens when an extraneous variable modifies the effect of the exposure of interest. Unlike confounding, effect modification is not an artifact that can (or should) be adjusted away or controlled. Instead, effect modification is a real aspect of the exposure-disease relationship under investigation. You could say that effect modification means this: rather than a single exposure-disease relationship, there are multiple relationships.

When effect modification has occurred, there are multiple effects of exposure in different groups, and different measures of effect need to be reported separately.

An example of effect modification

Friedenreich et al[184] reported effect modification in a case-control study of metabolic syndrome and waist circumference as risk factors for endometrial cancer. Odds ratios in this analysis were stratified for menopausal status, creating 2 groups: pre/perimenopausal and postmenopausal. In the post-menopausal group, the odds ratio for metabolic syndrome as a risk factor for endometrial cancer was 1.61 and that for waist circumference ($\geq$ 88 cm) was 2.01. In the pre/perimenopausal group, stronger effects were seen: 1.96 and 2.98 for metabolic syndrome and waist circumference, respectively. Apparently, these exposures produce 2 sets of effects in the population: 1 in pre/perimenopausal women and 1 in postmenopausal women. Since there are 2 different associations, it would be wrong to present only 1. The unstratified estimates would be a mixture of both associations, and would apply to neither postmenopausal nor premenopausal women. The only solution is to report the stratum-specific effects separately.

Stratification and homogeneous versus heterogeneous estimates

An important skill of epidemiologists is differentiating confounding and effect modification. Stratification is a very useful tool for doing this. After stratification for a confounder, you expect to see 2 stratum-specific (adjusted) estimates that are similar to each another, but different from the unadjusted (unstratified, or crude) measure of effect. If there is effect modification, the 2 stratum-specific estimates will be different from each another, as in the study by Friedenreich et al, which stratified on postmenopausal versus pre/perimenopausal status.

This distinction between similar and dissimilar stratum-specific estimates is key to the analysis of epidemiological data—so key that it has its own terminology. When 2 stratum-specific estimates are similar to each another, they are termed *homogeneous* (or you can say they display homogeneity). When they are different, they are termed *heterogeneous*.

STATISTICAL TESTS FOR HOMOGENEITY

Epidemiological analysis must always consider the role of chance. Saying that 2 estimates are homogeneous does not mean the estimates are exactly the same, but rather that chance can account for their differences.

Statistical tools can help determine whether 2 stratum-specific estimates are homogeneous. In stratified analysis, the Mantel-Haenszel test for homogeneity is commonly employed. In modelling, tests for statistical interaction between exposure and potentially modifying variables are often used. The model-based tests are called *tests of interaction*.

Key point: Effect modification is not a form of bias and cannot be addressed using statistical adjustments. This a real effect and should be reported through presentation of stratum-specific estimates.

Thinking deeper

"Cooking up" some confounding

The ingredients leading to confounding are well known (an independent risk factor associated with an exposure leading to intermixing of effects), but the concept can be difficult to grasp. To clarify how these ingredients produce confounding, let's "cook up" some confounding.

Many cake recipes tell you to mix ingredients in 2 separate bowls and combine them at a later stage. Our recipe for confounding uses the same approach, except the 2 bowls are 2 × 2 tables.

One of these tables depicts the exposure-disease association in the absence of an extraneous variable, and the other depicts the exposure-disease relationship in the presence an extraneous variable. Mixing these tables together is the opposite of stratified analysis, and pursued here for exclusively illustrative purposes. In stratified analysis, the starting point is a crude estimate of effect and stratification unmixes the variables that contribute to the effect.

Imagine an analysis of a sample of 1000 people, and consider an exposure and an extraneous variable. To simplify things, we'll ignore the issue of random error. Let's also avoid confusing language such as "exposure to the extraneous variable": we'll call the exposure the *target variable*. Assume the following:

- The baseline risk of disease in a group not exposed to either the target variable or the extraneous variable is 5%, or 0.05.
- The frequency of disease in a group that is exposed to the target variable but not to the extraneous variable is 10% or 0.10. (In other words, the target variable is associated with a doubling of risk.) This is the true effect of exposure: the effect that the analysis is seeking to estimate. In the presence of the extraneous variable, the effect of exposure is the same doubling of risk (meaning that we are "cooking up" confounding and are saying that there is no effect modification).
- Twenty percent of the population is exposed to the extraneous variable.

These assumptions allow us to predict what the 2 × 2 tables will look like.

One table will contain 800 people, since 80% of the sample is not exposed to the extraneous variable. The other table will contain the 200 people who are exposed to the extraneous variable.

The table with 800 people (the stratum not exposed to the extraneous variable) can be divided into disease and exposure contingencies based on the assumptions stated above. In this stratum, 10% ($n = 80$) will be exposed to the target variable. This means that there must be 720 in the nonexposed group within this stratum. There will also be 5% of this 720 ($n = 36$) who will have the disease ($720 \times 0.05 = 36$), leaving $n = 684$ who do not have the disease. Since exposure to the target variable is associated with a doubling of risk, there will be 10% of the remaining 80 (n = 8) who are expected to have the disease, leaving 72 of those with exposure who do not have the disease. The 2 × 2 table for this stratum—not exposed to the extraneous variable—will look like Table 31.

TABLE 31. FIRST OF 2 STRATIFIED 2 × 2 TABLES: STRATUM NOT EXPOSED TO THE EXTRANEOUS VARIABLE

	Disease	No disease	Totals
Exposed	8	72	80
Nonexposed	36	684	720
Total			800

The other table comprises 200 people (the stratum exposed to the extraneous variable). Since confounding can only occur if the extraneous variable is an independent risk factor for the disease, and since our goal is to "cook up" confounding, it will be assumed that the extraneous variable is associated with a threefold increase in the risk of disease. The final ingredient for confounding is that the extraneous variable should be associated with exposure to the target variable. To fulfill this requirement, it will be assumed that exposure to the target variable is 3 times as common in the group exposed to the extraneous variable. At this stage, all of the ingredients needed to concoct the second 2 × 2 table have been assembled.

In the stratum exposed to the extraneous variable, we have assumed that exposure to the target variable is 3 times as common, so 30% of these subjects are exposed to the target variable. There will therefore be 60 (200 × 0.30) in the exposed group and 140 in the nonexposed group. In the subjects within this stratum who are not exposed to the target variable, the risk of disease will be 15%, because the risk of disease is 3 times higher due to the independent effects of the extraneous variable. You would then expect that n = 21 would develop the disease (140 × 0.15), leaving n = 119 in the no-disease group. In the exposed group, the risk is double this (30% instead of 15%) because there is a doubling of risk due to exposure. Since these are independent effects, the joint risk is therefore a sixfold elevation. This leads to an expectation that 18 (60 × 0.30) will have the disease. Consequently, 42 will not have the disease. The 2 × 2 table for this stratum—exposed to the extraneous variable—will look like Table 32.

TABLE 32. SECOND OF 2 STRATIFIED 2 × 2 TABLES: STRATUM EXPOSED TO THE EXTRANEOUS VARIABLE

	Disease	No disease	Totals
Exposed	18	42	60
Nonexposed	21	119	140
Total			200

Note that if an incidence proportion ratio is calculated from each table, the result is the same, an assumption that was built into these calculations:

$$\text{Incidence Proportion Ratio (Stratum 1)} = \frac{0.10}{0.05} = 2$$

$$\text{Incidence Proportion Ratio (Stratum 2)} = \frac{0.30}{0.15} = 2$$

But what if we mix the 2 × 2 tables for stratum 1 and stratum 2 by tossing them into the same 2 × 2 table? The result is presented in Table 33. Each cell of the separate 2 × 2 tables is simply added together to produce this.

TABLE 33. UNSTRATIFIED 2 × 2 TABLE*

	Disease	No disease	Totals
Exposed	26	114	140
Nonexposed	57	803	860
Total			1000

*formed by adding the values in each of the 4 cells in Table 31 and Table 32

If an incidence proportion ratio is calculated from this table, the result is 2.8! Even though the 2 stratified tables had the correct incidence proportion ratio of 2.0, adding them together and calculating the crude incidence proportion ratio results in an incorrect estimate. This is because the 2 × 2 tables were cooked up with all of the ingredients to produce confounding.

In real-world epidemiologic analysis, things would go the other way. Normally, the first calculation would be the crude incidence proportion ratio, which would then be stratified on the extraneous variable. The crude estimate would be about 2.8. The analyst would notice that the adjusted, stratum-specific, relative risks were similar to each other and that they were different from the crude estimate, since they would only be about 2.0—thereby identifying the occurrence of confounding.

If you enjoy this kind of methodological unpacking, you could take this exercise further by setting up a spreadsheet to make all these calculations. This would make the calculations less tedious and would allow you to explore numerous scenarios.

Questions

1. List 3 conditions that must be present for a variable to act as a confounding variable according to (a) traditional and (b) DAG-based definitions of a confounding variable.

2. A case-control study by Weintraub et al[167] on the association between impulse-control disorders and dopamine-agonist exposure reported an unadjusted odds ratio of 2.72. Dopamine-agonists are drugs that mimic the effects of the

neurotransmitter dopamine. To explore confounding effects, a multivariable logistic regression model was produced. This model contained age, marital status, smoking, family history of gambling problems, and levodopa treatment (as well as the exposure variable: dopamine-agonist use). The adjusted odds ratio from this model was 2.72.

   a. What was the β coefficient for dopamine-agonist use in the logistic regression model?

   b. What does this model have to say about the issue of confounding?

3. A case-control study by Hackam et al[170] examined the association between ACE inhibitors and rupture of aortic aneurisms. It reported an odds ratio of 0.82. After adjustment for demographic characteristics, risk factors for rupture, comorbidities, contraindications to ACE inhibitors, health care use, and aneurism screening (in a logistic regression model), an adjusted estimate of 0.83 was found. What are the implications of this finding for confounding?

4. A case-control study by Rothwell et al[174] examined chiropractic manipulation as a risk factor for stroke. It found a significant association in those younger than 45, but not in older subjects.

   a. Is this an example of confounding?

   b. How should this result be reported?

5. Depression may be a risk factor for mortality. This condition is more common in young people who are, of course, less likely to die than older people. A Canadian study using data from the National Population Health Survey found an unadjusted hazard ratio of 1.0, suggesting no association of depression and mortality. However, with adjustment for age and sex, the hazard ratio doubled.[199]

   a. How can you explain this effect?

   b. When adjusted for other variables that may predict mortality (such as smoking), the association of depression with mortality again disappeared. Can this be explained in terms of confounding?

6. A case control study by de Gage et al[175] examined the role of benzodiazepines (a class of sedating medications) as a risk factor for Alzheimer disease. The study used Quebec administrative data sets and found a 50% higher odds of Alzheimer disease in benzodiazepine users. As is often the case with such studies, some potential confounding variables could not be measured. One of these was wine consumption, which may be a protective factor. The authors cited evidence that benzodiazepine users were more likely to be wine drinkers. What impact might the lack of control for wine consumption have on the study estimates?

7. Mente et al[205] analyzed pooled data from 4 studies to explore the possibility of a "U-shaped" relationship between sodium intake, on the one hand, and increased systolic blood pressure and cardiovascular outcomes, on the other. A U-shaped pattern would imply that both low and high levels of sodium intake are associated with increased risk. They concluded that: "Compared with moderate sodium intake, high sodium intake is associated with an increased risk of cardiovascular events and death in hypertensive populations (no association in normotensive populations), while the association of low sodium intake with increased risk of cardiovascular events and death is observed in those with or without hypertension. These data suggest that lowering sodium intake is best

targeted at populations with hypertension who consume high sodium diets." Is this an example of effect modification or confounding?

8. According to the Strengthening the Reporting of Observational Studies in Epidemiology (STROBE) statement,[206] P values are not appropriate criteria for selecting the confounders to adjust for in an analysis. Do you agree with this assertion?

9. Demoury et al[207] investigated the possible association between residential greenness and risk of prostate cancer using a case-control study design. The authors stated that residential greenness "has been associated with increased physical activity, lower odds of being overweight or obese, and lower exposure to air pollution." Are these variables possible confounders of the association in question?

10. Nonrandomized studies of treatment effectiveness are subject of a variety of biases. Suppose, for example, that physicians are more likely to prescribe a particularly potent treatment to patients with more severe disease. What type of bias would this cause: selection bias, misclassification bias, or confounding?

Stratified analysis and regression modelling in analytical studies

---

OBJECTIVES

- Explain the key importance of analysis-stage techniques to control confounding.
- Describe the following aspects of stratified analysis: fit with noncontinuous variables; pooling of estimates for better precision; identification of effect modification; and detection and adjustment for confounding variables.
- List the steps of stratified analysis.
- Describe the advantages of regression modelling over stratified analysis.
- List the steps of regression modelling.

The context for a deeper discussion of stratified analysis and regression modelling

Chapter 14 looked at design-stage and analysis-stage techniques to control confounding, and discussed them in the context of categorical variables, such as sex.

This chapter looks at analysis-stage techniques—stratified analysis and regression modelling—in more detail, and in the context of continuous variables, such as age.

Why provide a deeper discussion of stratified analysis and regression modelling? These techniques play a role in almost every analytical study, even in studies that have also used design-stage techniques to control confounding.

If you want to understand most of the empirical studies published in the clinical and public health literature, you need to understand the goals and strategies of stratified analysis and regression modelling.

Why do studies use design- and analysis-stage techniques to control confounding?

Design-stage techniques to minimize confounding include randomization, restriction, and matching (see pages 204–209). None of them are foolproof (and not all studies use them). So, analysis-stage techniques—stratified analysis and regression modelling—add confidence to conclusions about exposure-disease associations.

Randomization aims to ensure an equal distribution of all confounders, whether measured or unmeasured, between the groups in a study. This strategy even diminishes the effects of unknown confounders. It is the best way to control confounding, when it is feasible. However, it is not always completely effective. An unbalanced distribution of a confounding variable may occur by chance during randomization. This is unlikely, particularly if the sample size is large, but poses problems if it does occur. For these reasons, randomized studies usually strive to measure all potential confounding variables, so that confounding can be detected and appropriate adjustments can be made through stratification and/or modelling, if necessary.

Key point: Randomization is the best way to control for confounding (when feasible), but it is not foolproof. Analysis techniques to address confounding are sometimes necessary when chance imbalances occur during randomization.

Detection of, and adjustment for, confounding remain important in the other design-stage strategies, too.

Restriction eliminates extraneous variables by restricting who can participate in a study. A restricted (eliminated) variable cannot be a confounding variable. However, other variables in a restricted study could still confound exposure-disease associations.

Matching eliminates the effect of extraneous variables by balancing their presence in the groups a study compares. Matched variables cannot act as confounders. However, again, other variables can continue to confound results.

Stratified analysis

The principle underlying the use of stratification is straightforward. Confounding is an intermixing of the effects of an exposure with those of an extraneous variable. The goal of stratification is to unmix these effects.

Stratified analysis and categorical variables

Let's review sex as a confounding variable. If sex is a confounder, conducting the analysis separately in men and women will unmix the effect of an exposure from the effect of sex. An independent effect of sex can no longer be mixed up with effects of exposure if the effect of exposure is examined separately in men and women.

Procedures used to control confounding must also be capable of detecting confounding. (After all, there is no need to control confounding that does not exist.) A popular definition of confounding posits that the detection and control of confounding are related. This definition states that confounding occurs when an appropriate adjustment for confounding leads to a change in the estimated effect. Stratification unveils confounding when it leads to stratum-specific estimates that are different from the crude estimate and similar to each another. When an estimate is stratified (into 2 or more estimates), the stratified estimates are a type of adjusted estimate. If they differ from the unadjusted estimate and are similar to each other, then the occurrence of confounding has been demonstrated through stratification.

With sex as a possible confounding variable, stratification would involve: dividing the sample into male and female strata; calculating the stratum-specific estimates; and comparing the stratum-specific estimates first to themselves and then to the crude estimate. This procedure—stratification for

FIGURE 22. PROCESS OF STRATIFIED ANALYSIS

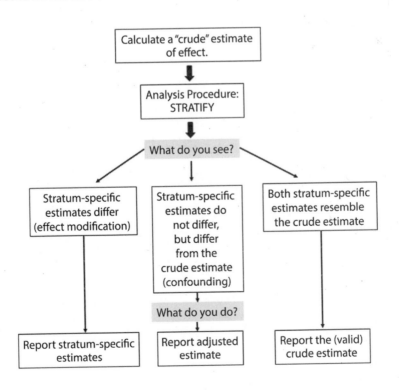

sex—figures frequently in analytical studies, because sex is a risk factor for many health problems, potentially associated with many exposures, and usually viewed as an extraneous variable since it is not modifiable. For example, Vinceti et al[208] used a case-control study to examine whether elevated levels of inorganic selenium in drinking water was a risk factor amyotrophic lateral sclerosis in a region of Italy. They reported a crude odds ratio of 4.2, which was found to be 4.3 in males and 4.0 in females. As the stratified estimates resemble each other and also resemble the crude estimate, this stratified analysis shows that sex does not confound the reported association. The process of stratified analysis is depicted schematically in Figure 22.

Key point: Stratified analysis is used to identify confounding variables and to adjust for their confounding effects.

Stratified analysis and continuous variables

To stratify for a continuous variable, such as age, you begin by creating age categories, and then examine the association within the resulting strata.

There are some practical considerations involved in creating categories for continuous variables.

If there are too many strata, the number of study participants in each stratum will be small and subject to random variation. As a result, if the study sample is divided into too many strata (e.g., age categories), stratum-specific estimates show wide variation simply due to chance. This can make it very difficult to detect whether effect modification or confounding has occurred.

If strata are too large, another problem arises. In the case of age, larger strata will contain more observations, but there may also be a larger variation of age within each stratum. For example, 5-year age strata may be too narrow to provide decisive evidence of confounding, but 25-year age strata may be too broad because age can vary so much within each stratum. The variation in age within broad strata increases the possibility that confounding effects occur within these strata (broad strata fail to fully control the confounding). A failure to fully adjust for the effect of a confounding variable due to excessively broad strata is called *residual confounding*.

Where continuous variables are potential confounders, stratified analysis must walk a fine line between the problems of residual confounding (when strata are too broad), and random variation of the stratified estimates (when strata are too narrow). This difficult reality means studies prefer modelling over stratified analysis, and almost all published studies now emphasize the use of models. Even so, it is important to be aware of stratified analysis: studies still use it even if they report it less and less frequently.

Stratum-specific estimates and pooling

Stratification breaks down a crude estimate into a series of stratum-specific estimates. These stratum-specific estimates are then adjusted for confounding. But because they are based on subsets of the larger sample, stratum-specific estimates are often imprecise. Precision is important, so techniques have been developed to pool these stratified estimates in a way that preserves control over confounding.

Pooling increases precision because the pooled estimates reflect all of the data. Note that pooling involves combining the stratified estimates, which maintains control of confounding. The pooled estimate is a weighted average of the stratum-specific estimates, which are adjusted for confounding. The parameter classically used for this purpose is the Mantel-Haenszel family of estimators. These pooled estimators can be easily calculated across a series of strata. The family includes pooled versions of the risk difference, risk ratio, rate ratio, and odds ratio. (Note that there is also a Mantel-Haenszel test for homogeneity, which is discussed later in this chapter. This test is used for a different purpose than the Mantel-Haenszel pooled estimators, but caution is required since it has a similar name.)

Pooled estimates are only meaningful if the stratum-specific estimates comprise a single underlying effect. Such consistency of effect across strata is called *homogeneity*. A lack of homogeneity—heterogeneity—implies that there are different effects of exposure in different strata—in other words, effect modification (see page 214). Effect modification makes pooling inappropriate.

Key point: While stratification typically results in a major loss of precision of stratum-specific estimates, much of the precision can be regained through pooling procedures. However, pooling should not occur in the presence of heterogeneity. Pooling is a procedure for achieving greater precision while controlling for confounding, whereas heterogeneity suggests effect modification.

The steps of stratified analysis in summary

Stratified analysis follows a classic series of steps.

First, you estimate a crude effect using a risk difference, risk ratio, odds ratio, hazard ratio, or other parameter.

Next, you examine the association within strata formed by levels of the potential confounding variable.

Then, you assess whether the resulting estimates are similar to each another (exhibit homogeneity)—you could do this with a statistical test for homogeneity.

If the estimates are dissimilar (heterogeneous), effect modification has been identified and the stratum-specific effects should be reported.

If they are similar (homogeneous), you assess whether they differ from the crude estimate. If they do differ, then confounding has been demonstrated. At this stage, you should report an adjusted estimate of effect, such as one of the Mantel-Haenszel family of parameters. If the estimates do not differ from the crude estimate, then there was no confounding and it is not necessary to report an adjusted estimate. The crude estimate is good enough.

A STEP-BY-STEP EXAMPLE OF STRATIFIED ANALYSIS

A classic example of confounding from the history of epidemiology is an investigation of Down syndrome published in 1966 by Stark and Mantel.[209]

A component of this work, which was conducted in the state of Michigan, explored the relationship between birth order and Down syndrome.

The study made a detailed tabulation of the data. The data table cross-referenced:

- birth order: first, second, third, fourth, or fifth and above
- maternal age: < 20, 20–24, 25–29, 30–34, 35–39 and 40+
- number of births with Down syndrome and the total births in the population

Dividing the exposure variable (birth order) into 2 categories for reasons of simplicity leads to the 2 × 2 table shown in Table 34.

TABLE 34. BIRTH ORDER AND DOWN SYNDROME

	Down syndrome	No Down syndrome
Birth order (third or more)	1547	1 328 554
Birth order (first or second)	877	1 400 752

A crude odds ratio calculated from this table is 1.86 (95% CI 1.71–2.02), suggesting that higher birth order is positively associated with this outcome. However, there is the possibility of confounding by maternal age, because birth order also reflects increasing maternal age: a woman's first child marks her youngest maternal age, and she is older with each subsequent child. An apparent effect of birth order may merely reflect an intermixed effect of maternal age. Table 35 shows the odds ratios for birth order calculated within each of the 6 strata for maternal age.

None of the 6 stratum-specific estimates suggest that birth order is associated with increased odds of Down syndrome. The elevated crude odds ratio was evidently due to an intermixing of the effect of maternal age with birth order.

However, the possibility of heterogeneity in these stratum-specific effects has not yet been addressed. With application of the Mantel-Haenszel test for heterogeneity, the result is nonsignificant ($P = 0.82$: a P value less than 0.05 is most often used for rejecting the hypothesis of homogeneity). A final step

TABLE 35. ODDS RATIOS FOR BIRTH ORDER STRATIFIED BY 6 RANGES FOR MATERNAL AGE

Maternal age category	Odds ratio	95% CI
< 20	0.53	0.14–1.39
20–24	0.85	0.67–1.07
25–29	0.97	0.79–1.20
30–34	0.80	0.65–1.00
35–39	0.89	0.72–1.10
40+	0.90	0.69–1.20

would be to calculate a pooled odds ratio—the Mantel-Haenszel combined odds ratio—to regain precision of the adjusted estimate. The value for this odds ratio is 0.88 and the 95% CI is 0.80–0.97.

You can practise calculating a Mantel-Haenszel pooled odds ratio with the following formula. The a, b, c, and d values are the usual values from the 2 x 2 table, and the subscript i has values of 1 to 6 for the 6 age strata in Table 35.

$$\text{OR}_{MH} = \frac{\sum_{i=1}^{i=6}\left(\frac{a_i \times d_i}{n_i}\right)}{\sum_{i=1}^{i=6}\left(\frac{b_i \times c_i}{n_i}\right)}$$

Table 36 breaks the odds ratios in Table 35 into their constituent a, b, c, and d values. This table provides all the values that you would need to calculate your own Mantel-Haenszel pooled odds ratio, using the formula above.

TABLE 36. CONTINGENCY TABLE VALUES FROM TABLE 35

Age Group		a_i	b_i	c_i	d_i	n_i
< 20	i = 1	4	129	17012	290920	308065
20 to 24	i = 2	101	283	264876	631464	896724
25 to 29	i = 3	226	162	445567	311339	757294
30 to 34	i = 4	287	120	351734	118014	470155
35 to 39	i = 5	485	119	187563	40966	229133
40 plus	i = 6	443	64	61802	8049	70358
Total		1546	877	1328554	1400752	2731729

The example shows very strong confounding effects. The direction of estimated effect changes with adjustment for maternal age from a crude odds ratio of 1.85 to an adjusted one of 0.88. Such effect reversals due to strong confounding are examples of the so-called Simpson's paradox.[210]

A final note about the Mantel-Haenszel family of statistics, which is the most common set of statistical tools for conducting stratified analysis: when frequency matching has been used, it is standard practice to preserve the matched categories as strata in the data analysis, and the Mantel-Haenszel family of statistics can be used for this purpose. The procedure can even be used to analyze individually matched data, where each matched group (e.g., 1 case and 5 controls) is treated as a stratum.

VARIATIONS IN TERMINOLOGY RELATED TO CONFOUNDING

Confounding effects, when uncontrolled, can make an association appear stronger or weaker than it actually is. When confounding makes an association appear weaker, some authors call the confounding variable a *suppressor variable*.[211] However, this terminology remains fairly uncommon in the health science literature.

Recall that another variation in terminology comes from literature describing directed acyclic graphs.[212,213] Here, the term *confounder* is restricted to variables that cause both the exposure and disease. This is different than the more standard definition provided above, which merely specifies that the confounder must be associated with the exposure and be an independent risk factor for the disease. In the development of a detailed causal model, the question of why a confounder is associated with exposure needs to be answered. However, for most epidemiological studies, it is sufficient to show that an exposure has an independent etiological effect, and the standard definition of confounding is sufficient for this purpose.

Effect modification in stratified analysis

We have already discussed the distinction between confounding and effect modification several times. It's repeated here because the distinction is so important to the analysis of epidemiological data.

The pooling strategies employed in classic stratified analysis are predicated on the presence of a single effect of exposure in different strata after stratification for an extraneous variable. If this is not the case—if the stratum-specific estimates are not homogeneous—then something other than confounding is at play.

If the stratum-specific estimates are different to an extent that cannot reasonably be attributed to chance, this means that they are actually providing evidence of differing effects of the exposure in the different strata. Such heterogeneity of effect indicates effect modification. In other words, the effect of exposure is modified by the effect of the extraneous variable.

> *Key point:* Effect modification is distinct from confounding, both conceptually and in the way it appears during data analysis.

The occurrence of effect modification precludes any assessment of confounding. Recall that confounding can be defined according to whether some form of adjustment alters the effect of exposure. If there is effect modification, there is no longer a single effect of exposure on which to make such a determination.

AN EXAMPLE OF EFFECT MODIFICATION IN STRATIFIED ANALYSIS

Tjepkema et al[214] used data from the Canadian census mortality and cancer follow-up study (1991 to 2006) to explore the association between socioeconomic indicators and both all-cause and cause-specific mortality.

When they looked at all-cause mortality, the hazard ratio associated with less-than-high-school education was 2.16 (95% CI 1.95–2.39) in their youngest age stratum (25–34), whereas it was only 1.52 (95% CI 1.46–1.59) in the oldest (55–64) age stratum. This suggests effect modification by age.

The 2 intermediate age strata had intermediate hazard ratios, suggesting that the effect declined across the studied age range.

It would be a mistake to obscure this kind of relationship by averaging the hazard ratio across these age strata. The authors appropriately presented the stratified estimates.

Unlike confounding, which is an artifact that can be corrected by adjustment, effect modification is something real, not to be hidden or minimized. Effect modification often has implications for public health and clinical practice.

For example, think back to the study that reported stroke as an adverse outcome following chiropractic manipulation (see page 160).[174] This study found a significant effect, but only in those younger than 45. If this study led to clinical recommendations, the recommendations might apply only to the specific age groups where an association occurred.

Another example comes from the previously discussed study by Friedenreich et al[184] (see pages 214–215) investigating the association of metabolic syndrome and waist circumference with endometrial cancer. This study found a stronger association in pre- or perimenopausal women as compared to postmenopausal women (effect modification by menopausal status). This finding may have implications for priority setting, or in the development of clinical interventions and guidelines.

> *Key point:* Effect modification is a real effect that should be described when it occurs. There is no basis for attempting to control or adjust for effect modification, which is a real effect rather than an artifact.

A NOTE ABOUT TERMINOLOGY: EFFECT MEASURE MODIFICATION

So far, we have used *effect modification* to describe the situation where an extraneous variable changes the strength of an exposure-disease association, manifesting as heterogeneity across strata.

The simplicity of this term is appealing, but it has a weakness.

Consider this hypothetical example. Imagine a stratified analysis with 2 strata. One stratum has a risk of 6% in its exposed group and 2% in its nonexposed group. The other stratum has a risk of 20% in its exposed group and 16% in its nonexposed group. An analysis based on risk differences would conclude that there is no effect modification, since the risk difference in each stratum is 4%. By contrast, a study using risk ratios would find a risk ratio of 3 in the first stratum and 1.25 in the second, strongly suggesting heterogeneity of effect.

So, the determination of whether an effect is modified often depends on the measure of effect used in the analysis—a stratified analysis based on the risk difference might uncover heterogeneity where a ratio-based measure of association would not, and vice versa.

For this reason, many epidemiologists prefer the term *effect measure modification* over the simpler, but less precise, *effect modification*.

Regression models

Chapter 10 introduced regression models in the form of linear equations with or without a log transformation (see pages 144–146). You can use statistical software to identify the equations that best fit an epidemiological data set. These statistical models are very useful for identification of confounding and effect measure modification.

Advantages of regression models

Regression modelling assists with some of the difficulties that arise in stratified analysis.

Regression models deal more effectively with the sparse-data problems that afflict stratified analysis. They are more capable of simultaneously controlling for multiple confounding variables and joint confounding (where several variables act together to produce confounding).

They also deal better with continuous variables, such as age. In stratification, continuous variables must be broken down, often arbitrarily, into categories. Regression modelling can often work with them directly, as continuous variables. This allows a more sophisticated assessment of effect measure modification and confounding while avoiding residual confounding.

Key point: A key advantage of regression modelling over stratified analysis is that continuous variables can be included in the model, and thereby adjusted for, without the necessity of imposing artificial categories onto ranges of continuous variables.

The steps of regression modelling

The steps for stratified analysis also apply to regression modelling.

The purpose of presenting these steps is to outline analytical strategies involved in statistical modelling, so that you can better interpret analyses reported in published studies. The purpose is not to demonstrate how to conduct analyses using statistical models—something that requires advanced training. In addition, the approach to modelling described here may differ from what you have encountered in other fields of study. Epidemiology emphasizes the use of statistical models as tools for handling the issues of effect measure modification and confounding. Other areas of research emphasize the use and development of statistical models to predict outcomes or explain variability in outcomes—a topic not discussed in this chapter, because it plays a smaller role in epidemiological modelling.

In regression modelling, you usually begin by making an estimate of the crude measure of association. This can be done using a statistical model that includes only 1 predictor variable: the exposure. Chapter 10 covered this kind of model (see page 146). Here, for example, is a model of the logistic form from chapter 10:

$$\text{Log Odds} = \alpha + \beta X_e$$

where X_e is an indicator variable for exposure with a value of 1 or 0

This model describes a log odds of α for the nonexposed (where $X_e = 0$) and a log odds of $\alpha + \beta$ for the exposed (where $X_e = 1$). In this type of model (since it predicts the log odds, it is a logistic regression model), β is a log odds ratio—so, you can use this kind of model to calculate the crude estimate.

Next, you use a model to assess the possibility of effect measure modification. This kind of model has 3 terms: the exposure variable, the extraneous variable, and a term that represents exposure both to the exposure variable and the extraneous variable—something called an *interaction term*. Here's the example from chapter 10 with these additional terms:

$$\text{Log Odds} = \alpha + \beta_e X_e + \beta_c X_c + \beta_i X_i$$

where X_e is an indicator variable for exposure, X_c is an indicator variable for the extraneous variable (a potential confounder or modifier), and X_i is an indicator variable for joint exposure (interaction) to X_e and X_c

Interaction terms serve the same purpose as the statistical tests for homogeneity routinely employed in stratified analysis. Where the variables are binary—for example with a value of 1 representing exposure to the exposure variable or the extraneous variable, and 0 representing nonexposure—interaction terms are calculated by multiplying the indicator variables together. As a result, interaction terms are often called *cross-product terms*.

The significance of such a term (a significant interaction) is the model-based test of heterogeneity. Statistical software identifies the β parameters that best fit the data. Such models also produce confidence intervals and evaluate the statistical significance of the coefficients, including interaction terms. Note that the same strategy of multiplying the 2 variables is used when the extraneous variable is a continuous variable, such as age.

If effect measure modification is identified, you report stratum-specific estimates. Or, you can report the model that contains the interaction term, since this model depicts differing effects across the strata.

If there is no effect measure modification, you should assess for confounding.

To assess for confounding, the model is regenerated without the interaction term. The output will be of the form:

$$\text{Log Odds} = \alpha + \beta_e X_e + \beta_c X_c$$

Now that X_c is in the model, β_e is adjusted for its effects—it is adjusted for confounding. If β_e from this type of model is different than β_e from a model that did not include the potential confounding variable, there is confounding. In this specific type of model—a logistic regression model—the inverse logarithm of β_e (from a model containing a term for the confounding variable) provides an odds ratio for the exposure that is adjusted for the effect of the confounding variable. In assessing for confounding, the unadjusted and adjusted odds ratios are easier to compare than the β coefficients from models. If there is no confounding, an adjusted estimate does not need to be reported: the unadjusted estimate is appropriate to report.

TWO STEP-BY-STEP EXAMPLES

Let's return to the study of Down syndrome by Stark and Mantel.[209]

A logistic regression model containing no extraneous variable or interaction terms has an α coefficient of −7.4 and a β coefficient (for being third or higher in the birth order) of 0.62. Recall that in an equation this type, the β coefficient is a log odds ratio (see pages 145–146). Taking the inverse log of this value yields the same odds ratio seen in the tabular analysis: exp(0.62) = 1.86.

Testing for interactions—by adding terms for maternal age and the relevant cross-product terms (the test was performed in this case using a likelihood ratio test)—finds no significant interactions: $P = 0.82$. Note the similarity of this value to that arising from the Mantel-Haenszel test for homogeneity in the stratified analysis.

As there is no evidence of effect measure modification, the next step is to determine an adjusted estimate using a model that includes the birth order variable and the maternal age indicators. Since there is homogeneity, the interaction term can be removed. The β coefficient for the birth-order variable in this model is −0.13, indicating an odds ratio of 0.88, the same as the Mantel-Haenszel combined odds ratio from the stratified analysis.

Key point: Regression modelling, as it is applied in epidemiology, is not fundamentally different from stratified analysis, either in terms of the logic that it follows or the purposes for which it is applied.

Here's another example, from a study covered in chapter 14 (see page 212). Modgill et al[128] investigated whether migraine increased the incidence of major depression using data from the Canadian National Population Health Survey. The investigators used a time-to-event analysis and therefore estimated hazard ratios. A hazard ratio from a model containing no extraneous variables was 2.1. No significant interactions between migraine and age or sex were found. However, when age and sex were included in the model, the effect of migraine diminished to 1.9, a change that provided evidence of confounding. In a model adjusting for sex alone, the adjusted hazard ratio was 1.9, suggesting that sex was the main confounder. This finding was not unexpected, because more women than men have migraine and female sex is a risk factor for depression. You may notice that 1.9 is not very different from 2.1, which is true. Some epidemiologists think that an estimate should change by a particular amount, such as 10%, to be interpreted as evidence of confounding. However, such rules are arbitrary. The real decision is about the best estimate to report: the adjusted or the unadjusted estimate. In this case, since confounding is expected to occur in the direction observed, it seems reasonable to conclude that the adjusted estimate more accurately reflects the independent effect of migraine.

Other examples of studies using regression models

Cheng et al[215] conducted a case-control study of the association between diabetes and colorectal cancer. These investigators identified several genetic variants associated with colorectal cancer risk. When they included these variables in a logistic regression model, they found that the odds ratio for diabetes diminished from 1.2 to 1.15, which (despite being a small change) was interpreted as evidence that the genetic variants confound the relationship between diabetes status and colorectal cancer risk.

Another case-control study evaluated the role of benfluorex (a psychostimulant derivative) as a risk factor for otherwise unexplained valvular heart disease.[216] The study found the crude odds ratio was huge: 40.4. No interactions with extraneous variables were identified during logistic regression analysis. With inclusion of body mass index and diabetes in the logistic regression model, the odds ratio was unchanged, indicating that its elevation was not an artifact due to confounding by these variables.

CRITICAL APPRAISAL AND REGRESSION MODELS

In critical appraisal, you need to be able to understand analyses that present modelling results to discern whether the data collected in a study advances the state of knowledge about an exposure-disease association.

The most common models encountered in the epidemiological literature are, like logistic regression, based on linear equations.

Models use different transformations so that their parameters reflect different types of epidemiological estimates. Models are available to adjust estimates of incidence rate ratios, risk ratios (including incidence proportion ratios and prevalence ratios), risk differences, hazard ratios, and odds ratios. They produce adjusted estimates when extraneous variables are added.

Thinking deeper

Regression analysis without a log transformation

Let's revisit a scenario from chapter 10.

In this scenario, there is a binary exposure variable (with 1 representing exposure and 0 representing nonexposure) and there is an extraneous variable coded in the same way (1 meaning exposed to it and 0 meaning not exposed to it).

A linear form of an equation including only an exposure and outcome, and without a log transformation—something like the basic unadjusted, or crude, 2×2 table of classic analysis—is as follows:

$$\text{Risk of Disease} = \alpha + \beta_e X_e$$

where X_e is an indicator variable for exposure and β_e is a risk difference associated with exposure

The fact that β_e is a risk difference indicates that this is not a log-transformed model. In other words, when a subject is not exposed ($X_e = 0$), the term on the right-hand side of this equation disappears and the risk of disease in the nonexposed is represented by α. When a subject is exposed ($X_e = 1$), the risk of disease is modelled as $\alpha + \beta_e$.

To say "β is a risk difference" alludes to the reality that the modelled risk in the exposed subjects minus the modelled risk in nonexposed subjects is $\alpha + \beta - \alpha = \beta$. Since the equation above takes a linear form, it would also be reasonable to regard β as a slope term: it is the change in risk of disease that occurs with each unit of exposure. In this scenario, there is only 1 unit of exposure since the exposure here is treated as a binary variable.

This revisited scenario is relatively simple. What if we add an extraneous variable?

This new variable produces a slightly expanded linear equation:

$$\text{Risk of Disease} = \alpha + \beta_e X_e + \beta_c X_c$$

where X_e is an indicator variable for exposure, β_e is a risk difference associated with exposure, β_c is a risk difference associated with the potential confounder, and X_c is an indicator variable for exposure to the confounding variable

In this equation, X_c has a value of 0 or 1 depending on exposure to the potential confounding variable.

The logic of stratified analysis points to a problem with this equation. The risk of disease in those not exposed to the confounder and also not exposed to the risk factor is modelled as α, since all of the other terms reduce to 0 in this scenario. When the risk factor is present but not the potential confounder, the risk of disease is modelled as $\alpha + \beta_e$. When there is exposure to the potential confounder but not exposure to the risk factor, the risk of disease is modelled $\alpha + \beta_c$. Finally, among those exposed both to the risk factor and the potential confounder, the risk is modelled $\alpha + \beta_e + \beta_c$.

This yields Table 37—a sort of parallel to the situation in which a 2 × 2 table is stratified according to the presence or absence of a confounding variable.

TABLE 37. TWO STRATIFIED TABLES

		Disease	No disease	Risk of disease*
Stratum 1 (not exposed to the potential confounder)	Exposed	a	b	a / (a + b)
	Not exposed	c	d	c / (c + d)
Stratum 2 (exposed to the potential confounder)	Exposed	e	f	e / (e + f)
	Not exposed	g	h	g / (g + h)

*The term *risk* assumes that the study design is capable of determining risk.

Each of the 4 risks of disease depicted in the far-right column of Table 37 would be predicted by the linear equations shown in Table 38.

In a stratified analysis, you would begin by calculating a measure of effect—say, the risk difference for the stratum not exposed to the confounder. However, the modelled values for the 2 risk differences here are the same:

$$\text{Risk Difference}(\text{Stratum 1}) = \alpha + \beta_e - \alpha = \beta_e$$

$$\text{Risk Difference}(\text{Stratum 2}) = \alpha + \beta_e + \beta_c - \alpha + \beta_c = \beta_e$$

TABLE 38. LINEAR EQUATIONS FOR THE RISKS DEPICTED IN TABLE 37

		Risk of disease*	Linear predictions*
Stratum 1 (not exposed to the potential confounder)	Exposed to risk factor	$a / (a + b)$	$\alpha + \beta_e$
	Not exposed to risk factor	$c / (c + d)$	α
Stratum 2 (exposed to the potential confounder)	Exposed to risk factor	$e / (e + f)$	$\alpha + \beta_e + \beta_c$
	Not exposed to risk factor	$g / (g + h)$	$\alpha + \beta_c$

*where risk of disease $= \alpha + \beta_e X_e + \beta_c X_c$

This means that the linear equation as stated above equates to a stratified 2×2 table analysis, but it does so with a constraint. The equation constrains the value of the risk difference to a single value—β_e—in both the stratum with exposure to the confounding variable and the stratum without.

So, the problem lies with the assumption that the 2 risk differences are homogeneous. They should certainly not be constrained to be identical, if they are in fact heterogeneous. The question of heterogeneity is an empirical question that must be answered. This means that there must be a different starting point that is able to accommodate the possibility of effect measure modification.

The solution is a cross-product interaction term. Such a term should be included early in the determination of whether interaction between the exposure and the potential confounding variable exists. This term is denoted i for *interaction*.

Adding this variable—X_i—and its estimated coefficient from the model—β_i—leads to the following expanded linear equation:

$$\text{Risk of Disease} = \alpha + \beta_e X_e + \beta_c X_c + \beta_i X_i$$

where X_e is an indicator variable for exposure, β_e is a risk difference associated with exposure, β_c is a risk difference for a confounding variable, X_c is an indicator variable for exposure to the confounding variable, β_i is the risk difference between the joint exposures and the sum of their effects, and X_i is an indicator of the joint exposure

This equation predicts each of the 4 risks of disease depicted in the far-right column of Table 39.

The 2 risk differences can now be different. The risk difference for stratum 1 has not changed: it is still β_e. However, the risk difference for stratum 2 is now $\beta_e + \beta_i$.

This expanded model that includes an interaction term, therefore, can incorporate an assessment of whether the interaction term is important. If the interaction term is important, then $\beta_e + \beta_i$ will be different than β_e.

TABLE 39. LINEAR EQUATIONS FOR THE RISKS DEPICTED IN TABLE 37: INTERACTION TERM INCLUDED

		Risk of disease	Linear predictions*
Stratum 1 (not exposed to the potential confounder)	Exposed to risk factor	a / (a + b)	$\alpha + \beta_e$
	Not exposed to risk factor	c / (c + d)	α
Stratum 2 (exposed to the potential confounder)	Exposed to risk factor	e / (e + f)	$\alpha + \beta_e + \beta_c + \beta_i$
	Not exposed to risk factor	g / (g + h)	$\alpha + \beta_c$

*where risk of disease = $\alpha + \beta_e X_e + \beta_c X_c + \beta_i X_i$

The test for statistical significance of the interaction term is a way of operationalizing this question, similar to the Mantel-Haenszel test for heterogeneity in stratified analysis. If β_i is determined not to be important, then the more basic model—including a single term for β_e, as summarized in Table 38—is sufficient. Furthermore, the risk difference from this model (β_e) is adjusted for the effect of the potential confounder, because the linear equation includes β_c.

The next step, assuming the interaction term is not significant in the model, would be to determine whether the inclusion of β_c results in a change to β_e. This amounts to an assessment of whether there is confounding.

Questions

1. Ideally, studies should measure all potential confounding variables. This allows confounding to be detected during data analysis. How can this be done? What principles are applicable to the challenge of identifying all potential confounding variables?

2. Jadidi et al[217] were interested in whether there might be an elevated risk of cardiovascular disease after a diagnosis of multiple sclerosis (MS). To address this question, they conducted a retrospective cohort study using linked Swedish databases (an inpatient register, a total-population register, and a cause-of-death register). They identified 8281 people admitted to hospital with MS between 1987 and 2009. They also selected a control cohort of 76 640 patients, matched for sex and date of birth, who did not have MS at the time of MS diagnosis in their matched case. An elevated incidence rate ratio (IRR) was identified for stroke (IRR: 1.7). Subsequently, the IRR was stratified by sex. The stratified estimates for men (IRR: 1.6) and women (IRR: 1.7) remained similar to each another and were also similar to the crude estimate. Keeping in mind that sex is associated with MS (this disease occurs more often in women), state a possible explanation for the lack of confounding.

3. In the Jadidi et al study, the IRR for heart failure, unstratified by sex, was 2.0 (rounded here from the reported value of 1.98). Upon stratification, this was found to be 1.4 in men and 2.3 in women. Does this provide evidence of confounding?

4. List examples of the advantages of modelling over stratified analysis.

5. Do you think that stratified analysis still has a role in epidemiology?

6. Part of the process of designing a study involves deciding what variables to measure. A study that does not measure effect-modifying variables cannot evaluate the effects of these variables in an analysis. In designing a study, how would you decide what variables to measure as potential effect modifiers?

7. The following table describes 3 possible outcomes of a stratified analysis or regression-model analysis.

Study finding	Interpretation	What should be reported
No heterogeneity, stratified estimates resemble crude	a	d
Heterogeneity	b	e
No heterogeneity, stratified estimates differ from crude	c	f

How would you interpret each of the scenarios depicted in the 3 rows of the table? Provide an interpretation for a, b, and c.

8. Each of the scenarios depicted in the 3 rows of the table require different reporting of results. What should be reported in these scenarios? Provide an answer for d, e, and f.

9. An advantage of modelling over stratified analysis is that modelling can include continuous variables without the need to create artificial categories. Suppose that age (in years) is included as a continuous variable in a logistic regression model. Exponentiation of the ß coefficient for age produces an odds ratio. Use words to state what this odds ratio means.

10. As part of a study, an epidemiologist includes age and sex in a logistic regression model. Inclusion of these variables results in a large change in the estimated odds ratio for exposure in the study. However, neither age nor sex is statistically significant in the model, so the epidemiologist decides to remove these variables from the logistic regression model. Do you agree with the decision to remove them?

Other study designs

OBJECTIVES

- Describe important features of the following study designs: nested case-control studies, case-crossover studies, retrospective cohort studies, randomized controlled trials, case-cohort studies, and ecological studies.
- Discuss advantages and disadvantages of these designs over other designs.

Study designs so far

So far, we have covered the "classic" epidemiologic study designs: cross-sectional studies, case-control studies, and prospective cohort studies.

This chapter looks at other common study designs in epidemiology.

It's important to know these. Identification of study design—through identifying a study's key features—is an early step in the process of critical appraisal: it begins the process of thinking through a study's vulnerability to error.

> *Key point:* Classification of study design is an important step in critical appraisal. While classification does not say anything definitive about the validity of a study, it helps to organize information about the study and to focus critical appraisal on likely vulnerabilities.

Nested case-control studies

Nested case-control studies are not very different from classic case-control studies. They have a special name because of the way they are conducted.

A nested case-control study is a case-control study situated within a prospective cohort study.

To review: case-control studies have a backward logical direction of inquiry (they start with the selection of cases—effects rather than causes) and a retrospective temporal direction (they "look back" to assess past exposures). The case-control design is vulnerable to selection bias, and the appropriate selection of cases and controls is often difficult.

Sometimes, a prospective cohort study provides an excellent framework to facilitate valid case-control studies. In these situations, there is a cohort being followed prospectively. This cohort generates cases and potential controls. This provides a well-defined source population from which cases and controls both arise, and a strong context for conducting a case-control study. For example, whenever a case occurs, a control can be selected from among the cohort members who do not have the disease at that point in time (the risk set), providing a firm procedure for control selection.

Key point: A nested case-control study is an ideal kind of case-control study because the source population for the cases and controls is well defined.

A nested case-control study often addresses a research question not posed at the beginning of its "host" prospective cohort study. The exposure variable at issue for the nested study may therefore not have been measured at the time of selection into the prospective cohort study. A nested case-control study can obtain these extra exposure measurements by assessing exposure in the case group and in a sample of the noncase group (controls). By assessing a sample of the noncase group—instead of the entire noncase cohort—the nested case-control approach applies the familiar efficiency of the case-control design in general: samples of controls generally provide comparable precision whether they are smaller (3 or 4 controls for every case) as when they are larger (10 or 20 controls, or more, for every case).

Nested case-control studies have other advantages over classic case-control studies. They can make selection of cases and controls easier, because the cohort is being actively followed and is presumably strongly engaged in research. They can achieve high response rates: in some prospective cohort studies, participants provide consent to be contacted for related studies. They can benefit from work already done by the host study, which may have already measured many relevant confounding or effect-modifying variables. They may find it easier to ensure that cases are incident cases, because of close follow-up in the host study—this leads to greater clarity of the temporal relationship between exposure and disease.

Nested case-control design also makes risk set sampling feasible. During prospective follow-up, specific members of the cohort will develop the outcome at specific times. At the time of emergence of each new case, the risk set consists of the case and all of the noncases at risk of the outcome at that specific time. In risk set sampling, a random sample of 1 or more controls is selected from this risk set, with replacement, as they remain in the population at risk and can become a member of other risk sets as additional cases emerge. This results in a data set that resembles a typical matched data set and must use analysis techniques consistent with this. The odds ratio from a nested case-control study that uses risk set sampling can be directly interpreted as a rate ratio and is not subject to the rare disease assumption.[218]

Verhave et al[219] studied the risk of thromboembolism in a cohort of 913 renal transplant patients. They observed an increased risk of thromboembolism relative to the general population (as assessed using Quebec administrative databases). To investigate the determinants of this increased risk, they nested a case-control study within their cohort of renal transplant patients. They used all 68 members of the cohort who had experienced thromboembolism (cases), and a matched group of 260 cohort members free of thromboembolism (controls). The nested study required that the controls were alive at the time of the thromboembolic event in their corresponding matched case. In other words, they used risk set sampling. The investigators calculated univariate odds ratios and conducted a multivariable analysis using a form of logistic regression that accounted for the matching (conditional logistic regression—recall that matching has implications both for study design and data analysis to assess the effects of covariates on their estimates). The study found that increased risk of thromboembolism was associated with low hemoglobin levels, use of sirolimus (a drug used to prevent rejection), and hospitalization. It found lower risk was associated with use of drugs inhibiting the renin-angiotensin system.

Case-crossover studies

Case-crossover studies are another variant of case-control studies.

Like case-control studies, they have a backward logical direction of inquiry. The investigation begins with the identification of a series of cases and then (this is the logically backward part) assesses exposure.

Unlike case-control studies, case-crossover studies use the same people for cases and controls.

The focus of a case-crossover study is the timing of exposure. Instead of comparing a group with disease to a group without the disease, a case-crossover study assesses the frequency of exposure in the cases immediately before the onset of disease, and compares this to another time when the same people did not develop the disease. In this sense, these studies also have a retrospective temporal direction. The underlying logic is this: if an exposure precipitates disease, that exposure should occur more frequently during the interval before disease onset than during some other interval when disease did not occur.

The case-crossover design is used to study outcomes that rapidly, and typically temporarily, follow exposure—for example, the transient risks that follow alcohol consumption.[220]

Key point: Case-crossover studies are a case-control variant that emphasize the timing of exposures within people, rather than the differences in the frequency of exposure between groups of people.

In a classic case-control study, the cases and controls are different people and the observations made by the investigators of the frequencies of exposure in cases and controls are independent observations. In situations where they are not independent, such as when pair matching has been implemented, different methods of analysis are required to account for this (e.g., conditional logistic regression, described in the previous section). In some ways, the case-crossover design is the ultimate form of matching. Because the comparisons occur within individuals, all of the individual characteristics that don't change over time and might contribute to the outcome are "matched" and, therefore, cannot act as confounders of the exposure-disease relationship. This eliminates confounding that arises from fixed characteristics such as genetic factors, stable psychological characteristics (personality), education, and stable aspects of health status.

Key point: Analysis of data from a case-crossover study closely resembles that of a pair-matched case-control study.

Redelmeier et al[221] used the case-crossover design to investigate whether driving convictions were effective in preventing traffic fatalities. They identified licensed drivers in Ontario who had been involved in fatal crashes, and examined whether these drivers had received traffic convictions in the month before their fatal crashes, as compared to the same month a year prior. They also examined additional referent periods. They used analysis procedures for matched data and determined that a conviction within the previous month was associated with fewer fatal accidents.

Retrospective cohort studies

Prospective cohort studies have a forward logical direction and a prospective temporal direction. They start with exposure, measuring this in the present, and then follow participants into the future and determine their disease outcomes.

Retrospective cohort studies have a forward logical direction—starting with exposure and asking whether an increased risk of disease follows exposure—but they have a retrospective (backward) temporal direction.

Some cohort studies are neither prospective nor retrospective. These studies start in the past, retrospectively, and follow the respondents to the present, but also follow respondents prospectively into the future. This type of study is called *ambispective*.

Key point: Retrospective cohort studies have the same logical direction as prospective cohort studies, but differ in temporal direction. Retrospective cohort studies look back in time.

Retrospective cohort studies require exposure data from the past. Many use data from occupational settings. Some occupational exposures can be defined by participation in a particular industry (e.g., uranium mining). Sometimes, exposure data may have been measured routinely for safety purposes (e.g., radiation exposure badges). In other instances, a group may have been exposed to a disaster or accident (e.g., a nuclear meltdown), which qualifies the group as an exposed cohort.

After finding a data source, a retrospective cohort study must then find a way to measure the relevant health outcomes from the time of exposure to the present day. This can often be accomplished through record linkage.

Because retrospective cohort studies are often conducted in occupational settings, the selection of referents (the nonexposed group) is challenging. In occupational retrospective cohort studies, researchers often use the general population as a referent. This choice of referent means selection bias may occur: working people (in occupational studies, the exposed group comprises only working people) may differ in many ways from nonworking people (possible members of the nonexposed group). The most obvious concern is that jobs require good health, since workers must be able to function at their jobs. Workers, therefore, tend to be healthier than people who are not working—a phenomenon called the *healthy worker effect* (we also discussed this effect on page 130).

Workers are likely to differ from the general population in many ways other than the healthy worker effect. For example, some occupational groups tend to be dominated by young people. Some may have an imbalanced sex ratio. This produces an obvious vulnerability to confounding by the nonmodifiable variables of age and sex. Typically, occupational retrospective cohort studies use indirect standardization to address this vulnerability: they most commonly report measures of effect as standardized mortality ratios (SMRs), standardized morbidity ratios (also SMRs), and standardized incidence ratios (SIRs).

Key point: Retrospective cohort studies are very useful for studying occupational cohorts. These studies often use indirect standardization to support comparison to general population referents.

Retrospective cohort studies do not always rely on general population referents. Some use referent cohorts consisting of other workers—for example, people employed by the same company who worked in a different setting (e.g., front-office workers at a mining company, as opposed to miners themselves). In the best-case scenario, the study uses the same exposure measures to assess the exposed and referent cohorts, and can track both cohorts effectively over (past) time. These studies employ the same measures of association typical of prospective cohort studies: incidence proportion ratios (risk ratios), incidence rate ratios, and hazard ratios.

In Canada, retrospective cohort studies are a particularly important study design because Canada has rich sources of administrative data, which are often used in epidemiologic research. Previous chapters presented examples of administrative data sets, including hospital discharge data, ambulatory care data, and physician-billing data. Administrative data are also available for drug exposures, such as drug claims that are eligible for reimbursement from government sources, or prescription-dispensing data collected by governments from pharmacies when a prescription is filled. In the field of pharmacoepidemiology, pharmaceutical data typically define exposures; subsequent hospitalizations, emergency-department visits, or physician visits can be used to define outcomes. A national network, called the Canadian Network for Observational Drug Effect Studies, or CNODES,[222] has emerged a leader in such studies. The next section provides an example of a CNODES retrospective cohort study.

Examples of retrospective cohort studies

An early retrospective cohort study examined cancer risk and mortality in Air Canada pilots[223] using SMRs and (for cancer incidence) standardized incidence ratios. For all cancers, the SMR was 0.63, likely indicating a healthy worker effect. The study identified an elevated standardized incidence ratio for acute myeloid leukemia and an elevated SMR of 26 for aircraft accidents.

Dimich-Ward et al[224] examined cancer mortality and incidence among nurses in British Columbia. They found low SMRs and standardized incidence ratios for most cancers. Malignant melanoma, however, had a standardized incidence ratio of 1.3.

Villeneuve and Morrison[225] studied a cohort of fluorspar miners in Newfoundland to examine a possible association between radon exposure (which had been measured in the cohort) and subsequent coronary heart disease mortality. To account for the healthy worker effect, these investigators based their analysis on relative risks associated with different levels of radon exposure within the same cohort. The results suggested a possible association: the relative risk for the highest level of radon exposure was 1.5, but the 95% CI included the null value (the reported CI was 0.77–2.75)—so the result was not statistically significant. The investigators extended the follow-up for another 10 years and eventually concluded that there was no evidence of association.[226]

CNODES investigators from 7 provinces used administrative pharmaceutical data to identify a retrospective cohort exposed to atypical antipsychotic drugs.[227] They compared various drugs to a common comparator (risperidone) to explore the incidence of hyperglycemic emergencies in the 365 days after initiation of the medications. The analysis was conducted separately in each of the provinces (and also in a UK database) and then combined using meta-analysis techniques. The primary hypothesis was that a drug with strong metabolic effects (olanzapine) was associated with a greater risk of hyperglycemic emergency than risperidone. This hypothesis was not confirmed. However, in a secondary analysis, they reported that another drug (quetiapine) was associated with a significantly lower risk of hyperglycemic emergency than risperidone.

Randomized controlled trials

Randomized controlled trials have a forward logical direction: they start with an exposure and then determine outcome. They also have a forward temporal direction: they follow their participants from the present into the future. So, they are similar to prospective cohort studies in these ways, but they are fundamentally different in a key way.

Randomized controlled trials, unlike prospective cohort studies, are not observational studies: they are interventional studies. The investigators assign subjects to the exposure, and they do this by a random process.

All randomized controlled trials are interventional studies, but not all interventional studies are randomized controlled trials. Interventional studies that use nonrandom procedures to assign exposure are called *quasi-experiments*. In classifying studies, you need to be careful about the concepts of random and nonrandom because investigators use terminology inconsistently. Some authors describe randomization as a key feature of experimental studies. This is not a good use of terminology. The term *experiment* typically connotes a study conducted in a highly controlled setting, such as a laboratory. In an experiment, the effect of an independent variable on a dependent variable is examined with everything else held constant. Such studies are really the antithesis of epidemiological research, which usually seeks to investigate real-world problems in real-world settings. It is better to classify studies as interventional if the investigator assigns the exposure, and also to specify whether this assignment occurred randomly (randomized controlled trial) or nonrandomly (quasi-experiment).

Key point: Randomized controlled trials are a form of interventional prospective cohort study in which the exposure is randomly assigned.

What is so special about randomization? Recall that confounding occurs when an independent risk factor is unequally distributed between exposure groups. Randomization helps to ensure that there is no inequality in the distribution of extraneous disease determinants. The law of large numbers helps to ensure that all extraneous variables will be equally distributed among the exposure groups. Restriction is another strategy to control confounding. By simply eliminating participants exposed to a potential disease determinant, the possibility of confounding by those determinants is eliminated. Randomized controlled trials tend to liberally employ restriction, before randomization. Other methods to detect and control confounding variables—stratification and modelling—may also be used in such studies during data analysis. However, they can only be used for variables that are known to be potential confounders and that were consequently measured. As stated previously, the unique power of randomization is its ability to control for the confounding effects of variables that are not measured, including those that are not even known.

Key point: The unique power of randomization is its ability to control for the confounding effects of variables that are unmeasured and perhaps not even known.

Selection bias in randomized controlled trials

It is sometimes said that randomization controls for selection bias. There is some truth in this assertion.

For selection bias to occur, a process affecting participation in a study must unfold in a way that depends both on exposure and disease.

Normally, a prospective cohort study is protected from such bias because the outcome has not occurred at the time of selection.

Randomized controlled trials are usually conducted to evaluate treatments, putting a different twist on this situation. The treatment is administered in such trials by clinicians working in clinical settings. A methodological concern is that this allocation of exposure may occur in a way that depends on the expected treatment outcomes. For example, in a placebo-controlled randomized controlled trial, clinicians might try to get patients whom they think will respond well to a treatment into the treatment arm, rather than the placebo-controlled arm, of the trial. They could do this, for example, by gaming or distorting the allocation procedure. If the allocation is randomized, this is—in theory—impossible to do. Since randomization ensures that the allocation of exposure cannot depend on outcome, it should prevent such selection bias from occurring. However, in practice it is important not only that a study be randomized, but also that the procedure used for randomization be of sufficient quality that it cannot be subverted. Some of the early efforts to conceal randomization codes were easy to subvert. For example, someone could "transilluminate" sealed envelopes to see the allocation codes they contained,[228] or they could simply open several envelopes and select allocations they wanted for particular patients. In most contemporary trials, random allocation is done using a computer-generated sequence of random numbers. To produce reliable results, this sequence needs to be concealed from those involved in the trial, and ideally it should be generated and applied at a remote location. Next, it needs to be communicated to investigators by some subversion-proof means (such as an interactive voice response system or a secure website). In addition, the allocation needs to occur after the participants have provided consent, to avoid selective nonconsent depending on assignment. The procedures used in random allocation should be accessible to audits and have strong quality control. The procedures must also be reported in archived study protocols and publications, so they are open to critical appraisal.

Key point: Randomization can prevent selection bias and confounding if it is implemented properly.

In addition to key advantages for the control of confounding, the randomized controlled trial also incorporates a way of controlling for nonspecific aspects of treatment, such as the placebo effect, regression to the mean, and the Hawthorne effect.

In the placebo effect, people who believe they are receiving treatment for a condition tend to experience better outcomes than people who believe they are not receiving treatment. This is especially true for subjectively reported outcomes.[229] In regression to the mean, people tend to volunteer (or be recruited) for trials when they are more ill than usual and, over time, return closer to their baseline level of clinical severity.

In the Hawthorne effect, people who are enrolled in research studies, and who are undergoing heightened levels of scrutiny as a result, tend to have better health outcomes than those who are not enrolled in studies and are less closely observed. The Hawthorne effect gets its name from a famous study conducted at the Hawthorne Works, an electrical company near Chicago.

The control group in a randomized controlled trial helps to address all of the pitfalls of nonspecific effects, but only if its members receive exactly the same scrutiny and care as those receiving active treatment. Of note, the need for identical scrutiny and care also applies to comparative clinical trials, which evaluate a new treatment against an existing standard treatment, rather than against a placebo.

Critical appraisal and randomized controlled trials

Well-established standards of methodology and reporting are available for randomized controlled trials.[230] These can be helpful as guides to critical appraisal.

In addition, randomized controlled trials have methodological resemblances to prospective cohort studies, so critical appraisal follows familiar principles.

Even though randomization provides protection against selection bias, attrition can still lead to the occurrence of such bias. Attrition must therefore be minimized in randomized controlled trials. An interesting way to deal with potential bias due to attrition in randomized trials is to conduct an intention-to-treat analysis. This means that everyone randomized is included in the analysis, even if they do not actually comply with the treatment or if they leave the study. This requires the use of an imputation procedure to complete the data set, such as carrying forward the last available observation. This strategy is believed to help prevent the occurrence of selection bias resulting from attrition, but is sometimes criticized as being excessively conservative.

Measurement bias can also compromise the validity of randomized trials: trials must use blinding to prevent raters who are classifying outcome status from knowing treatment status. Trials should be double blind, which means that both participants and the trial staff are blinded. This will prevent the type of differential misclassification bias that could otherwise occur if outcome raters tended to rate randomized groups differently.

Often, randomized controlled trials occur in closely monitored settings and with highly selected participants. For example, trials often exclude individuals who have serious medical conditions other than the target condition, or who are very old or on other medications. In the real world, however, such individuals may be candidates for the treatment in question. As a consequence, the generalizability of trial results to real-world populations is often questionable. For this same reason, randomized controlled trials tend to most often assess *efficacy* (effect of a treatment under ideal conditions) rather than *effectiveness* (the effect in a real-world setting). Some trials, called *pragmatic clinical trials*, seek to address this problem. Pragmatic trials employ randomization, but are conducted in realistic samples of participants and in conditions that resemble real-world clinical practice. These trials are intended to assess the effectiveness of treatments rather than their efficacy.

Darsaut et al[231] compared 2 surgical treatments for unruptured intracranial aneurysms using a pragmatic-trial design. The 2 treatments were surgical clipping and endovascular coiling. The study, called CURES, enrolled patients from neurosurgical centres in Calgary, Edmonton, Montreal, Ottawa, and a study centre in Belgium. These were all real-world centres offering both treatments. The eligibility criteria were basic, and clinical personnel in the study centres collected the data. The study used a clinically relevant definition of treatment failure (i.e., failure of the allocated treatment, hemorrhage during follow-up, or residual or recurrent aneurysm detected by brain imaging) and the odds ratio to compare the 2 groups. No significant differences between the 2 treatments were found.

Examples of randomized controlled trials

Randomized controlled trials are among the most frequently published studies. A typical example is the Can-SAD trial by Lam et al[232] at the University of British Columbia. These investigators compared bright light therapy for winter depression to a standard antidepressant medication in 4 Canadian centres. They used the following procedures: a computer-generated code for random allocation, centralized allocation to treatment, double-blinded outcome assessment, and an intention-to-treat analysis. They found few differences in the effectiveness of the 2 treatments.

The Women's Health Initiative Randomized Controlled Trial was an important randomized controlled trial from the point of view of public health.[233] This study sought to clarify uncertainties in a literature of observational studies that had evaluated combined estrogen and progestin (hormone replacement therapy) in postmenopausal women for prevention of heart disease and certain cancers. The trial included 16 608 women between the ages of 50 and 79, randomized either to hormone treatment or placebo. The results indicated that health risks (an elevated risk of cardiovascular disease) exceeded the benefits of treatment. Because equipoise was lost, the trial was stopped after 5 years when these risks became evident to a monitoring committee.

The trials described above are examples of phase 3 trials. They have the clear objective of evaluating the efficacy (or effectiveness) and safety of a treatment. A phase 3 trial of a proposed treatment always uses a randomized controlled trial study design. The process of developing a new drug, procedure, or vaccine does not start with phase 3 trials. The process usually starts with preclinical work conducted in laboratories using animal models. This is followed by phase 1 trials, which are conducted with healthy volunteers. Phase 1 trials often use low doses of a drug with the primary objective of confirming safety. Phase 2 trials use participants with the disease to be treated and administer the new treatments at dosages that are expected to be effective. These studies provide preliminary evidence about safety and efficacy or effectiveness, setting the stage for the more definitive phase 3 studies. Phase 4 studies come after the phase 3 trials are completed and a product has received regulatory approval for use. Phase 4 studies are typically observational studies that seek to understand beneficial and adverse effects in real-world populations engaged in real-world health care.

Chakraborty and Parvez reviewed the state of knowledge about treatments and vaccines for COVID-19 in mid-2020.[4] They conducted a review of published studies indexed in PubMed (https://pubmed.ncbi.nlm.nih.gov/) and ongoing studies registered in ClinicalTrials.gov (a widely used archive of protocols for trials). Their search uncovered 1515 intervention trials for treatment of this disease, which is amazing when you consider that COVID-19 had been first described only about 6 months earlier. They classified these studies in terms of phase, finding that 197 of them were phase 1 trials, 598 were phase 2 trials, and 350 were phase 3 trials. They reported that 75 were phase 4 trials.

Case-cohort studies

A drawback of the prospective cohort study design is its inefficiency. It needs a large investment of resources to track cohorts over time—and, typically, only a small proportion of a cohort will ever develop the outcomes under investigation. The case-cohort study design seeks to improve efficiency by making a subcohort its focus, rather than the entire cohort.

A case-cohort study compares a series of cases to a subcohort. The subcohort is drawn from the larger cohort that gives rise to the cases. As the name suggests, the study design is a kind of hybrid between case-control and cohort methodologies.

To make the design clear, let's compare it to the nested case-control study design. In a nested case-control study, the controls are selected from cohort members who do not have the disease at the time when each case develops the disease (the risk set). In a case-cohort study, the subcohort represents the entire cohort from which the cases arose. This is done by selecting the subcohort from the population at risk at the start of the cohort's follow-up interval. Typically, such studies are analytic in their orientation and therefore select incident cases for their case groups. The subcohort is representative of the larger cohort comprising people at risk of developing the disease. The subcohort does not include prevalent cases, but because the subcohort is selected at the beginning of follow-up, some of its members may develop the disease during follow-up.

Unlike a nested case-control study, a case-cohort study can use the same subcohort as a referent in analyses of many different outcomes. This makes the design especially efficient: it provides the flexibility of a prospective cohort study to examine multiple outcomes, while also delivering the special efficiency of a case-control study.

Because of the way in which the sample is collected, case-cohort studies must use specially adapted statistical techniques.

Van Lonkhuijzen et al[234] used a case-cohort design to investigate meat consumption and endometrial cancer risk. They identified 26 024 residents of Ontario who had participated in a prospective cohort study called the

Canadian Study of Diet, Lifestyle, and Health. They linked their study data, which included a dietary questionnaire assessing meat consumption, to the Ontario Cancer Registry and the national mortality database to determine outcome. The study included 116 cases diagnosed with endometrial cancer during, on average, 11 years of follow-up. The subcohort consisted of a random sample of the entire at-risk cohort and included 1830 respondents. Notably, 19 members of the subcohort were also cases because they developed endometrial cancer during follow-up. Van Lonkhuijzen et al used modified proportional hazards models to estimate hazard ratios for the exposure. The hazard ratio for a comparison of the highest-to-lowest quartile of red meat consumption was 1.6, but the result was not statistically significant. The 95% CI was 0.86–3.08.

Another case-cohort study examined associations between dietary intake of B vitamins and the incidence of various types of cancer. It used data from the Canadian Study of Diet, Lifestyle and Health. This was a large study ($n = 73\ 909$) that recruited participants who were alumni from universities in Alberta and Ontario in the mid-to-late 1990s. Exposure was assessed using a 166-item food frequency questionnaire, from which vitamin intake could be estimated. Since the coding of dietary and lifestyle questionnaire data is complex and resource intensive, this was done for random samples of the study cohort with a view to using data from these subcohorts in subsequent case-cohort studies.[235] Cancer incidence was determined by linking the survey data to the Canadian Cancer Registry, the Ontario Cancer Registry, and the national mortality database. The food frequency questionnaires of participants who developed cancer, as determined via follow-up, were coded, and researchers used a case-cohort analysis to compare the case groups to the subcohort. Quartiles and tertiles were used to identify low levels of B vitamin consumption. A modification of the Cox proportional hazards model was used in the analysis to compare case groups to the control cohort. One such case-cohort analysis found that high intake of folic acid protected against endometrial and ovarian cancers, and high intake of vitamin B6 was protective against ovarian cancers.[236]

Ecological studies

Ecological studies are a distinct type of study design, differing from all of those discussed so far. They use a unit of analysis not based on individual people. The unit of analysis in ecological studies consists of groups of people, such as the population of neighbourhoods, cities, or countries.

Ecological studies assess correlation between exposure and disease, both measured at an aggregate level. Because correlation is so often the method of analysis in such studies, they are sometimes called *correlational studies*. Examples of aggregate measures of exposure include mean sodium consumption per person in different countries, and average number of grams of fish consumed in different provinces. Typical aggregate outcomes might be age-standardized mortality rates in different countries or cancer incidence in different provinces.

Examples of ecological studies and data sources

Ecological research mainly focuses on hypothesis generation. It is also a way to engage aggregate statistics. Many suitable aggregate statistics are routinely available. For example, the World Health Organization reports mortality statistics for almost every country in the world.[237]

Cheng et al[238] used mortality data for 193 countries in an ecological study showing that country-level measures of water sanitation were negatively correlated with infant and maternal mortality.

Durbin et al[239] correlated hospital admission rates for psychosis and mood disorders with the percentage of immigrants in the population of 507 census-derived geographic areas in Ontario. They found a positive correlation (Pearson correlation coefficient: 0.22) for the percentage of first-generation immigrants in these areas and rates of first admission for psychotic disorders. However, the association was attenuated when adjustments were made for population density and average income—2 potential confounders—in the geographic areas.

Stieb et al[240] used data about fine particulate matter (a form of air pollution consisting of particles less than 2.5 micrometers in diameter) combined with incidence estimates of COVID-19 cases from the Canadian COVID-19 Data Portal.[112] They found that health regions with more fine-particulate-matter pollution had a higher incidence of COVID-19 disease. Note that this study did not assess the amount of exposure at the individual level, but rather examined both pollution and incidence in health regions. Information about health region characteristics that might confound this association was obtained from the Canadian Community Health Survey. In keeping with the goals of an ecological study, the authors concluded: "While our results generate hypotheses for further testing, they should be interpreted with caution and require further examination using study designs less prone to bias."

Canada has several sources of important ecological data, including the Canadian Urban Environmental Health Research Consortium, or CANUE for short.[241] CANUE's mission is to facilitate research that increases knowledge about the impact of the urban environment on health. They do this partially by creating shared data sources and tools that can advance this understanding. CANUE produces data sets with information on topics such as air pollution, greenness, nighttime light, and social and material deprivation.

Social and material deprivation are important social determinants of health. These are examples of variables that are sometimes thought about as individual characteristics (e.g., having a personal income below the poverty line), but they also apply to the social and material environment in which people live. Deprivation is a situation of disadvantage, which can apply to individuals or communities. (Social deprivation refers to disadvantages in social connectedness; material deprivation refers to disadvantages in material goods.[242]) Pampalon et al have developed area-level indices of deprivation that can be applied to small geographical areas called *census dissemination areas*,[242] using data routinely available from the census for each dissemination area in the country. With these indices, it is possible to conduct ecological studies, or to link information about social and material deprivation to individual data from sources such as national surveys or administrative data that contain geographical information, such as an address or postal code.

Strengths and weaknesses of ecological studies

Most ecological studies have descriptive aims. If suitable aggregate data are available, ecological studies provide an inexpensive study design for generating hypotheses. However, these studies are not entirely limited to descriptive aims. Some investigators are interested in evaluating etiological hypotheses through ecological studies. In other words, they are not merely concerned with aggregate statistics as an easily accessible proxy for individual exposures, but with characteristics that are best conceptualized at an aggregate level, as described above for social and material deprivation. Other examples are the extent of income inequality in a particular community, or its walkability, or its availability of green space. For example, Auger et al[243] examined the extent of income inequality in 143 Quebec communities, using a variety of indicators, and examined the relationship of this variable to mortality rates in those communities. Although the correlations differed depending on the definition of income inequality, alcohol-related mortality was found to be significantly associated with income inequality.

When it comes to causal reasoning, ecological studies have notable deficiencies. A particularly important concern is the ecological fallacy. This concept emphasizes the danger of making inferences about individual people based on correlations between aggregate units of individuals. For example, the observation that higher rates of admission for psychotic disorders tend to occur in areas with a higher percentage of immigrants does not necessarily mean that immigrants have higher rates of admission. It could be nonimmigrants who are being admitted more often. Individual-level data would be required to clarify this.

Ecological studies also have a very limited ability to address the issue of confounding, owing to their lack of individual-level data.

A large drawback to ecological studies is that their target of estimation, usually a correlation, is not easily interpreted in terms of risk and probability.

A correlation between aggregate exposures and outcomes does not have the same intuitive meaning as many of the other parameters encountered in the epidemiological literature. A correlation coefficient simply describes the tendency of 1 variable to vary with another.

Key point: The most prominent methodological concern with ecological studies is their vulnerability to the ecological fallacy. However, some exposures are ecological characteristics (e.g., income inequality) and here, the concern does not apply.

Thinking deeper

Statistical analysis in case-crossover studies

Most standard approaches to statistical analysis assume that the observations in a sample are independent of each another.

In case-control studies, observations often consist of matched pairs, which are nonindependent. Specialized statistical procedures have been designed for this situation.

Case-crossover studies also have nonindependent observations, since they compare exposures during different time periods within the same person. For example, Di Bartolomeo et al[220] compared the following in the same people at different times of day:

- the frequency of alcohol consumption in the 6 hours before an episode of driving ending in a crash
- the frequency of alcohol consumption in the 6 hours before an episode of driving without a crash

The data consisted of pairs of observations and the approach to analysis needed to reflect this. Table 40 presents a 2 × 2 table for a paired analysis. Note that the table differs from usual 2 × 2 tables: the counts within its cells are pairs of observations rather than individual people. The table shows the results for 752 observations made in 326 people recorded by Di Bartolomeo et al.

TABLE 40. 2 × 2 TABLE FROM A CASE-CROSSOVER STUDY BY DI BARTOLOMEO ET AL[220]

		Alcohol consumption in 6 hours before driving episode without a crash	
		Yes	No
Alcohol consumption in 6 hours before driving episode with a crash	Yes	3	24
	No	18	281

Note that Table 40 resembles the table used for pair-matched case-control studies. In pair-matched case-control studies, however, each cell contains a count of pairs of people rather than pairs of observations within a single person.

Table 40 contains paired observations of 2 types: concordant and discordant.

The concordant pairs include the 3 respondents who reported consuming alcohol before both of the driving episodes and the 281 respondents who did not drink before either driving episode. These pairs provide no information about the association under investigation.

The discordant pairs, however, do provide information. Drinking before the occurrence of a crash, and not drinking before an episode of incident-free driving, suggests an etiologic role for alcohol. By contrast, drinking before an episode of incident-free driving, and not drinking before an episode with a crash, gives the opposite impression. If drinking contributes to the risk of a crash, then the former type of pairing should be more common than the latter. As it turns out, the ratio of these 2 discordant pairs is the odds ratio for this association. In this case, the odds ratio is 24/18 or 1.33, as reported in the original study.[220]

Questions

1. What is the main difference between a nested case-control study and a case-cohort study? Identify key advantages of case-cohort studies over:
   a. nested case-control studies
   b. prospective cohort studies

2. Reich et al[244] sought to determine whether the introduction of better options for medical management of ulcerative colitis (e.g., ciclosporin and tumour-necrosis-factor alpha inhibitors) had reduced the frequency of colectomy surgery (a type of treatment reserved for patients whose disease cannot be managed medically). They used administrative data in Alberta to address this question. They determined the rate of surgery per year, before and after the new treatments were introduced. An increasing rate of surgery was seen up to the introduction of the new medications, followed by a decline. The investigators concluded that the rate of surgery was declining as a result of improved medical therapies.
   a. What kind of study design is this?
   b. Do you believe that showing a decline that starts at the introduction of a new treatment confirms a causal impact of that treatment?

3. What are the key differences between a retrospective cohort study and a case-cohort study?

4. Describe the main advantage of the case-crossover design compared to other study designs.

5. What, in your opinion, is the biggest advantage of randomized controlled trials over nonrandomized interventional studies and observational studies?

6. The case-crossover design would appear to have the best possible means of controlling for confounding. Since comparisons are made within individual

people, all possible confounders would seem to be matched between the 2 time intervals being compared. In your opinion, does this preclude the occurrence of confounding? Can you think of a way in which confounding could nevertheless occur?

7. Randomized controlled trials typically apply stringent selection criteria. For example, they may restrict eligibility to people free of diseases other than the target disease. They may also apply age or gender restrictions. These restrictions may be applied to control confounding, for safety reasons, or to help prevent other threats to validity such as bias arising from attrition. It has been argued that this may reduce the generalizability of randomized controlled studies, since patients in real-world settings are no longer fully represented. Is it illogical to sacrifice some degree of generalizability to achieve better validity?

8. If you accept that a lack of generalizability is a problem with randomized controlled trials, what might be a suitable methodological approach to deal with this problem?

9. Minaker et al[165] analyzed data from the 2014–2015 Canadian Student Tobacco, Alcohol and Drugs Survey to describe patterns of driving under the influence of alcohol and cannabis. However, they also included 2 area-based variables: school region socioeconomic status (as assessed using data from the 2011 census) and school location (urban or rural). Is this study best classified as cross-sectional or ecological?

10. What measure of association is most commonly used by ecological studies?

Other measures of association in epidemiology

- Define the following measures of association: attributable risk among the exposed, attributable risk percent, population attributable risk, population attributable risk percent, number needed to treat, and number needed to harm.
- Describe how to interpret these measures of association.

Measures of association so far

So far, we have discussed the measures of association most often used in classic epidemiological studies. These include:

- prevalence differences, prevalence ratios, and prevalence odds ratios in cross-sectional studies
- odds ratios in case-control studies
- risk differences, risk ratios, incidence odds ratios, incident rate ratios, and hazard ratios in prospective cohort studies

We have also discussed several composite measures including QALYs and DALYs.

This chapter covers other measures of association that convey important and useful epidemiological information. Most of these measures are estimates based on risk differences, but they seek to quantify more than just an association. They seek to quantify the causal impact of a risk factor on a population. They comprise types of attributable risk.

Attributable risk among the exposed

You can quantify an association by subtracting a frequency from another frequency. The proper interpretation of the resulting difference depends on the nature of the frequencies.

If the frequencies are incidence proportions, which quantify risk, the difference would be a risk difference. If a risk difference is believed to represent a causal effect, you could call it an *attributable risk among the exposed*—a member of the family of attributable risk parameters.

$$\text{Attributable Risk}_{exposed} = \text{Incidence Proportion}_{exposed} - \text{Incidence Proportion}_{nonexposed}$$

Labelling this risk difference an *attributable risk* clearly gives it a causal interpretation. There are situations where this is not justified. For example, if the difference between the 2 incidence proportions could arise from a confounding variable, the risk may not be attributable to the exposure.

If the exposure truly is causal, however, the attributable risk among the exposed reflects the extent of risk in exposed subjects due to the exposure. The formula makes the basis of this interpretation evident: if the difference in risk is attributable to the exposure, removing the effect of that exposure would render the 2 incidence proportions equal to each another. The risk difference, therefore, quantifies the extent to which risk in exposed subjects could be diminished if the effects of the exposure were eliminated.

Attributable-risk measures have value in public health because they help quantify the impact of a risk factor. Attributable risk among the exposed and several related parameters (discussed below) are therefore measures of impact as well as measures of association.

Attributable risk percent

Some epidemiologists prefer to present estimates of attributable risk among the exposed as percentages rather than simple risk differences. It would be accurate to call this parameter *attributable risk among the exposed percent*— but the shorter name (*attributable risk percent*) is easier.

Instead of quantifying how much risk of disease could be diminished by eliminating (or ameliorating) the effect of exposure in the exposed subjects (attributable risk among the exposed), the attributable risk percent quantifies the percentage of risk among the exposed that could be eliminated by doing so.

The first step is to change the risk difference into a proportion of the incidence among the exposed, and then to multiply the proportion by 100 to create a percentage.

$$\text{Attributable Risk } \% = \left(\frac{\text{Incidence Proportion}_{exposed} - \text{Incidence Proportion}_{nonexposed}}{\text{Incidence Proportion}_{exposed}} \right) \times 100$$

Note that attributable-risk measurement has importance for primary prevention. Primary prevention involves eliminating an exposure or ameliorating its effects (e.g., through reducing rates of smoking, correcting lipid imbalances, implementing appropriate occupational safety measures, etc.) to diminish incidence of disease. In other words, it targets risk factors with the goal of reducing incidence. Attributable-risk measurement helps quantify the potential impact of primary preventive interventions.

A small amount of algebra provides another formula for the attributable risk percent among the exposed:

$$\text{Attributable Risk \%} = \left(\frac{\text{Risk Ratio} - 1}{\text{Risk Ratio}} \right) \times 100$$

This is a handy formula because it allows attributable risk percent to be calculated from an approximation of the risk ratio, such as an incidence odds ratio from a case-control study (see "Thinking Deeper" in this chapter).

There is a lot of variability in the terminology for attributable risk. Some epidemiologists refer to the attributable risk percent as the *attributable fraction*, and do not necessarily express it as a percentage. Or they may use a similar term: *attributable proportion*. Others use *attributable fraction for the exposed* to clarify that it reflects impact on those who are exposed and not the entire population. When you read a study that reports these parameters, it is important to look carefully at the how the study uses the term *attributable risk*.

Key point: Attributable risk parameters combine risk differences with a judgement that those differences reflect a causal effect. They help to predict the potential impact of primary prevention on the health status of an exposed population.

Preventive fraction

Some exposures decrease risk, rather than increase risk. For example, a diet high in fruits and vegetables has many health benefits, leading to a lower incidence proportion for several outcomes (e.g., heart disease and cancer) among those exposed. In this scenario, the formula we have presented for attributable risk percent would result in a negative number—which could complicate its interpretation. The preventive fraction is a way of calculating an attributable fraction for a protective association:

$$\text{Preventive Fraction} = \frac{\text{Incidence Proportion}_{\text{nonexposed}} - \text{Incidence Proportion}_{\text{exposed}}}{\text{Incidence Proportion}_{\text{nonexposed}}}$$

The formula for the preventive fraction differs in 2 ways from the formula for the attributable fraction. First, in the numerator, the order of the incidence proportions is reversed. This means that the preventive fraction will be positive for a protective association. Second, the demominator has changed and now contains the incidence in the nonexposed, rather than the exposed.

Epidemiology has different goals for risk factors versus protective factors. For protective factors, the goal is to increase exposure among those not exposed. We want to quantify the reduction in incidence that would occur through increased exposure to the protective factor. Attributable risk answers the question: How much disease could be prevented among the exposed by removing a harmful factor (risk factor)? Preventive fraction answers the question: How much disease among the nonexposed could be prevented by adding an exposure?

This fraction may also be expressed as a percentage, according to preference. Here's another way to state this formula (see "Thinking Deeper" in this chapter):

$$\text{Preventive Fraction} = 1 - \text{Risk Ratio}$$

Population attributable risk

It is sometimes valuable to understand the effect of primary-prevention interventions on an entire population. This requires a parameter beyond attributable risk among the exposed, which can only quantify the effects of primary prevention among the exposed.

Elimination of a risk factor, even a factor strongly associated with disease, will not prevent very many cases of disease if only a small subset of the population is exposed to the risk factor. For example, due to strict regulation, the frequency of exposure to asbestos is low in developed countries. As a result, even though asbestos is a strong risk factor for lung cancer among those exposed to it, asbestos does not have a large impact at the population level. Weaker risk factors that are more prevalent (e.g., smoking) can have a larger impact.

Population attributable risk is a composite parameter that incorporates the prevalence of exposure and its strength of association. The most intuitive formula is:

$$\text{Population Attributable Risk} = \text{Incidence Proportion}_{total} - \text{Incidence Proportion}_{nonexposed}$$

Here, the effect of exposure in the population is represented as the difference between incidence in the total population (which in turn reflects the effect of the exposure in question and all other factors) and incidence in the nonexposed (which reflects the risk of all other factors in the absence of the exposure). If the exposure could be eliminated, or all of its effects ameliorated, the incidence in the total population would be that of the nonexposed. Population attributable risk represents the extent of change in incidence that would occur in a population if the effects of the exposure were eliminated.

Population attributable risk percent

Population attributable risk can also be expressed as a fraction or a percentage:

$$\text{Population Attributable Risk \%} = \left(\frac{\text{Incidence Proportion}_{total} - \text{Incidence Proportion}_{nonexposed}}{\text{Incidence Proportion}_{total}} \right) \times 100$$

A cautionary note: some epidemiologists use *attributable fraction* to refer to population attributable risk percent. It is always important to understand what investigators actually did in an analysis: don't assume that all investigators use terms the same way.

Another formula for population attributable risk percent is this:

$$\text{Population Attributable Risk \%} = \frac{(\text{Risk Ratio} - 1) \times \text{Proportion Exposed}}{1 + (\text{Risk Ratio} - 1) \times \text{Proportion Exposed}} \times 100$$

This formula is useful because it does not depend on incidence rates. Case-control studies, for example, can produce estimates of relative risk even when they cannot produce incidence estimates. A case-control study with a suitable control group—a control group that represents the general population—may allow estimation of the proportion exposed to a risk factor in the population. However, it is not easy to see how this formula works. A helpful graphic is proposed by Hanley.[245] Figure 23 shows a population of which half is exposed to a risk factor (shaded grey in the graphic) but where the risk factor does not elevate the risk. In other words, the risk ratio is 1. Half of the cases will occur in the exposed group and half in the nonexposed group. Now look at Figure 24. Here, the risk ratio is 1.8, leading to excess cases in the exposed group. The excess cases are the product of the risk ratio minus 1 (see the right-hand side of Figure 24) multiplied by the proportion exposed (the width of the grey area), divided by this quantity plus the nonexcess cases. In Figure 24, this is the product of 1 (which is the null value of the risk ratio) and 0.5 + 0.5 (which is the sum of the proportions exposed and nonexposed). Note that the sum of the proportions exposed and nonexposed will always equal 1: they are complementary. Figure 24 therefore shows the origin of the 1 that appears in the denominator of the equation. In this example, the population attributable risk percent is 28.6%.

FIGURE 23. POPULATION ATTRIBUTABLE RISK PERCENT FOR AN EXPOSURE (PROPORTION EXPOSED = 0.5) WITH A RISK RATIO OF 1

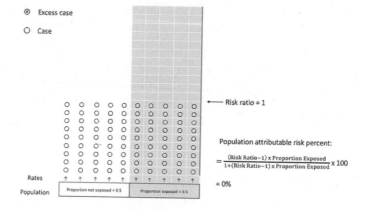

FIGURE 24. POPULATION ATTRIBUTABLE RISK PERCENT FOR AN EXPOSURE (PROPORTION EXPOSED = 0.5) WITH A RISK RATIO OF 1.8

Key point: Population attributable risks are a family of parameters that combine risk differences with judgements about causation to predict the potential impact of primary prevention on the health status of the total population.

Numbers needed to treat and harm

The efficacy of a treatment should be assessed in comparison to placebo in a randomized controlled trial. Consider a treatment that produces a positive outcome twice as often as placebo does. Suppose that the placebo response rate for this particular condition is 33% and, with this treatment, 66% achieve a positive outcome. It would be correct to state that the treatment doubles the probability of a positive outcome. Another way to quantify the effect of this treatment is to use a difference: you could assert that the treatment increases the probability of a positive outcome by 33%. A third way is to calculate the number needed to treat, which is the reciprocal of the absolute difference—in this case 1/0.33, or approximately 3. The implication is that 3 people must be treated to achieve 1 positive outcome due to treatment.

Freedman et al[246] reviewed the literature for oral-disease-modifying treatments in multiple sclerosis in order to determine the numbers needed to treat for several such treatments. For example, they looked at published outcome data from 2 trials (together including $n = 1540$ respondents) of dimethyl fumarate. In the placebo group, the risk of relapse was 0.37, whereas in the intervention group it was 0.19. The absolute risk difference was therefore 0.18. The number needed to treat is the reciprocal of this value, or 5.6.

The number needed to harm is a related parameter. Consider a rare adverse medical event that occurs with a frequency of 1 in 100 000 in the general population over the course of 1 month. Suppose that a new drug is reported to be associated with a fivefold increased frequency of this event. The number needed to harm is again the reciprocal of this absolute difference of 4 per 100 000, which is $n = 25\ 000$. This is the number of people that would need to be treated with this drug before 1 adverse event was created.

Slobogean et al[247] studied ulnar nerve injuries in patients receiving 1 of 2 surgical procedures for supracondylar fractures of the humerus. They reviewed studies of closed-reduction and percutaneous pinning that used either a crossed-pin or lateral-pin procedure. They identified 32 such studies, reporting data on 2639 patients. They used meta-analysis to derive an estimated 0.035 risk difference, which was higher with the crossed-pin procedure. This led to an estimated number needed to harm of 28. The authors concluded that there is an ulnar nerve injury for every 28 patients treated with the crossed-pin versus the lateral pin procedure.

Thinking deeper

Estimating attributable risk without incidence data

The formulas presented in this chapter are standard for dealing with incidence data and best convey the meaning of the parameters.

However, it may be useful to estimate such parameters even in situations where incidence data are not available. For example, a case-control study may produce a valid approximation of a risk ratio that reflects a causal association. Nevertheless, it is not obvious how to calculate the attributable risk percent from the case-control data.

In considering this problem, the basic formula for attributable risk percent is a good place to start:

$$\text{Attributable Risk \%} = \left(\frac{\text{Incidence Proportion}_{\text{exposed}} - \text{Incidence Proportion}_{\text{nonexposed}}}{\text{Incidence Proportion}_{\text{exposed}}} \right) \times 100$$

Next, recall the basic formulation of the risk ratio as the ratio of 2 incidence proportions:

$$\text{Risk Ratio} = \frac{\text{Incidence Proportion}_{\text{exposed}}}{\text{Incidence Proportion}_{\text{nonexposed}}}$$

This means that the incidence proportion for the exposed can be written a different way:

$$\text{Incidence Proportion}_{\text{exposed}} = \text{Risk Ratio} \times \text{Incidence Proportion}_{\text{nonexposed}}$$

Then, substitute this expression for *incidence proportion*$_{exposed}$ in the equation for attributable risk percent:

$$\text{Attributable Risk \%} = \left(\frac{[\text{Risk Ratio} \times \text{Incidence Proportion}_{\text{nonexposed}}] - \text{Incidence Proportion}_{\text{nonexposed}}}{\text{Risk Ratio} \times \text{Incidence Proportion}_{\text{nonexposed}}} \right) \times 100$$

Incidence proportion$_{nonexposed}$ can now be factored out of the numerator of the equation:

$$\text{Attributable Risk \%} = \left(\frac{\text{Incidence Proportion}_{\text{nonexposed}} \times (\text{Risk Ratio} - 1)}{\text{Risk Ratio} \times \text{Incidence Proportion}_{\text{nonexposed}}} \right) \times 100$$

Finally, *incidence proportion*$_{nonexposed}$ cancels out, leading to a formula for calculating the attributable risk percent from the risk ratio:

$$\text{Attributable Risk \%} = \left(\frac{\text{Risk Ratio} - 1}{\text{Risk Ratio}} \right) \times 100$$

As an intuitive confirmation of the formula, note that the equation indicates that when the risk ratio is 2—indicating that the exposure doubles the risk—the attributable risk percent will be 50%. Attributable risk percent can be estimated from a case-control study in situations where the odds ratio is considered a good estimate of the risk ratio.

In the case of the preventive fraction, it is possible to follow the same reasoning. Consider this formula for the preventive faction:

$$\text{Preventive Fraction} = \frac{\text{Incidence Proportion}_{\text{nonexposed}} - \text{Incidence Proportion}_{\text{exposed}}}{\text{Incidence Proportion}_{\text{nonexposed}}}$$

You can write this formula as 2 fractions:

$$\text{Preventive Fraction} = \frac{\text{Incidence Proportion}_{\text{nonexposed}}}{\text{Incidence Proportion}_{\text{nonexposed}}} - \frac{\text{Incidence Proportion}_{\text{exposed}}}{\text{Incidence Proportion}_{\text{nonexposed}}}$$

This leads to the alternative formula:

$$\text{Preventive Fraction} = 1 - \text{Risk Ratio}$$

Questions

1. Shiue et al[248] estimated that the population attributable risk percent was 9% for the effect of low indoor room temperature (< 18 degrees) on high blood pressure. They based their calculation on an odds ratio derived from the 2010 Scottish Health Survey, a cross-sectional study.

    a. Taken at face value, what does this estimate mean?

    b. Do you have any reservations about the estimate?

2. Kuendig et al[249] used hospitalized cases and controls to estimate odds ratios quantifying the association of alcohol exposure and injury. They estimated what they called the alcohol attributable fraction (AAF) using the formula:

$$\text{AAF} = \frac{\text{Odds Ratio} - 1}{\text{Odds Ratio}}$$

    What type of parameter is the AAF?

3. Based on case-control data, Yusuf et al[250] estimated a population attributable risk of 35.7% for currently smoking versus never having smoked as a risk factor for myocardial infarction. Assume that the estimate is valid. Explain the meaning of this parameter in plain language.

4. Here is a table from a study describing incident depression in medical inpatients in relation to a set of drugs believed to contribute to depressive symptoms.[251]

	Depressed	Total Cohort
Exposed to a potentially depression-causing drug	17	86
Not exposed to such a drug	5	92

    a. Using the formula provided in this chapter, calculate attributable risk among the exposed.

    b. Calculate attributable fraction among the exposed (express the parameter as a percentage).

    c. Calculate the population attributable risk.

    d. Calculate the population attributable risk percent.

e. The data presented in the table are unadjusted, yet associations between drugs and depression are likely to be confounded by the severity of the illness being treated. In pharmacoepidemiology, this phenomenon is called *confounding by indication*. How does this affect your interpretation of the parameters calculated from the table?

5. Arseneault et al[252] followed a birth cohort to determine whether cannabis use increased the risk of psychosis. They assessed a particular psychotic disorder, schizophreniform disorder, which is often a precursor to schizophrenia. They categorized 730 children who reported no use or minimal use as nonexposed. Of these, 22 developed a psychotic disorder by age 26. Among 29 exposed subjects, 3 developed psychosis. What is the population attributable risk?

6. What type of parameter does the following type of statement refer to? "Elimination of exposure X could reduce the incidence of cancer Y by 50% in the Canadian population."

7. The term *attributable* risk clearly implies causality. Yet, outside of the laboratory, it is very difficult to confirm a causal effect. Philosophically, can epidemiological data ever accurately estimate attributable risk?

8. Ninety percent of people with upper respiratory infections will recover within 1 week of antibiotic treatment. However, 80% will recover without any treatment. What is the number needed to treat?

9. Freedman et al[246] assessed the number needed to treat for several multiple sclerosis outcomes, including the outcome discussed in this chapter: any relapse. This question is about another outcome the study assessed: relapse leading to hospitalization. In the dimethyl fumarate group, the estimated risk of relapse leading to hospitalization was 0.031. In the placebo group, it was 0.048. Calculate the number of patients that must be treated to prevent relapse leading to hospitalization.

10. Do you perceive any shared properties of population attributable risk and the number needed to harm? What, if any, are these commonalities?

Evaluating epidemiological studies

18

Causal judgement in epidemiology

OBJECTIVES

- Describe the role of judgement in causal reasoning in epidemiology.
- Describe causal reasoning in the context of primary, secondary, and tertiary prevention.
- List classic criteria for weighing judgements about causality.
- Describe how greater-than-additive risk helps identify causal mechanisms.
- Describe the philosophy of the potential outcomes model of causation.
- Present a directed acyclic graph to depict a causal mechanism.

Critical appraisal and causal judgement

This chapter presents criteria for evaluating findings of causality in epidemiological studies—a key and complicated task in critical appraisal.

Findings of causality first require valid epidemiological estimates—estimates, in other words, that arise from properly conducted, well-designed studies. This book has described the characteristics of properly conducted, well-designed studies.

Findings of causality also require judgement. Causal significance is never self-evident—so, in critical appraisal, judgements about causation must always be carefully weighed.

In weighing judgements about causation, thousands of specific considerations could come into play. You risk paying too much attention to certain issues, and not enough attention to others.

The criteria in this chapter help clarify issues of concern. They do not provide a method or formula for determining causality, and they should not be regarded as a source of evidence for causation. Rather, they provide a framework to guide the task of weighing.

This chapter takes direction from the most widely used criteria, which appear in 2 classic sources: a 1965 paper by British epidemiologist Bradford Hill,[253] and a 1964 report on smoking and health from the US surgeon general.[254]

Key point: Causality in epidemiology is an issue of judgement. These judgements are complex and can be facilitated by a framework.

Causation and validity

In critical appraisal, you start by assessing the validity of a study's estimates of epidemiological effect before you consider any claims it makes about causality. This is a hierarchical relationship: valid estimates of exposure-disease association precede conclusions about exposure-disease causality (disease etiology).

It's important not to be too dogmatic about this, though. Many studies are vulnerable to nondifferential misclassification bias. The direction of the resulting bias is predictable and towards the null value (see page 162). A study vulnerable to this type of bias, and reporting a strong association, needs careful consideration. The estimate may not be valid in the strictest sense, but it may be clear that it underestimates an effect that exists—so, in this case, the association is stronger than the estimate suggests.

As a task of critical appraisal, assessing a study's conclusions about causality differs from assessing its vulnerability to random error and bias. Random error and bias are relatively objective concepts: confidence intervals quantify vulnerability to random error, and concrete mechanisms link methodological features (e.g., classification error rates and selection probabilities) to systematic error.

Causality, however, is more subjective. Critical appraisers often find themselves taking issue with investigators' judgements about the causal implications of their findings—even findings based on valid estimates. For example, investigators sometimes overlook the limitations of their work, and critical appraisers sometimes conclude such investigators are "biased." This is a different use of *bias* than in the technical context of systematic error and internal validity.

Key point: Validity and etiology are hierarchical considerations. Consideration of causality cannot move forward until the existence of an association has been confirmed through a valid estimate.

THE CONCEPT OF CAUSATION IN EPIDEMIOLOGY

The concept of causation, as it applies in epidemiology, differs from concepts of causation encountered in other types of scientific research. Rather than searching directly for the underlying pathophysiological events that lead to disease, epidemiologists seek modifiable links in specific causal chains of events that ultimately lead to diseases and other adverse health outcomes.

The ultimate test for an epidemiological finding is its ability to make a difference in clinical practice or public health—so, in terms of primary, secondary, and tertiary prevention.

Primary prevention

Primary prevention seeks to interrupt a destructive chain of causal events. For example, if people are becoming sick from drinking contaminated water, it may seek to provide clean drinking water, because the quality of drinking water is a modifiable link in a causal chain. Chains of causality leading up to this modifiable link may explain why a population has become exposed to unclean water: these may involve war, or a lack of effective civil institutions, or a faulty monitoring system. Additional links in the causal chain may also explain why the unclean water makes people sick: these links may involve reproduction of microbes in the gastrointestinal tract and the molecular actions of toxins produced by those microbes. But primary prevention focuses on links in chains of causality it can modify.

Secondary prevention

Secondary prevention, which involves screening for diseases, also brings a narrow focus to chains of causality. The links between screening activities and improved health depend on many factors—for example, whether people participate in screening, whether screening tests are accurate, and whether follow-up treatments are effective. So, secondary prevention identifies and fosters chains of causality that may make screening activities effective in improving the health of populations: administration of accurate screening tests, leading to earlier detection, leading to earlier treatment, leading to better outcomes.

Deciding whether to screen is often controversial. This is because screening often seems to make sense, but is actually only a preferred strategy in specific situations. Wilson and Jungner, in a 1968 World Health Organization publication, made the first and most famous attempt to identify situations in which population screening can be beneficial.[255] Their list of 10 principles became very influential: in a 2018 paper, Robert Smith called them the "10 commandments" of screening.[256] An update of these principles by Dobrow et al appeared in the *Canadian Medical Association Journal* (in the same issue as Smith's commentary).[257] This was based on a systematic review and a consensus-seeking "Delphi" process, from which 12 principles emerged, paraphrased below:

1. The epidemiology should be understood, and the screening program should target a condition of importance.

2. The natural history of the disease or condition should be understood, and there should be a detectable preclinical phase. This means that there should be a way of detecting the disease before it becomes evident clinically (in which case, the issue is that of clinical care, not screening).

3. The target population (the population targeted by the screening program) needs to be clearly defined, and can be reached by the testing and following intervention.

4. An accurate (e.g., highly sensitive, highly specific, strong positive predictive value) and safe screening test should be available. The test needs to be acceptable to the target population and must be very safe.

5. The screening test needs to be clearly interpretable in terms of what results indicate a need for further testing (to confirm the diagnosis) or a need for care.

6. There should be a clear and widely accepted course of action for what should be offered to participants with positive screening tests. Whatever this course of action is, it must modify the natural history of the disease, and be accessible and acceptable to the participants.

7. There must be an adequate infrastructure (such as financial and human resources) to provide timely access to all aspects of the screening program, including the testing, and postscreening testing and follow-up care.

8. The screening program must be coordinated or integrated with the health care system, so that optimal care (including provision of information, counselling, referrals, management, etc.) can be offered to the participants.

9. The program must be clinically, socially, and ethically acceptable to all involved.

10. Both the benefits and harms (including the possibility of overdiagnosis and overtreatment) must be well understood. The overall benefit must outweigh the harms.

11. There should be an economic evaluation to confirm that the costs of the program are warranted in view of its benefits. This evaluation should take a health system or societal perspective. This is because the costs of screening must superior to the outcomes that would be achieved if the funding were invested in some other aspect of health care.

12. The screening program should be planned as a program, and its outcomes should be monitored and evaluated with dedicated information systems and funding, and with ongoing quality control.

Tertiary prevention

Tertiary prevention—reducing negative impacts of established disease—targets specific links in chains of causality that lead to better outcomes for clinically established diseases (e.g., the administration of drugs or delivery of other treatment or rehabilitative practices). The effectiveness of a treatment—a drug, for example—depends on chains of causal events including regulatory and economic issues (both strongly related to availability of a drug), prescription of the drug by a physician, purchasing the drug from a pharmacy, adherence to the treatment regime, absorption of the drug, interaction of the drug with biological processes, and subsequent actions that diminish the impact of the disease or cure it. Tertiary prevention targets modifiable factors within this chain of causality such as whether a treatment is administered or not.

Chains of causality link together into causal webs. Within this universe of causality, epidemiological studies tend to be opportunistic. They look for best opportunities to intervene in processes of causation.

Criteria for weighing causality

A popular approach to making decisions about causality is to consider sets of criteria. These cannot confirm criteria, but they represent concepts around which relevant judgements and decisions can be supported. This section presents the most widely used causal criteria: the Bradford Hill criteria.

Temporality

Temporality refers to the question of whether exposure to a risk factor precedes the disease outcome. Temporality is the most important criterion for weighing causality, because a cause must precede an effect. Studies that fail to clarify the temporal relationship between exposure and disease therefore fail to quantify a necessary feature of a causal relationship.

Some study designs are inherently better at clarifying the issue of temporality than others. Cross-sectional studies and ecological studies tend to be particularly weak in this regard. Case-control studies can be just as weak on temporality if they fail to use truly incident cases.

Key point: Temporality is the most important and useful causal criterion, since a cause must logically precede an effect.

Strength of association

Strength of association is a causal criterion identified by Hill. It says that strong associations are more likely to indicate causality than weak associations.

This criterion draws attention to some of the practical realities of epidemiological research. Epidemiological studies are almost always subject to some source of error, such as random error, bias, or confounding. The possibility always exists that data indicating a weak association could arise by chance, or from some minor defect in study design or analysis. However, it is less likely that data indicating a strong association would arise from such circumstances. So, although a weak association does not preclude causality, a strong association is more strongly suggestive of causality.

Note that strength of association does not reflect a single metric. Associations can be measured using either difference or ratio-based measures, and a strong association on 1 scale may be weak on another.

Key point: The value of strength of association as a determinant of causality reflects practical realties of epidemiological research. Strong associations are less likely to arise from minor defects in study design.

Also note that precision affects this criterion. You need to check the confidence intervals of a study reporting a strong association. If the point estimate is large, but the lower limit of the confidence interval is near the null value (a value of 1 for a relative measure and a value of 0 for a difference-based measure), it is not possible to be confident that an association really is strong.

Consistency

The criterion of consistency refers to consistent findings among many studies investigating a possible association (i.e., within a literature of studies), not to the findings of any particular study.

Again, this criterion reflects some of the practical realities of epidemiological research. No single epidemiological study is perfect. All studies are vulnerable—in varying ways and degrees—to random and systematic error. However, different studies are likely to have somewhat different vulnerabilities to error. For example, case-control studies tend to have different vulnerabilities than prospective cohort studies. Also, different populations may embody different distributions of potentially unknown or unmeasured confounding variables. They may also differ in factors that affect the probability of recruitment, consent, and participation. Measurement instruments may perform differently in different populations because of language and culture. For all of these reasons, a result consistent across different types of studies conducted in different times and places is more likely to be a causal effect.

> *Key point:* The casual criterion of consistency does not refer to the results of a particular study, but rather to the level of consistency seen in a literature of studies.

Like assessing strength of association, assessing consistency requires nuanced consideration. For example, inconsistency within a literature of studies may result from inconsistent quality among the studies (e.g., some studies are better resourced than others, some use more accurate measures of disease and exposure). In this situation, it would be a good idea to look for consistency in the highest-quality studies, rather than the entire literature. Another concern is that a literature of studies may appear more consistent than it really is. For example, if a drug company conducts multiple studies, some of which are positive and some of which are negative, it may choose to publish only the studies with the most favourable results. This would make the literature look falsely consistent.

Specificity

This criterion is rarely used. However, it was included in Hill's paper and also in the surgeon general's report.

The specificity of an association refers to whether a risk factor is associated specifically with a disease outcome, or nonspecifically with several or many outcomes. This criterion relates to important ideas early in the history of epidemiology about linking infectious agents to disease (see Koch's criteria, page 6).

When an infectious agent causes a disease, it may be possible to find that agent in all cases of the disease, and not in people without the disease, as Koch postulated. This idea no longer has power for causal reasoning. Some examples illustrate why:

- Infectious agents that cause serious disease in vulnerable individuals (e.g., the immunocompromised) may exist as normal flora in healthy individuals.
- The most important risk-factor associations for chronic diseases tend not to be in any way specific. For example, obesity is a risk factor for type 2 diabetes, but lots of obese people do not have diabetes and lots of people with diabetes are not obese. Obesity is also known to increase the risk of several negative health outcomes, not just diabetes.
- Carcinogens, such as those contained in cigarette smoke, increase the risk for multiple cancers (including cancers of the mouth, pharynx, larynx, and esophagus) and also chronic conditions such as coronary artery disease, emphysema, chronic bronchitis, and asthmatic bronchitis.

Even so, in a widely cited study discussing the evidence for causality in the association between human papilloma virus and cervical cancer, Bosch et al[258] identified lack of evidence for the virus's involvement in other cancers as evidence of specificity.

Key point: Hill's specificity criterion in not very important for causal judgement.

Biological gradient

Sometimes, biological evidence suggests that a higher level or intensity of exposure leads to greater incidence of disease. This effect is sometimes referred to as a *dose-response relationship*. In such cases, a biological gradient may provide supportive evidence for causation.

However, biological gradients pose many problems for identifying causal relationships. Most of these relate to situations where a biological gradient might not be seen even if there was a causal effect.

This would happen in a saturation effect. In this case, some level of exposure has a causal impact on risk, but higher levels of exposure do not create higher levels of risk. Presumably this happens because the underlying biological effect is occurring through a saturated mechanism.

It could also happen where a range of exposures occurs below a threshold demarcating a harmful level of exposure. There may not be a biological gradient below this threshold.

The US surgeon general's report did not include biological gradients among its criteria for weighing causality, and a biological gradient is not a strong indicator of causality. Epidemiological publications, however, frequently mention biological gradients as evidence supporting causal interpretation.

Key point: While a biological gradient may be viewed as supporting the idea of causation, particularly if biological theory suggests that such a gradient should exist, the absence of such a relationship does not usually provide evidence against causation.

Biological plausibility

This criterion links the interpretation of epidemiological information to biological data from basic science. If an epidemiological estimate suggests an effect that is not very plausible according to other elements of current biological knowledge, it is more likely that the finding represents an artifact rather than truth.

The biggest problem with this criterion is philosophical. Epidemiology is an empirical science that depends on the law of large numbers to produce informative estimates from samples representing populations. This is based on the fundamental assumption that the distribution of diseases in populations reflects the determinants of those diseases. It seems illogical, given this perspective, to discount estimates based on the supposition that they do not align with known biological mechanisms. Thinking back to the story of John Snow (see page 5), it would have been a mistake to dismiss the link between sewage-contaminated water and cholera just because the biological agent (the cholera bacillus) was unknown.

Like all causal criteria, this criterion requires careful consideration. A plausible association is less likely to be an artifact than an implausible association—but a biologically implausible finding, if replicated, requires biological investigation.

Coherence

This criterion is similar to biological plausibility, but engages a wider field of inquiry, beyond biology. Coherence refers to the fit of an epidemiological estimate with results from any type of scientific research or theory. As with the issue of biological plausibility, such considerations are important, but should not be viewed as necessary features of a causal association.

Experimental evidence

Hill's paper referred to experimental or "semiexperimental" evidence as a criterion for weighing causality.

In current epidemiology, researchers sometimes use the phrase *experimental evidence* to indicate that a study has employed randomization. Randomization is a uniquely powerful strategy for addressing the issue of confounding in epidemiological research. For this reason, judgements about causality from interventional studies—which use randomization—carry a lot of weight.

Ethics disallows the assignment of potentially harmful risk factors to study subjects, so interventional studies do not have routine use in epidemiological research. In the only area where they can be used (the evaluation of treatments), randomized controlled trials have become the most important type of epidemiological study.

All strategies to control confounding—not just randomization—are central to causal reasoning in epidemiology. These strategies seek to confirm that an observed effect arises from particular exposure-disease associations, and not other, independent risk factors.

Analogy

Analogy refers to causal inference drawn from comparison or correspondence to other causal associations. Hill listed this criterion, but its usefulness is questionable and it is rarely used.

Key point: Coherence, experimental evidence, and analogy are not very useful criteria for supporting causal judgements in epidemiology.

Other approaches to causality

Causal pie model

The causal pie model (see page 166) is built on the idea that diseases develop from multiple causes, rather than a single cause. A good way to understand this way of thinking is to contrast it with the idea of a single necessary and sufficient cause. To say that a risk factor is a necessary cause means that the risk factor must be present for the disease to occur. To say that a risk factor is a sufficient cause means that it alone is enough to cause the disease. The etiology of disease is never this simple: it is usually a combination of exposures that are sufficient to cause a disease. In the causal pie model, a set of component causes that are sufficient to cause a disease is a sufficient causal mechanism.

The causal pie model has some interesting implications for the interpretation of epidemiologic data, which are discussed in the Thinking Deeper section of this chapter. Stated briefly, the model predicts that a greater-than-additive interaction between 2 component causes implies that those 2 causes participate in a sufficient causal mechanism. However, it is not as widely referenced in discussions contained in published papers as the Bradford Hill causal criteria.

Potential outcomes model

The potential outcomes model is based on counterfactual reasoning. Counterfactual reasoning involves consideration of a situation that is counter to the facts—a situation, in other words, that does not in fact occur. Consider a randomized controlled trial of a treatment compared to placebo. According to the potential outcomes model, the treatment could be said to cause improved outcomes if the people who received treatment had better outcomes than they would have had without treatment. The "without treatment" situation is counterfactual: in reality, the people were treated.

You could say that causal inference in the potential outcomes model arises from comparing 2 groups, where only 1 group can actually be observed. The 2 groups are (1) the treated group, which is observed, and (2) the treated group had they not been treated, which cannot be observed. In a randomized controlled trial, there is reason to hope that the placebo control group is equivalent to the treated group on all determinants of outcome, even unmeasured ones. Consequently, the outcome observed in the placebo-treated group should approximate the potential outcome of the treated group had they not been treated and vice versa. A statistical comparison of treatment to placebo in a randomized controlled trial can therefore be understood as a statistical method of identifying a causal effect.

The potential outcomes model is easy to understand in the context of randomized controlled trials. It is less easy to understand in observational studies, where there is no reason to believe that outcomes observed in a control or referent group accurately represent the outcomes of an exposed group had they not been exposed. However, the potential outcomes model is implicit in many epidemiologic strategies. For example, matching on known confounders is a way of trying to ensure that differences between exposed and nonexposed cohorts reflect a causal effect of exposure as opposed to other characteristics that may differ between the groups. The model has also led to the emergence of specialized statistical techniques that seek to make causal inferences through counterfactual reasoning. One of these uses propensity adjustments to approximate the required counterfactual. A propensity score is an estimate of the probability of exposure. By matching an exposed and nonexposed group on the propensity of exposure, the counterfactual scenario is emulated. In addition to matching, propensity scores can be used in regression models or in the calculation of weights.

Directed acyclic graphs

Another approach to causality is based on graphic methods. A particularly popular approach uses directed acyclic graphs (DAGs), which were briefly introduced in chapter 15. These causal diagrams follow strict rules and allow complicated ideas about causality to be expressed without algebra. They can also be linked to statistical-analysis techniques, thereby supporting and clarifying the assessment of causal hypotheses.[212]

DAGs include variables (sometimes called nodes or vertices) connected by single-headed arrows (sometimes called edges or arcs). The arrows represent direct links from causes to effects. Figure 25 shows 5 simple examples of DAGs. In all the examples, E depicts an exposure variable and D depicts disease.

Graph 1 of the figure depicts a situation in which an exposure (E) is not a cause of a disease (D), but where a confounder (C) can cause both E and D. The single-headed arrows connecting C to E, and C to D, signify these causal effects. The lack of an arrow between E and D represents a strong statement that E does not cause D. The term path describes any route that follows the arrows connecting the nodes. In graph 1, only a single path connects E to D, which can be written E-C-D. Paths are called *directed* if the arrows that form them connect in a series that points the same way (in other words, the head of the first arrow points to the tail of the subsequent arrow, and so on). But paths do not need to be directed, as in the case of E-C-D.

FIGURE 25. SIMPLE EXAMPLES OF DIRECTED ACYCLIC GRAPHS (DAGs)

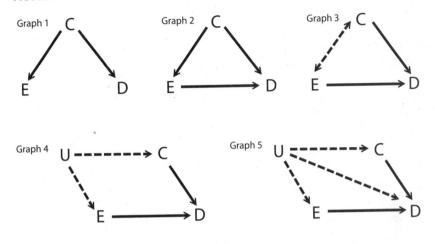

In graph 2 of Figure 25, E causes D, as indicated by the 1-headed arrow connecting these 2 nodes. There are now 2 paths connecting E and D. The first is the direct causal effect of E on D, and second is the nondirected E-C-D path. Graph 2 also depicts confounding by the variable C. DAGs can be used to identify variables that need to be controlled in order to make an unbiased estimate of the exposure-disease relationship. In graph 2, controlling for C (e.g., by adjustment in a regression model) blocks the E-C-D path (the second of the 2 paths connecting E to D), providing control of the confounding effect.

The classic definition of confounding initially presented in this book did not stipulate that a confounder must be a cause of exposure, only that a confounder and exposure must be associated. Indeed, the 2-headed arrow depicted in the confounding triangle (see Figure 20, page 201) is sometimes used in DAGs to indicate that both exposure and the confounder have common causes, explaining their association. Graph 3 of Figure 25 illustrates this approach (note that it resembles Figure 20). Graph 4 shows a confounder that is not a direct cause of exposure: here, an unknown variable or variables (U) is a cause of both of E and C. Note that adjustment for C continues to block the biasing paths, such that an estimate with this adjustment would control the confounding attributed to C. Now look at graph 5: U is now also a cause of D, so that 3 paths connect E to D. In graph 5, adjustment for C will not fully control the confounding because the E-U-D path remains open.

Effective use of DAGs engages rules and terminology beyond the simple examples in Figure 25. For example, DAGs must be acyclic (which is what the A in DAG stands for): they can have no closed loops. DAGs clarify complex causal connections and can guide decisions about when to adjust for specific variables during regression analysis. They can also provide guidance on when not to adjust for specific variables. For example, when 2 arrows converge on a single node, the variable is called a *collider variable*. Adjustment for such variables can sometimes introduce, rather than reduce, bias.

Figure 26 depicts the variable C as a collider variable rather than a confounding variable. Note that there are no causal effects of C on E or D. Instead, both E and D cause C. Their causal effects collide in C. In this situation, the path E-C-D is naturally blocked by the collider. In data analysis, a lesson from this DAG is that adjustment for C is not necessary to obtain a valid estimate of the effect of exposure. However, if an investigator were to adjust for variable C, the path would be opened and bias would be introduced into an estimate of the effect of E on D. This type of bias, caused by an attempt to control for a variable that is (in this case) caused both by exposure and disease is called *collider bias*.[213] This example illustrates that DAGs can identify variables that should be and should not be adjusted for in regression models. Also note that the term *adjusted* does not imply inclusion of the variable in a regression model: adjustment could also take some other form, such as restriction or matching. When using DAGs, authors often use the term *conditioning* instead of *adjustment* to keep this clear.[213]

Consider the case series as a study design. A case series is a group of cases of the same disease. The purpose of a case series is to describe characteristics of the disease in detail. Consequently, a case series is restricted to cases, or you could say that is it conditioned on disease status. Typically, many variables cause a disease, so the disease outcome is a collider variable. In a case series, the restriction means that there has been conditioning on that collider variable by design. Consequently, associations between all of the various causes of that disease are distorted by collider bias. Case series that describe associations between risk factors for a disease based on case-series data are reporting invalid estimates.

This is not to say that case series are useless. The frequency of specific features in a case series can be important. For example, a 1981 case series described 4 cases of previously healthy gay men with pneumocystis pneumonia and candidiasis— infections that typically occur when the immune system is suppressed. The researchers confirmed the immunosuppression using laboratory tests and noted the occurrence of a rare cancer (Kaposi sarcoma) in 1 of the cases.[259] These observations contributed to the later identification of an emerging disease, acquired immunodeficiency syndrome (AIDS).

DAGs can also depict mediation. Figure 27 shows the variable C as a mediator of the exposure-disease relationship. Remember that, since all of the arrows go in the same direction, this is a causal path, and remember that adjustment for a variable on such a path blocks it. Consequently, adjustment for the mediating variable would eliminate the effects of the exposure. This would be a mistake because this is a causal path. The correct approach would be to obtain a valid estimate of the causal effects of exposure by not adjusting for this variable.

Figure 28 shows a situation in which exposure has a total effect that is partially mediated by another variable. Here, by blocking 1 of 2 causal paths, adjustment for the mediator would lead to an underestimation of the total effect of exposure.

For a detailed description on how to draw and interpret DAGs, see Greenland, Pearl, and Robins.[212] Another good resource is the freely available software DAGitty, which provides an easy to use interface for drawing DAGs.[260] The online version of DAGitty (http://www.dagitty.net/) was used to produce some of the DAGs presented in this chapter's figures.

FIGURE 26. CAUSAL GRAPH DEPICTING A COLLIDER VARIABLE

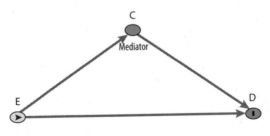

FIGURE 27. CAUSAL GRAPH DEPICTING C AS A MEDIATOR OF THE EFFECT OF E ON D

FIGURE 28. CAUSAL GRAPH DEPICTING C AS A PARTIAL MEDIATOR OF THE EFFECT OF E ON D

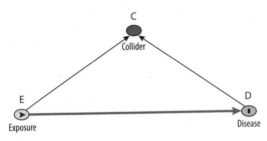

EPIDEMIOLOGICAL INVESTIGATION OF OUTBREAKS

Determination of causality is a particularly urgent matter in the investigation of outbreaks. Traditionally, the process of investigating an outbreak follows a series of steps. The *Communicable Disease Management Protocol Manual* from Manitoba Health[261] summarizes 10 steps as follows:

1. Establish the existence of an outbreak.
2. Confirm the diagnosis.
3. Establish a case definition and count cases.
4. Relate the outbreak to time, place, and person.
5. Determine who is at risk of becoming ill.
6. Formulate a tentative hypothesis.
7. Compare the hypothesis with the established facts.
8. Plan a detailed epidemiologic investigation.
9. Prepare a written report.
10. Implement control and prevention measures.

These steps are illustrated in a 2017 investigation of multiple *Salmonella* serotype infections.[262] The occurrence of an outbreak was first established on May 6, 2014 by PulseNet USA: 9 *Salmonella* isolates were identified that had an indistinguishable pattern on a test called *pulsed-field gel electrophoresis* (this corresponds to step 1 and step 2 of the Manitoba manual). The same pattern was then found in PulseNet Canada. Case definitions were then developed (step 3). In Canada, the case definition was as follows: a culture-confirmed case with *Salmonella* Newport, *S.* Hartford, *S.* Oranienburg, or *S.* Saintpaul on or after December 1, 2013, indistinguishable on pulse-field gel electrophoresis from the outbreak strains. Questionnaires were developed and deployed to identify exposures of the cases (step 4), supplemented by a more focused questionnaire to better identify those at risk (step 5). This was based on a tentative hypothesis (step 6). Initially a pattern of healthy eating among the respondents was identified in response to open-ended questions. Follow-up questions focused on health foods such as smoothies, supplements, seeds, and fruit. Guided by the responses to the follow-up questions, investigators formulated a hypothesis, which they assessed (step 7) in a series of iterative steps using more and more refined questionnaires. Those at highest risk were found to be people who consumed chia seeds and chia seed powder. Among those with the illness, 86% reported consumption of 1 or more of these products. By good fortune, the Public Health Agency of Canada was conducting a nutrition survey at the same time, and the investigators were therefore able to determine that only 6.4% of the general population was exposed to chia seeds (and less than 1% to chia seed powder). The frequency in the cases was thereby confirmed as much higher than the frequency in the general population (step 8). It was possible to trace all of the cases back to a single supply firm located in Canada. Reports were submitted to proper authorities in accordance with international regulations (step 9), and, in Canada, 9 public recall warnings and product recalls occurred (step 10), terminating the outbreak.

Thinking deeper

Greater-than-additive risk and causality

Kenneth Rothman's causal pie model (see page 166) has some interesting implications for causal reasoning. Other names for the causal pie model are the *Rothman model* and the *sufficient-component cause model.*[263]

The core concept of the causal pie model is this: diseases arise from component causes that, in various combinations, form a causal mechanism that leads to disease onset.

Component causes are exposures or risk factors. Rothman calls them *component causes* because, as a graphic, his model presents exposures or risk factors as "pieces of pie" in a causal mechanism presented as a "whole pie." There may be several combinations of component causes that can lead to a disease. If 1 of these component causes is present in all possible causal mechanisms, it can be regarded as a necessary cause. If there is a necessary component cause, it will be seen as an exposure in every person with the disease.

The causal pie model views the induction period of a disease as the time between exposure to a component cause and the completion of the causal mechanism through addition of other component causes. The model simplifies the ideas of "triggering or precipitating events," and "vulnerability or predisposing factors." In the causal pie model, a triggering or precipitating event is a final component cause that completes a causal mechanism. Vulnerability and predisposing factors are component causes that have not yet (and may never) participate in completed mechanisms.

In epidemiological studies, the causal pie model—though very interesting in theory—has much less currency than causal criteria in discussions of causality. Despite this, it has some interesting real-world implications.

Consider a study investigating the effects of 2 component causes (labelled A and B) on disease incidence. In this study:

- Some cases of disease may occur among people who are not exposed to either component cause. This would confirm that there are causal mechanisms that do not involve either A or B.
- Some cases may occur among subjects with exposure to A but not B. The incidence in this group reflects the existence of causal mechanisms that involve A and other, presumably unknown, component causes.

The risk difference for A is the difference between these first 2 groups. A similar situation would apply to those who have exposure to B but not A, and this also leads to a risk difference.

The interesting group is the group with exposure to both A and B. If there are no specific causal mechanisms that require A and B, the risk difference for this double-exposure group will equal the sum of risk differences for the single-exposure groups (A-not-B and B-not-A groups), because the cases of disease in this group will arise by 1 of these 2 types of mechanism. By contrast, if there are specific mechanisms that require both A and B, the risk difference for this double-exposure group will be greater than the sum of risk differences for the single-exposure groups.

Greater-than-additive effects would manifest as interactions in models based on risk differences, suggesting that such models, and interaction terms nested within them, may be particularly useful for exploring causal effects. Statistical tests based on this theory have been developed.[264]

The important link between absolute changes in risk and causality high-lights the importance of being able to translate relative measures into absolute measures. This can easily be done if the resulting absolute difference is reported as a percentage or fraction. Here is the formula:

$$\% \text{ Change in Risk} = \left(\text{Relative Risk} - 1 \right) \times 100$$

In other words, a relative risk of 2.0 indicates a 100% increase in risk, and a relative risk of 1.5 represents a 50% increase in risk.

Au et al[264] examined whether there was a greater-than-additive effect of elevated C-reactive protein and depression on diabetes incidence. They found no significant interaction. Their study reported that the hazard ratio (a relative measure of effect) for elevated C-reactive protein only was 1.43, that for depression only was 1.63, and that for both exposures was 2.03. Converting these relative measures to absolute change, the absolute change associated with C-reactive protein was 43%, that for depression was 63%, and that for both was 103%. Notice that the additive effects of the individual exposures (43% + 63% = 106%) are almost identical to the absolute effect of the double exposure. This suggests that both factors elevate the incidence of diabetes, but does not suggest that there are specific causal mechanisms for diabetes that require both factors to be present.

Questions

1. A review of the association between cannabis exposure and psychosis referenced a dose-response relationship as evidence in support of a causal connection.[252] How strong do you think this argument is?

2. Mente et al[265] sought to evaluate evidence for a causal association between dietary factors and coronary heart disease by conducting a systematic review of the literature. In general, do you feel that it is appropriate to address questions of causation with literature reviews?

3. In their review of dietary factors and coronary heart disease, Mente et al adopted a criterion-based strategy for their assessment of causation, but decided to emphasize only 4 of Hill's criteria: strength, consistency, temporality, and coherence. Do you agree with their choices? Can you guess their reasons for not addressing biological plausibility, analogy, and dose-response relationships?

4. Since Hill's classic paper,[253] biological plausibility has been viewed as a causal criterion. However, in that same paper, Hill seems to dismiss it: "It will be helpful if the causation we suspect is biologically plausible. But this is a feature I am convinced we cannot demand. What is biologically plausible depends upon the biological knowledge of the day."

   a. In your own words, state a reason not to include consideration of biological plausibility.

   b. Hill seems to argue that strength of association is the most important criterion for causation: "First upon my list I would put the strength of the association." Can you produce a counter argument?

5. Hill alludes to how causation is conceptualized in epidemiology with the following statement: "How such a change exerts that influence may call for a great deal of research. However, before deducing 'causation' and taking action we shall not invariably have to sit around awaiting the results of that research. The whole chain may have to be unravelled or a few links may suffice. It will depend upon circumstances." What does he mean by "links in a chain"?

6. A prospective cohort study by Gray et al[198] sought to determine whether exposure to a specific group of drugs mostly used to treat insomnia or anxiety (benzodiazepine and related drugs) increased the risk of developing dementia. Compared to nonusers of these drugs, low-level users had a 25% increase in their risk of dementia, moderate users had a 31% increased risk, and heavy users had a 7% increased risk. The authors concluded that this pattern did not support a causal association. Explain this conclusion.

7. List the 10 classic steps for investigating an epidemic.

8. Do you think it would be a good idea to develop a rating scale to assess causality from the various causal criteria listed in this chapter?

9. A particularly famous DAG is the "m diagram" originally presented by Greenland et al.[212] A version of this diagram is presented in Figure 29. Based on this diagram:

   a. How many paths connect exposure to disease?

   b. Which paths are directed/causal and which are not?

   c. Would a crude estimate of the exposure-disease association reflect a causal effect under this causal model?

   d. Would adjustment for the variable labelled Z be a good idea?

FIGURE 29. M DIAGRAM: A DIRECTED ACYCLIC GRAPH

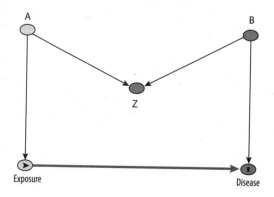

10. What single factor most strongly limits the extent of causal inference that can be made from cross-sectional data?

Steps in critical appraisal

OBJECTIVES

- Describe the goals of critical appraisal.
- List steps for critical appraisal, and describe their hierarchy.
- Explain critical appraisal as a skill honed with practice, feedback, and knowledge.
- Identify several structured tools to support critical appraisal.

The goals of critical appraisal

Critical appraisal forms part of the necessary work of researchers, clinicians, and public health professionals.

Researchers need to understand the existing state of knowledge before they can strive to add to that knowledge. They must be able to tell when a reported finding is completely wrong, when it needs further substantiation, or when it can reasonably be accepted as a fact.

Clinicians need to keep up with scientific developments in their fields of practice. They need to know when a new approach to treatment or a new method of assessment can be implemented or, perhaps even more importantly, when evidence in support of its implementation is lacking. They need to be able to see through exaggerated claims and distorted conclusions.

Public heath professionals need to identify solid, up-to-date information to shape decisions about public policy, regulation, health surveillance, prevention, and health promotion.

None of these challenges can be addressed by accepting what researchers claim to be true. They can only be accomplished by critical examination of the scientific literature. Making the right decisions depends on being able to determine which assertions are supported by evidence and which are not.

If it is accepted (as it should be, see page 16) that the law of large numbers is the main driving force for scientific progress in the health sciences, then critical appraisal safeguards its integrity. Real evidence comes from the processes described in this book: sampling, measurement, detection of effect measure modification, control of confounding, and appropriate interpretation of the resulting estimates (if they are valid) in terms of their causal significance and generalizability.

Research is a conduit for information and knowledge. Critical appraisal gauges the success of research in achieving this goal. Critical appraisal is, therefore, an important part of channelling the mathematical reality of the law of large numbers through observation and analysis, which delivers real scientific progress.

The process of critical appraisal unfolds at all levels of scientific inquiry, millions of times every day, all around the world.

Consider the typical process for undertaking a study, which often begins with a grant proposal. Researchers typically ask colleagues to read and criticize their grant proposals before submission. By providing criticism of research methods, this type of internal peer review helps to identify and correct study-design defects—for example, vulnerability to random error from inadequate sample size—that could otherwise lead to erroneous results. When proposals are submitted to funding agencies, peer reviewers again critically appraise proposed research methods, seeking defects that could render the results vulnerable to error. This critical peer review helps to ensure that studies likely to produce erroneous results (either as a result of random error or systematic error) are not funded. If funded and implemented, studies are written up and submitted to journals. Peer reviewers, again, critically appraise studies to assess whether the studies should be published. This ensures that the limitations of studies are openly acknowledged. If published, studies undergo assessment by those who read them—such as researchers, clinicians, and public health professionals. Study methods, analysis, results, and interpretations must again pass the test of critical appraisal.

The default position in critical appraisal is, of course, a critical stance. Results are not accepted as true because investigators assert that they are true. It is better to assume that results are false, and to only grudgingly accept them if vulnerabilities to random error, systematic error, and confounding cannot be uncovered. If the methods of a study allow the possibility of serious error, a critical appraiser should reject the results unless convinced that potential errors—whatever they might be—would not substantially distort the study results. If a study does not provide enough information to support critical appraisal—in other words, if the quality of its reporting is low—critical appraisers should question the veracity of the reported results.

Critical appraisal step by step

The parts of a published study

Published studies usually include a statement of purpose for the research they report. This is almost always supported by a discussion of relevant background literature, which aims to demonstrate that the study engages important questions that prior studies have not addressed, or have insufficiently addressed because of faulty methodology.

Next, there is typically a summary of the methods employed, perhaps with some words of justification for decisions about study design and procedures. This summary usually includes information about the selection of subjects, measurement of study variables, and procedures to assess vulnerability to random error and to control confounding.

This is followed by presentation of the study results and discussion of the implications of the findings for causality and generalizability, and for clinical practice and public health.

Finally, there is usually an acknowledgement of the limitations of the study.

The value of an organized approach to critical appraisal

Critical appraisal usually needs to address all aspects of published studies (although studies may assert they have already addressed all relevant issues). The exception is when a study flaw makes further appraisal irrelevant. For example, invalid estimates make questions of causality and generalizability unimportant.

Critical appraisal is a complex task: it is easy to get off track and miss important points. It helps to structure the task.

The steps presented here provide a coherent framework for the principles and strategies covered in this book.

Step 1: Identifying the study's research question or hypothesis

A study's topic of inquiry should be clearly stated in a form that aligns with an estimate or comparison.

It should be stated either as a hypothesis (e.g., that an exposure is significantly associated with a disease, that a treatment leads to better outcomes than placebo) or a question (e.g., Does this exposure increase the risk of this disease? Does this treatment lead to a better outcome than treatment with placebo?). Some research questions are descriptive, but they must still be stated clearly: "What is the distribution of deaths due to cerebrovascular disease in Ontario?"[266] An example of an analytical hypothesis is: "We hypothesized that COX-2 inhibitor use would be associated with increased bone mineral density (BMD) in postmenopausal women not using estrogen therapy."[267]

Some published studies are poorly conceptualized. Investigators (authors) may not express goals in a way that fits the needs of critical appraisal. For example, they may state that their goal was to "explore" or "look at" an issue. They may then present various estimates or models, and attempt to form conclusions based on interpreting these estimates and models. In this situation, it is it best to set aside the authors' narrative, and focus on a particular estimate or result reported in the study. Sometimes, you may need to state a coherent hypothesis or research question that the authors themselves did not state. At least then, the study can be critically appraised in a coherent fashion. In essence, this converts the authors' vagueness into real methodological issues: vulnerability to type I error or other problems that emerge with the selective reporting of exploratory or descriptive results. However, the lack of a clear question is a "red flag" since it implies a lack of discipline in the analysis, and leaves an open door for selective reporting. In the absence of a clearly stated question, study results are less reliable.

Let's consider an example. A study by Agrawal and Ebrahim[268] includes the following statement in the background section of its abstract: "It is postulated that a diet high in legumes may be beneficial in preventing diabetes. However, little empirical evidence on this association exists in developing countries. We aimed to examine the association." If critical appraisal took this vague statement as its focus, it would do no more than evaluate an opinion. As it turns out, though, this was a cross-sectional study that used the odds ratio as its measure of association—so, a coherent approach to critical appraisal would assess the validity of the prevalence odds ratio, and then critique the authors' conclusions about causality in view of the cross-sectional design. This orients critical appraisal towards the tractable goals of appraising the validity of a prevalence odds ratio and perhaps assessing the extent to which it can support a causal interpretation. However, a more clearly stated question would have been desirable.

Some studies state objectives in a way that serves as an excellent starting point for critical appraisal. Consider the statement of objectives in the abstract of a study by Cedergren and Källén: "This study determined whether obese women have an increased risk of cardiovascular defects in their offspring compared with average weight women."[269] Although the statement does not have a question mark, it clearly represents a research question: Do obese women have an increased risk of cardiovascular defects in their offspring? Critical appraisal can then evaluate how well the study answers that research question.

A study by Petitti et al[270] states this objective: "To assess the risk of environmental heat-associated death by occupation." Yet, the study was a case-control study, a design that cannot assess risk. Rather, the study reported age-adjusted odds ratios, which provide estimates of relative risk. In this case, critical appraisal should begin by noting the true focus of the study (estimating relative risk), and proceed by assessing the validity of the reported odds ratios and the causal interpretations associated with them.

> *Key point:* The results of a study generally relate to a research objective. Identification of a study's objective is a good early step in critical appraisal.

Guidance is available on developing good research questions. The PICO approach is particularly useful for analytical studies. Recall that the *P* in *PICO* stands for patient, population, or problem; *I* for intervention or outcome; *C* for the comparison of interest; and *O* for the outcome of interest. This framework is less useful for descriptive studies, such as those estimating prevalence. Here, the lack of an intervention or exposure and a comparison between exposed and nonexposed leads to an abbreviated version of PICO called *PO.*[271] Another acronym for assessing research questions is FINER, which stands for **f**easible, **i**nteresting, **n**ovel, **e**thical and **r**elevant.[271] FINER can help articulate a good research topic, but it is not as helpful as PICO on clarity of the research question.

Step 2: Identifying the exposure and disease variables

You can easily get off track in critical appraisal without a clear sense of the exposure and disease of interest.

For example, the stated objective of an analysis arising from the Women's Health Initiative was: "To assess the major health benefits and risks of the most commonly used combined hormone preparation in the United States."[233] This study examined many health outcomes—so, many possible exposure-disease associations. Critical appraisal, however, requires a more precise focus. A precise focus on specific exposure-disease associations allows evaluation of issues such as measurement accuracy, or attrition related to disease and exposure status. In the case of this study, it would be best to gain a clearer picture of the specific outcomes of interest before proceeding further with critical appraisal.

> *Key point:* Identify the exposure and disease variables early in the process of critical appraisal.

Step 3: Identifying the study design

Once you have identified the exposure and disease variables, it is usually quite easy to identify the study design.

If the study is observational and the measures are aggregate, the study is ecological. If the measures are individual, examining the temporal direction (cross-sectional, retrospective, or prospective?) and logical direction of the study's inquiry (forwards or backwards?) should help clarify the study design.

Often, of course, the authors have already classified the study design and made a statement about what sort of study they have conducted. However, a little skepticism makes sense here, because authors may use terminology incorrectly or choose terminology that they think will put a positive spin on their results.

While different study designs have different strengths and weaknesses, there are no absolute rules about what designs are better or worse overall. For a particular question, for example, a case-control design may lead to a more valid answer than a prospective cohort design, even though prospective cohort studies are often viewed as more robust in their methods. Even a randomized study, often regarded as the gold standard in study design, can be inferior to other types of studies if it is poorly conducted. So, classifying the design of a study should not lead directly to conclusions about the quality of the study. The point of classification is to add structure to the task of critical appraisal. As soon as you determine, for example, that a study is cross-sectional, you can immediately flag difficulties that the study may have in determining temporality—an issue with implications for causal reasoning. Other designs raise other red flags (see Table 41).

> *Key point:* Classifying study design does not in itself identify methodological problems, but it can help to organize critical appraisal and often points to potential methodological problems.

Although no specific study design has inherent superiority for all research questions, in general some study designs deliver superior evidence. The Oxford Centre for Evidence-Based Medicine has produced a hierarchy of

TABLE 41. "RED FLAGS" CLASSICALLY ASSOCIATED WITH PARTICULAR STUDY DESIGNS

Study design	Red flags
Case-control studies	Recall bias (differential misclassification of exposure)
	Selection bias
Cross-sectional studies	Lack of temporal clarity
Ecological studies	Ecological fallacy
	Difficulty detecting and controlling confounding
Prospective cohort studies	Bias due to attrition (selection bias)
	Differential misclassification of outcome
Randomized controlled trials	Diminished generalizability

levels of evidence.[272] The hierarchy places systematic reviews of homogeneous results at the top level of evidence, followed by randomized controlled trials, cohort studies, and case-control studies. Case reports and expert opinion rank lowest in the hierarchy.

Step 4: Assessing selection bias

Why selection bias first?

There are 2 main sources of error in epidemiological research—random error, and systematic error leading to bias. Which should you consider first in critical appraisal?

Systematic error comes first. The logic behind this assertion is that systematic error and random error have a hierarchical relationship. Random error is quantified using techniques such as statistical tests and confidence intervals—but if an estimate is invalid in the first place, these quantifications of the role of chance are pointless. No one cares whether an invalid (biased) estimate is statistically significant. Indeed, P values and confidence intervals have little meaning in the face of systematic error. Therefore, systematic error (bias) is the best place to start.

Of the 2 main categories of bias—misclassification bias and selection bias—selection bias is probably the best to consider first, since the subjects for a study must be selected before measurement can occur.

Key point: Selection bias is a good place to begin addressing the issue of bias, because—methodologically—selection occurs before classification of disease and exposure status.

To assess selection bias, you need to conceptualize the selection probabilities and apply the rules that determine when selection bias will occur. With selection probabilities, it is important to think broadly. Selection probabilities are influenced by more than just sampling. They are also influenced by factors such as provision of consent, provision of information, and attrition. Anything that affects participation must be considered.

Selection probabilities, however, are not usually known—not to critical appraisers, and generally not to researchers either. An exception is survey research, where selection probabilities are often known and factor into the planning and analysis of the survey data. Therefore, the assessment of selection bias usually involves a qualitative assessment of the likely values of selection probabilities.

In a study that is estimating a frequency such as prevalence, the rules governing the assessment of selection bias are simple. If the selection probability depends on the attribute whose frequency is being assessed, bias will occur.

The rules are more complex in analytical studies, in which the targets of estimation are population parameters such as odds ratios and risk differences. Here, the selection probabilities will often depend explicitly on disease (e.g., in a case-control study) or on exposure (e.g., in many prospective cohort studies). This in itself does not cause selection bias. However, selection bias will occur if the probability of selection of cases and controls—in a case-control study, for example—depends on exposure in some way that differs between the cases and controls. Similarly, in a prospective cohort study, attrition may introduce bias if it depends on disease in a way that differs between those with and without exposure.

Selection bias in schematics

Figures 30, 31, 32, and 33 express these principles in schematics. They use arrows to represent movement from the population (where disease-exposure contingencies are represented by uppercase letters) to the sample (where they are represented with lowercase letters). A formula for the odds ratio—at the bottom of each figure—shows another way to describe these principles.

Figure 30 and Figure 31 describe selection effects in a case-control study. In a case-control study, the selection probabilities for cases are much greater than controls (shown by more arrows for cases than controls). In Figure 30, these probabilities vary in exactly the same way for cases and controls. In an odds ratio calculated from this study, the arrows occur to the same extent in the numerator and denominator, cancelling out, and demonstrating that selection bias does not occur in this scenario.

FIGURE 30. SCHEMATIC OF AN UNBIASED CASE-CONTROL STUDY

In Figure 31, the selection probabilities for cases vary by exposure. This can happen if a case-control study has flawed methods that result in a greater probability of selection for exposed cases than nonexposed cases, and do not result in the same influence of exposure in selection of controls. The odds ratio ends up having too large a numerator, leading to bias. Figure 31 describes the process by which sets of selection probabilities translate into bias in an estimated odds ratio.

FIGURE 31. SCHEMATIC OF A BIASED CASE-CONTROL STUDY

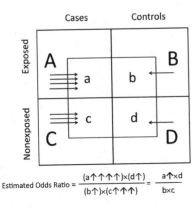

Figure 32 and Figure 33 describe selection effects in cohort studies. Note that in Figure 32—an unbiased cohort study—overrepresentation of exposed subjects does not result in bias. One of the advantages of cohort studies is that they can oversample from groups with a rare exposure. Figure 31 shows that this in itself does not cause bias.

FIGURE 32. SCHEMATIC OF AN UNBIASED COHORT STUDY

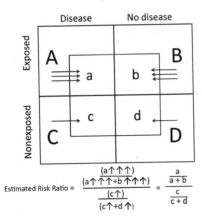

Figure 33 shows a biased cohort study, where attrition results in an underestimation of the effect of exposure: attrition has occurred to a greater extent among exposed subjects with disease than among exposed subjects without disease, whereas the same effect does not occur in the nonexposed cohort.

FIGURE 33. SCHEMATIC OF A BIASED COHORT STUDY

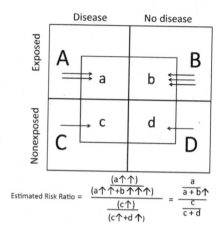

Figure 34 depicts selection bias in a risk difference. This mirrors the bias in Figure 33, except the measure of effect is now a risk difference rather than a risk ratio. In the risk difference in Figure 34, the first risk in the risk difference is too small, resulting in an underestimation of this effect.

FIGURE 34. SCHEMATIC OF A BIASED COHORT STUDY: RISK RATIO AS MEASURE OF EFFECT

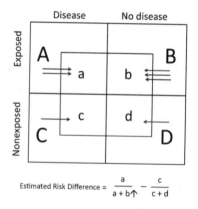

The 2 parts to bias assessment

Critical appraisal of selection bias—and all bias—has 2 parts. First, you determine if a source of vulnerability to bias exists. If a source exists, you then determine the expected direction and magnitude of bias.

Note that the schematics presented in this section can clarify the direction of bias. They can also indicate magnitude. For example, Figure 34 could have indicated bias of a greater magnitude by depicting the underrepresentation of exposed cases with 1 arrow rather than 2 arrows.

Decisions about the direction and magnitude of bias represent judgements made by critical appraisers. The representation of these judgements using visual aids such as the schematics presented here adds structure to the critical-appraisal process.

Key point: By considering probability of selection in relation to disease-exposure contingencies and study designs, the direction and magnitude of selection bias can be anticipated.

Step 5: Assessing misclassification bias

If a study is vulnerable to selection bias—and the vulnerability arises from a defect that would lead to serious over- or underestimation of the target parameter—then the task of critical appraisal might stop there. There's no point looking for more flaws if the flaw you've found is fatal. However, if the impact of selection bias is posited to be negligible or at least modest, then there is value in continuing.

For studies estimating a frequency, the rules governing misclassification bias are again fairly straightforward. Insensitivity of the measure used to classify the attribute will lead to false negatives, deflating the numerator and leading to underestimation of the frequency. A lack of specificity in such a measure will predictably lead to false-positive results. These can be expected to inflate the numerator of the frequency with a resulting systematic tendency towards overestimation.

Again, the situation is more complex when the goal of a study is to estimate a complex parameter such as a ratio or a difference between frequencies. Misclassification can then be differential or nondifferential. If nondifferential, the direction of bias is predictably towards the null value. If differential, you need to think hard to determine its expected direction and magnitude.

Differential misclassification bias in schematics

Figure 35 describes an unbiased study. It contrasts with Figure 36 and Figure 37, which describe the effects of misclassification bias.

Note that these schematics do not use uppercase and lowercase letters to distinguish populations and samples—after all, selection plays no role in the mechanisms leading to misclassification bias. Misclassification bias results from classifying members of the study sample into the wrong categories in the classic 2 × 2 contingency table.

Figure 35 represents the process of classification of exposure in a case-control study where there are no classification errors. The outer box of the schematic represents the actual status of the sample (depicted with lowercase letters since these are sample values). Here, all of the exposed subjects are true positives for exposure and all of the nonexposed subjects are true negatives for exposure. The contingencies according to the classification are the same as the real contingencies in the sample and there is no bias introduced into the estimate.

FIGURE 35. SCHEMATIC OF AN UNBIASED CASE-CONTROL STUDY: ODDS RATIO AS MEASURE OF EFFECT

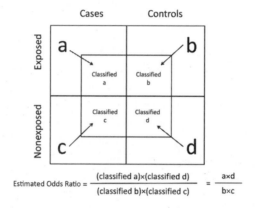

Figure 36 describes a case-control study where misclassification from recall bias has taken place. In recall bias, people with a disease tend to think harder about possible causes of their condition. They are more likely to recall

FIGURE 36. SCHEMATIC OF A BIASED CASE-CONTROL STUDY: RECALL BIAS, ODDS RATIO AS MEASURE OF EFFECT

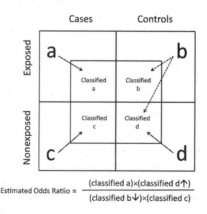

exposures than members of the control group. Here, the misclassification is due to a lower sensitivity for classification of exposure among the control group. So, some of the exposed persons in the control group are misclassified as nonexposed, moving people from the upper-right contingency cell to the lower-right cell (depicted as a dashed line in Figure 36). When the odds ratio is calculated, there will be too few in the upper-right cell and too many in the lower-right cell, leading to an overestimation of the odds ratio.

Key point: Critical appraisal must distinguish differential and nondifferential misclassification bias in analytical studies, because these different forms of bias have important implications for the direction of bias.

Figure 37 presents another classic form of differential misclassification bias: diagnostic suspicion bias (surveillance bias) in cohort studies. The idea is that the measure of disease status may be less sensitive in the nonexposed than in the exposed. Because there is a higher index of suspicion among the exposed, they are followed more closely or assessed more carefully. Some of those in the nonexposed group are sometimes misclassified as nondiseased because they are not followed closely enough for all cases to be detected.

FIGURE 37. SCHEMATIC OF A BIASED COHORT STUDY: DIAGNOSTIC SUSPICION BIAS

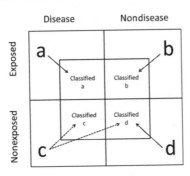

The risk ratio will be overestimated in the scenario in Figure 37 because the denominator of the risk ratio will be too small:

$$\text{Estimated Risk Ratio} = \left[\frac{\left(\dfrac{\text{Classified } a}{\text{Classified } a + \text{Classified } b} \right)}{\left(\dfrac{\text{Classified } c{\downarrow}}{\text{Classified } c{\downarrow} + \text{Classified } d{\uparrow}} \right)} \right]$$

As with selection bias, the assessment of misclassification bias should also include an assessment of the magnitude of bias. The assessment is again a matter of judgement, but the schematics can help structure it. For example, Figure 37 depicts the misclassification of nonexposed cases due to low sensitivity of diagnostic procedures in the nonexposed cohort. You can look up what is known about the accuracy of the diagnostic procedures used in a study. For example, if a diagnostic procedure is expected to achieve only 50% sensitivity in the nonexposed cohort, the arrow (dotted line) leading to the "classified d" cell will move half of those who should be in the "classified c" cell to the "classified d" cell. Assuming that other aspects of classification are accurate, this would make the value of c in the denominator of a risk ratio about half as large as it should be, thereby doubling the value of the risk ratio.

Step 6: Assessing confounding and effect measure modification

Effect measure modification first

The issues of effect measure modification and confounding always go together. Confounding cannot be considered unless effect measure modification has been assessed.

An obvious question for critical appraisal concerns whether a study has addressed these issues properly. If you are concerned that an extraneous variable may have modified the effect of the exposure variable in a study, then you will want to see that the study has assessed this possibility. A study would normally do this with a test for heterogeneity in a stratified analysis or with an interaction term in a regression model. If effect measure modification has not been assessed, then the study's estimates may be meaningless averages of the effect in people with or without the modifying variable.

Confounding next

If a study has addressed effect measure modification—or if effect measure modification is not a concern—then your next focus is how the study controls confounding.

There are usually 3 concerns about confounding.

The first common concern is that a potential confounder exists that the study has not addressed. Any independent risk factor for the study's outcome may act as a confounder, if it is also associated with the exposure in question. It is often not possible to find high quality information in the literature about associations between potential confounders and exposure variables, but many studies have identified risk factors for diseases. Any independent risk factor for a disease is a potential confounding variable, since it may also be associated with exposure (note, however, that this is unlikely in the case of a randomized study). Ideally, you would want to see every independent risk factor addressed in some way as a potential confounding variable, either at the design stage or in the analysis. If you can identify a potentially confounding variable that has not been addressed, you have identified a methodological weakness of the study. The term *omitted variable bias* is sometimes used for bias that arises from failure to control for the effects of a confounding variable.

The second common concern arises if confounding has been poorly dealt with in an analysis. When matching or stratification is used, confounding can persist if the matching characteristics are too broad or the strata are too broad. For example, if cases and controls are matched on age too broadly (e.g., within plus or minus 10 years instead of plus or minus 1 year), or if broad rather than narrow age strata are used, then the confounding effects of age may not be fully controlled. There may be enough variation in risk within these groups that confounding can occur. This is called *residual confounding*, and, when it occurs, pooling procedures such as the Mantel-Haenszel family of pooled estimators will not fully adjust for its effects. When confounding is addressed using adjustment in a regression model, inaccurate measurement of the confounder can also result in a failure to fully control the confounding effect. Even when randomization is used, a risk factor may still have an unbalanced distribution between groups. Consequently, confounding may still occur and authors should provide a careful comparison of the randomized groups to ensure that an imbalance has not occurred.

The third concern about confounding is whether the procedures used to control confounding in a particular study were adequate. A variety of problems may occur, including a failure to distinguish between a confounding variable and a mediating variable. Recall that a confounding variable must be an independent risk factor for the outcome under study. If an extraneous variable falls on a causal pathway linking exposure to disease—in other words, if they exist on the same causal chain of events—adjustment as if this variable were a confounder will attenuate the effects of the exposure, creating the false impression that the exposure is not causally related to the disease.

Recall that in epidemiology, the concept of causation is related to the general goal of epidemiologic research, which lies in informing public health or clinical action. If changing the exposure will prevent disease, for example, then the effect is important for public health, and its disappearance when a mediator is erroneously treated as a confounder is misleading. Discerning whether a variable is an independent risk factor or a mediator of the effects of the exposure must often come from the literature. An interesting example has unfolded in a debate about whether very strenuous physical activity may have negative health implications. O'Keefe et al[273] described a U-shaped relationship between running distance per week and all-cause mortality. Runners had lower mortality than nonrunners, but runners covering distances greater than 20 miles per week had increased mortality, similar to nonrunners. These estimates were adjusted for body mass index, blood pressure, diagnosis of hypertension, lipids, glucose, and psychological factors.[274] Pointing out that many of these variables are beneficial effects of running, Weber[275] later argued that the U-shaped curve may have been exaggerated because these adjustments may have removed (or adjusted away) many of the beneficial effects of running. Consistent with this, the authors subsequently repeated their analysis with adjustment only for age and sex. While a U-shaped pattern was still evident, it was "blunted" compared to what had been previously reported.[274]

Key point: Assessment of the control of confounding in a study should assess whether potential confounding variables were treated correctly (e.g., during stratification or modelling), and also whether all important potentially confounding variables were included.

Step 7: Assessing the role of chance

In epidemiology, the role of chance is assessed using either statistical tests or confidence intervals. Confidence intervals are the preferred procedure. Unlike P values, confidence intervals do not confound the effect of sample size with that of effect size. Instead, they provide a plausible range of values for an estimated epidemiologic parameter. However, P values continue to be commonly reported. This produces a temptation to interpret confidence intervals as if they were tests of significance. Keeping in mind, for example, that an odds ratio has a null value of 1, it may be tempting to interpret a 95% CI primarily by whether it crosses the null value, as this would indicate statistical significance. However, this would be a mistake because confidence intervals have much to say beyond statistical significance. To interpret a confidence interval, it is a good idea to look at 2 different things: the location of the interval and also its width. The location of the upper and lower confidence limits provides information about the smallest and largest population values that are consistent with the observed data. Anything between these 2 limits is a plausible value for the population parameter. The width of the interval quantifies the precision of the estimate.

When P values are reported in a study as indicators of statistical significance, critical appraisal needs to focus on the vulnerability of the study to type I or type II error, depending on the results the study reports.

If a study reports a significant result, the concern is with type I error. If a study has a small number of tests (ideally, 1 test to evaluate a single well-defined primary hypothesis), the P value quantifies the risk of type I error. However, if the analysis is poorly structured and there are multiple hypotheses, or ill-defined hypotheses, then the risk of type I error is decidedly higher. Remember that, when using tests based on a 5% level of confidence, there is a 5% chance of type I error. If a study uses multiple tests, there is a much higher probability of type I error: the risk for each specific test is 5%. There is no way to know which of the significant tests are type I errors, so a shadow is cast over all the results.

If a study reports a statistical test that is not significant, the possibility of type II error must be considered. The probability of type II error is related to the power of the study. It is therefore very helpful if studies report a justification for their chosen sample size, such as a power calculation.

Of course, if the estimate is biased then confidence intervals are of little interest—nor are P values. In this situation, confidence intervals do not quantify the role of chance properly, nor does their width reflect the precision of the estimate in a meaningful way. When an estimate is biased and the sample size for the study is very large, the confidence intervals are likely to be extremely narrow and are unlikely to include the actual population at all. Given this state of affairs, the naive interpretation of a 95% CI (or, of course, a P value) in the presence of bias is internally contradictory.

> *Key point:* Interpretation of a confidence interval involves consideration of the location of the confidence limits and the width of the interval.

Step 8: Addressing causality

The concept of causality is hierarchically related to the concept of validity. If an estimate is invalid, there is often no point in considering its causal significance. Note, however, that this is not always the case. For example, consider an estimate that suggests a strong effect, but that may be affected by non-differential misclassification bias—it is safe to say that the actual estimate is stronger than reported. Here, it may make sense to consider questions related to causation.

> *Key point:* If an estimate is unbiased, causation may be considered. A common approach is to consider causal criteria, as described—for example—by Bradford Hill.

The etiological effect of age poses some unique issues. Many diseases, including most cancers and cardiovascular diseases, have increasing incidence with increasing age. Age is measured in units of time (years since birth), but is usually regarded as a proxy measure for biological changes that occur, over time, in the body. As such, age is not a causal factor in its own right, but an indirect indicator of a large number of other causes. This is not a major problem for epidemiological research since age is a nonmodifiable variable anyway. Age is therefore treated as a potential effect modifier or confounder in most epidemiological analyses.

Age can also reflect other types of effects. Keyes[276] defines a *cohort effect* as "variation in the risk of a health outcome according to the year of birth, often coinciding with shifts in the population exposure to risk factors over time." Keyes argues that in epidemiology, cohort effects can be viewed as an interaction between the age of a particular birth cohort and the exposures they encounter during key periods in their lives.

Step 9: Assessing generalizability

If an estimate is judged to be invalid, then there is no point assessing its generalizability. Internal validity is a necessary precondition for any consideration of external validity.

Keep in mind the distinction between internal and external validity. Internal validity can be defined in a technical sense as the absence of bias—it is something you can assess objectively in critical appraisal. External validity is a study's applicability to populations beyond its target population—its assessment is entirely a matter of judgement.

If you are reading a study from the United States, for example, you can reasonably ask whether the study applies to Canada (as long as its estimates are judged valid). This assessment—as in all considerations of external validity—would be a matter of considered opinion, not fact.

In general, epidemiological findings that involve biological aspects of disease etiology (such as the increased risk of cardiovascular disease associated with smoking) are likely to be readily generalizable, whereas associations that involve culturally sensitive or health system–related estimates are less likely to be generalizable.

Key point: Consideration of *P* values and confidence intervals, as well as issues of causation and generalizability, is important when an estimate is internally valid. When an estimate is invalid, these considerations are not usually important at all.

Step 10: Reporting a critical appraisal

A critical appraisal can usually be written up in a few pages, or provided verbally in 5 to 10 minutes. It should normally follow the steps presented in this chapter. This means that it would often start with a brief summary of the work: the objectives of the study, the exposure and disease variables, and the study design. This would be followed by an examination of the key issues of bias, effect measure modification, and confounding, as outlined above. If the results of the study are considered invalid, the appraisal may end there. If the estimates are determined to be valid, a discussion of their causal significance and generalizability are often pursued.

Critical appraisal as a skill

This chapter has presented a series of steps to guide critical appraisal, but critical appraisal is too complex to be simply a technical procedure.

Critical appraisal is a skill and, like all skills, requires practice and feedback.

It also requires knowledge. For example, consideration of biological plausibility often depends on knowledge of physiology, and judgements about external validity require knowledge of different populations.

The best way to develop the skill of critical appraisal—to build your fluency with study designs and types of error, to identify critical gaps in your knowledge—is to apply it in settings where feedback is available, such as peer-review groups and journal clubs.

Checklists to support critical appraisal

Some organizations have designed tools to support the goals of critical appraisal. The Critical Appraisal Skills Programme, or CASP[277]—among the most widely used—has developed educational materials based on a "Users' guides to the medical literature,"[278] a series of articles spearheaded by Dr. Gordon Guyatt of McMaster University and published the *Journal of the American Medical Association* starting in 1993.

CASP has critical-appraisal checklists for a variety of study designs. The checklists have 3 sections, each focused on an important consideration: (1) whether the results of the study are valid; (2) what the results are; and (3) whether the results help locally. The CASP checklist for case-control studies—as an example—has 11 questions that break down these considerations into specific issues. The CASP checklists, and others like them, cannot be completed without a good working knowledge of epidemiology. For example, the case-control study checklist includes the question: "Were the controls selected in an acceptable way?" Answering this question requires careful consideration and focused thinking, as we have seen. So, while critical-appraisal checklists provide guidance on issues to consider when critically appraising a study, they will never replace informed judgement based on knowledge of epidemiology.

CASP specifically disavows using its checklists as assessment tools, but other critical-appraisal tools, such as the Downs and Black scale, have been adopted for exactly this purpose. Systematic reviews often use these tools to quantitatively grade the quality of studies in a literature. The Downs and Black scale[279] consists of 27 items covering topics such as clarity of reporting, internal and external validity, and power. Although the instrument is designed for case-control and cohort studies, many of the items fit best with nonrandomized studies of interventions. Also, as with CASP, the items do not seek to replace the judgement of a knowledgeable rater. For example, item

21 asks: "Were the patients in different intervention groups (trials and cohort studies) or were the cases and controls (case-control studies) recruited from the same population?" Clearly, the item is concerned with the issue of selection bias, but a single item cannot in itself address the subtleties of such an issue.

Another instrument—the Newcastle-Ottawa scale—was developed by the University of Newcastle in Australia in collaboration with the University of Ottawa. The goal of the scale is to assess study quality for use in systematic reviews that include observational studies. The scale is consistent with the approach to critical appraisal presented in this book. It emphasizes 3 domains related to selection bias, confounding, and misclassification bias: "selection of the study groups; the comparability of the groups; and the ascertainment of either the exposure or outcome of interest for case-control or cohort studies respectively."[280]

The Newcastle-Ottawa scale has separate versions for cohort and case-control studies, and offers a manual on scoring. It breaks down the 3 domains into multiple items, all of which require judgement and a working knowledge of epidemiologic concepts. In other words, the scale doesn't make critical appraisal any easier or more accurate, but it does quantify the risk of bias in a study in a way that can be used for stratification or sensitivity analysis in meta-analysis.

For randomized controlled trials, the Cochrane Collaboration's risk-of-bias (RoB) tool is most commonly used, an updated version of which was published in 2019.[281] This tool assesses risk of bias in domains that are most relevant to the randomized controlled trial study design, using terminology such as "bias due to deviations from intended interventions" and "bias due to missing outcome data."

Other sources of checklists for critical appraisal include the Clarity Group at McMaster University[282] and the Joanna Briggs Institute at the University of Adelaide in Australia.[283]

Standardized reporting of studies

Published studies do not always report enough information to allow for critical appraisal, which means that it is not possible to tell whether their results are valid. Fortunately, reporting standards are available to investigators. Reporting standards help ensure that published studies provide enough information about their methods for readers to make strongly informed decisions about the validity of study results. The most widely used reporting standards in epidemiology come from the Strengthening the Reporting of Observational Studies in Epidemiology (STROBE) statement.[284] provides checklists for reporting cohort, case-control, and cross-sectional studies. Another reporting standard—the RECORD statement and checklist—provides key reporting standards for epidemiologic research in Canada, particularly because epidemiological research in Canada often uses administrative data sources.[285] (RECORD stands for **RE**porting of Studies **Co**nducted Using Observational **R**outinely Collected **D**ata.) Various reporting standards applicable to different types of studies have been collected through an initiative called the EQUATOR Network (EQUATOR stands for enhancing the **qu**ality and **t**ransparency of **health research**).[286]

Questions

1. Identifying a study's design can help to focus critical appraisal on the potential vulnerabilities of a study because specific methodological vulnerabilities tend to be associated with specific study designs. Identify the single most notorious vulnerability of each the following study designs:
   a. ecological studies
   b. cross-sectional studies
   c. randomized controlled trials
   d. prospective cohort studies
   e. case-control studies

2. Do you think there are any situations in which an invalid estimate can be generalized to another population? What are the implications of your opinion on this question for critical appraisal?

3. Can a study conducted in Newfoundland be generalized to British Columbia?

4. Many contemporary studies present complex models that simultaneously adjust for multiple potential confounding variables.
   a. These studies often fail to report whether they evaluated interactions between these variables and the exposure of interest. In your opinion, is this a problem?
   b. Sometimes, the authors defend the inclusion of variables in these models based on whether they are statistically significant. Does this seem to you like the best way to decide what variables should be included in a regression model?

5. All major medical journals have web pages where they post online versions of studies. It is usually possible for authors to publish supplementary materials relevant to their studies. In your opinion, what kinds of materials would be most helpful to critical appraisers?

6. Pampalon et al[242] have developed and validated a social-deprivation index for Canada. The index uses census information to characterize the extent of social deprivation in geographically defined areas. The index has been found to predict several adverse health outcomes. Since the index describes social deprivation in a geographical area rather than an individual person, are all of these results vulnerable to the ecological fallacy?

7. Describe what is wrong with the following statement: "Cross-sectional studies are always less informative than prospective studies."

8. A disadvantage of prospective cohort studies is their expense. Imagine a hypothetical situation in which costs were not an issue. You have unlimited funds
to support your research. Would it always be better to conduct a prospective
cohort study than a case-control study?

9. Many journals endorse reporting standards, such as those provided through
the EQUATOR Network, as a way to ensure the quality of published studies. Can
you think of any potential disadvantages of such reporting standards?

10. If a flaw (e.g., a vulnerability to random or systematic error) is identified in a
study, should this preclude its publication in the peer-reviewed literature?

Answers to questions

Chapter 1

QUESTION 1

a. There are different types of administrative data. In Canada, provincial public health insurance plans are widely available sources of data. These data include diagnostic codes that fee-for-service physicians submit to provincial plans to get paid, and summaries that are completed by hospitals when discharging patients. These data may not be accurate for some conditions—for example, for conditions where people do not seek assistance from physicians or hospitals. They may also lack accuracy where several diagnoses might be relevant. For example, physicians often only need to report a single diagnosis to receive payment, yet many people have more than a single disease. Also, some provinces require only "rough" diagnostic codes (e.g., the first 3 characters of the 5-character International Classification of Disease, or ICD—codes which sometimes represent a group of diseases rather than a single disease).

b. The study seeks to quantify the amount of disease in the population, so it has primarily descriptive aims.

c. For a condition that may have a different prevalence in different provinces, pooling estimates from different provinces to produce a national prevalence estimate would be a major concern. Extending results that are based on 5 provinces to all 10 provinces would amount to assuming that the prevalence is the same in all provinces.

d. This kind of information is important for 2 main reasons. First, those planning health services need to know how much disease is in a population, so they can anticipate the quantity of resources needed. However, if differences were observed among provinces, this might generate hypotheses about risk factors for the disease. In turn, this might lead to additional studies (analytical studies) seeking to determine why the prevalence is higher in some regions of the country than in others.

QUESTION 2

a. The study does not target a population that is entirely geographically based, but it still targets a well-defined population. This is a population-based study.

b. This study is concerned with the distribution and determinants of health issues (pain, undertreatment of pain) in a defined population, so it is an epidemiological study. Some might call this *health services research* to emphasize that it is focused on a health-system performance issue—the proper management of pain—but it is not necessary to make this distinction.

c. Epidemiological studies need large samples so that they can see patterns of disease and exposure in populations. The "noise" of random variation often obscures these patterns when samples are small.

d. They have identified a problem. Further understanding the basis of this problem, or doing something about it, will improve the health of members of this population.

e. Like all descriptive studies, this study has value in identifying a problem, which makes it possible for health services to address the problem. The study has also quantified the extent of the problem—another valuable piece of information for administering health services. The study may also lead to analytical studies that investigate why the problem is happening.

QUESTION 3

a. This study is concerned with whether a particular risk factor (fewer years of education) increases the risk of Alzheimer disease. The study is evaluating a hypothesis about disease etiology, so it is an analytical study.

b. In this case, it is not easy to discern how this information would be useful for prevention through public health action. However, identification of this association could prove valuable for understanding the disease, and a better understanding of the disease could ultimately play a role in prevention.

QUESTION 4

These studies share the following focus with the work of John Snow: examining patterns of distribution of diseases in populations. They seek to identify the burden of disease, generate hypotheses about disease etiology, or test hypotheses about disease etiology.

QUESTION 5

a. If this association can lead to actions that will diminish mortality due to cholera, then those actions are valuable. This kind of information can lead to fruitful public health actions, saving lives and preventing suffering. Such actions do not always (indeed they rarely) depend on a full understanding of each step in the pathophysiology of a disease.

b. Diseases occur as a result of an intermixing of many component causes. *Vibrio cholerae* is obviously a key component cause, but it is only 1 step on a causal chain of events. Intervening at other places along that chain (e.g., the safe disposal of fecal waste and protection of drinking water supplies) can effectively control cholera.

QUESTION 6

a. Most epidemiologists would not consider a case report to be an epidemiological study design. A case report only describes the experience of a single person and therefore cannot provide information about the distribution and determinants of disease in a population.

b. A case series has more than 1 case, so in this respect it has a superficial resemblance to a descriptive epidemiological study. Indeed, it is sometimes classified as such. However, it is not really an epidemiological study because the characteristics of a particular group of people who happen to have been seen in a particular clinical setting say very much about the distribution or determinants of disease in a population. The lack of connection to patterns seen in a population means that case series are not epidemiological study designs.

QUESTION 7

Most epidemiological studies examine the distribution and determinants of chronic diseases. These conditions have many contributing causes, some of which are unknown. Individual differences would make it impossible to learn very much about the disease by describing the characteristics of individual people. However, comparing large groups of people can still yield very useful comparisons, such as the frequency of disease in people with or without an exposure. Epidemiological studies are very useful in the study of chronic diseases.

QUESTION 8

It is very unlikely that epidemiology will become obsolete. One reason is that no matter what new treatments, diagnostic tests, and so on come out of laboratory research, there will still be a need to explore their safety and usefulness in human populations. This requires epidemiological methods. Also, as progress is made in public health and clinical practice, the remaining problems become more and more difficult to deal with. They also require increasingly sophisticated epidemiological analysis. As society progresses more and more deeply into the "information age," the availability of data increases and becomes more complex, requiring the skills of people with training in epidemiology.

QUESTION 9

On the surface, precision medicine's emphasis on individual outcomes and tailoring of preventive and therapeutic strategies to individual people seems quite different than epidemiology's emphasis on populations. However, the advent of precision health care actually makes epidemiological information more important than ever. In order to predict individual outcomes, it is usually necessary to have a lot of information about the determinants of disease, including those determinants that differentiate between subgroups of patients. This information must almost always come from epidemiological sources.

QUESTION 10

The distinction between health services research and epidemiology is artificial in at least this sense: in epidemiology almost any characteristic that differs between people can be viewed as an exposure. Also, any unintended outcome of health services or a bad, as opposed to a good, outcome can be regarded as a disease. As such, health services researchers work in a specialized subdiscipline of epidemiology. However, they may also have special skills in areas such as economic analysis or policy analysis that are not components of mainstream epidemiology.

Chapter 2

QUESTION 1

The prevalence is 2,273,800 /30,378,269, or 0.075, or 7.5%.

QUESTION 2

a. The prevalence is 9/401, or 0.022, or 2.2%.

b. The standard error is 0.007.

QUESTION 3

Point prevalence estimates the proportion in a population with a disease. This parameter is of clear value for descriptive epidemiology because it quantifies the burden of disease. If point prevalence is particularly high or low in a particular population, it may also generate hypotheses about etiology, another important descriptive goal. However, point prevalence is less useful for analytical epidemiology because it does not quantify the risk of developing a disease—it is merely the proportion having a disease.

QUESTION 4

Basic epidemiological parameters are intended to quantify probabilities and risks. When a risk does not apply to a segment of the population, such as women in this case, that segment would not usually be included in the calculation.

QUESTION 5

In principle, there is no reason to quantify the precision of an estimate that actually is the population estimate. In practice, when a parameter such as prevalence is measured at several different times, some degree of random variation will likely affect the estimates. This is especially true for rare diseases. As a result, procedures such as confidence intervals are commonly used to assess the "stability" of proportions and rates in entire populations.

QUESTION 6

Prevalence is a descriptive parameter that helps to quantify the burden of disease in a population. Expressing prevalence as a count links directly to the number of people needing health care for that condition, which is an advantage for planning and administration. Expressing prevalence as a count also has a disadvantage: since populations are usually of different sizes, a mere count is not very good for comparing 2 estimates.

QUESTION 7

Even though the cause of the error may be, in a sense, random, the net effect is that some people without diabetes will be incorrectly classified as having it. This will cause the estimate to be systematically too high.

QUESTION 8

If this random pattern of responding caused the estimate to be erroneous, it would be a form of systematic error. Random error arises due to sampling variability, not to inaccurate measurement.

QUESTION 9

It is not unfair. Critical appraisal helps to clarify whether reported results are vulnerable to errors.

QUESTION 10

a. Estimates that arise from samples are always vulnerable to random error, but if the sample size is large, such error will be minimal.

b. It is true that removal of 1 person from the population would slightly change the underlying proportion that applies to the next person's selection. Each observation is therefore not entirely independent. Some statistics include finite population correction factors to deal with this problem. However, in a practical sense, it is rarely an issue since epidemiologists typically deal with large populations and their samples are usually a small proportion of those populations, a situation in which this nonindependence becomes trivial.

Chapter 3

QUESTION 1

a. Of the 10 people, there are 4 who become ill during the observation period. Therefore, the annual period prevalence is 4/10.

b. In August, there are 3 people with the disease. The population at this point in time consists of 9 people, since 1 has died. The point prevalence is therefore 3/9.

c. This is the proportion of people at risk of the disease who develop the disease during the defined interval of follow-up. There are 2 people that have the illness at the baseline time point and who are therefore not at risk. Two of those who are at risk develop the disease, which makes the cumulative incidence proportion 2/8.

d. Since this is a mortality rate, all 10 subjects contribute person-time observations to the calculation, regardless of whether they have the disease at baseline. Everyone alive is at risk of death. However, person-time after death is not counted because it does not exist. The total person-years of observation is 105 (the grid potentially holds $10 \times 12 = 120$ person-months of observation, but there are 15 white squares) and there are 3 deaths, so the rate is 3 per 105 person-months, or 0.029 per person-month, or 0.029 $month^{-1}$. To convert this value to person-years, multiply it by 12 (months per year): 0.343 $year^{-1}$.

e. Since the disease is a recurrent disease, people reenter the population at risk after they recover. Therefore, even person number 4 provides person-time at risk starting in April. The only person contributing no person-time is person number 9, because that person is ill throughout the entire interval. However, people who are ill do not contribute to person-time at risk. The total person-time at risk is 83 person-months. Since the disease is recurrent, there can be more than 1 episode of illness in a given person. Therefore, person number 7 contributes 2 episodes to the numerator of the incidence rate. So, there are 3 incidents per 83 person-months, or 0.036 $month^{-1}$, or 0.434 $year^{-1}$.

QUESTION 2

a. Of the 10 people, there are 3 who become ill during the observation period. Therefore, the annual period prevalence is 3/10.

b. In August, no one has the disease. The point prevalence is therefore 0.

c. Of 9 persons at risk at the baseline time point, 2 develop the disease during follow-up. The incidence proportion is therefore 2/9.

d. There are 85 person-months of observation and 4 deaths, so the mortality rate is 4/85 person-months, or 0.047 $months^{-1}$. This corresponds to 0.565 $years^{-1}$.

e. There are 82 person-months at risk of the disease, contributed by the 9 people free of disease at the baseline time point. Two incident cases arise from this person-time at risk. The incidence rate is therefore 2/82 person-months, or 0.024 months^{-1}, which is 0.293 years^{-1}.

QUESTION 3

a. There are 2 people affected during the 1 year of observation. Therefore, the period prevalence is 2/10.

b. The point prevalence is the same in each month: 1/10.

c. Eight of the 10 people contribute 12 person-months of observation. The other 2 contribute 6 person-months each. The incidence rate is therefore 12/108 person-months, or 0.111 months^{-1}, or 1.33 year^{-1}. Note that it is possible for an incidence rate to have a value greater than 1: this is a rate, which can be associated with different units, not a proportion.

d. The prevalence odds is equal to the incidence rate multiplied by mean duration. Each episode has a 1-month duration. So, the prevalence odds are the same as the incidence rate, except that the units disappear during the process of multiplying 1 month by 0.111 month^{-1}. Of course, you could also calculate the prevalence odds by dividing the number of people with an episode by the number of people without an episode: 1/9 = 0.111. In addition, you could calculate the prevalence odds from the prevalence proportion using the formula for this purpose (odds = proportion / 1 − proportion), which is 1/10 / (1 − 1/10) = 0.111.

QUESTION 4

a. 0.0009

b. 0.0091

c. 0.0989

d. 9

QUESTION 5

Prevalence (which quantifies how common a disease is) is approximately equal to incidence (expressed as a rate with time^{-1} units) multiplied by the duration of illness (in time units). Since insulin is a life-saving treatment for people with insulin-dependent diabetes, its discovery lengthened the duration of illness and has increased its prevalence.

QUESTION 6

There is no such formula. A formula exists for calculating period prevalence from an incidence rate and a mean duration of illness, but not for calculating period prevalence.

QUESTION 7

Incidence rates have arbitrary time units. To convert a per-month rate to a per-year rate, simply multiply by 12. This works because there are 12 months per year— nothing has changed, only the units.

QUESTION 8

The calculation is correct. Because the time units in an incidence-rate calculation are arbitrary, the value of the parameter can assume any value. Unlike an incidence proportion, there is no reason an incidence rate must have a value of less than 1.

QUESTION 9

Point prevalence is definitely the "default" version of prevalence. Unless otherwise specified, "prevalence" means "point prevalence." A real advantage of point prevalence over period and lifetime prevalence is its clear meaning—the proportion of a population at a point in time that has a disease. Other forms of prevalence usually come into use because of the special characteristics of the disease in question. For example, the point prevalence for migraine is the proportion of the population at a point in time having migraine, which doesn't do a good job of quantifying the proportion of the population burdened by migraine or the proportion in need of migraine management. A period prevalence estimate might be more meaningful in the context of migraine for this reason. Lifetime prevalence is usually reserved for conditions that a person is considered to have permanently, based on their personal health history, such that remission of symptoms is not taken to mean that the disease has "gone away." An example is schizophrenia. The proportion of the population that has schizophrenia is the proportion that has had characteristic episodes of this illness during their lifetime—hence, for this type of condition, lifetime prevalence may be the preferred parameter.

QUESTION 10

This interpretation of the parameter is incorrect. The proportion of the population that has had a condition up to a point of time at which prevalence is assessed is the lifetime prevalence. The sample used in a prevalence study includes people of various ages, but the question is always whether they have had that condition in the past. It is not usually possible to measure the proportion of a population that will have a condition at any time in their lives, since this would need to be assessed at the very end of their life, near the time of their death, which is not usually practical.

Chapter 4

QUESTION 1

Approximately 300 000 people die in Canada from all causes each year. This is the numerator of a crude prevalence calculation. Statistics Canada produces annual population estimates—the 2020 population projection for Canada on July 1 was 38 005 238, or approximately 38 million. Crude mortality in Canada is therefore approximately 300 000 divided by 38 005 238 or approximately 789 per 100 000. Roughly consistent with this, Statistics Canada reported a 7.6 per 1000 population crude mortality rate for 2019. This can properly be called a rate, because the midyear population (July 1) was used in the calculation. The midyear population is a good approximation of person-years of life within the population during that year.

QUESTION 2

The cause-specific mortality rates for tuberculosis and malignant neoplasms can be estimated using the same procedure described for question 1. You also need to decide how to report the estimate. Dividing 70 by 38 005 238 (see answer to question 1) leads to a cause specific mortality of 0.0000018 year^{-1} or 0.0018 per 1000 year^{-1}. However, this is a difficult number to digest. It would perhaps be better to report this as (roughly) 1.8 per million year^{-1}, since this immediately suggests the number of expected deaths in a country of approximately 38 million. Seventy thousand deaths lead to a mortality rate of 0.0018 year^{-1}, or 1842 per million year^{-1}.

QUESTION 3

a. In Canada, age 75 is most often used as the index age against which to determine potential years of life lost (PYLL). In this collision, 2 people died, losing 55 and 53 potential years of life, respectively. The total lost is therefore 108 PYLL. The vulnerability of young people to traumatic deaths, particularly motor vehicle–related deaths, accounts for the major contribution of trauma to PYLL in Canada.

b. Since this person was more than 75 years old, his or her death is not considered to have caused any premature mortality. The contribution to PYLL is 0.

QUESTION 4

a. The conditions that kill the most people in Canada are cancer, heart disease, and stroke.[287] To find more detailed information, look up Table 13-10-0394-01.

b. According to a 2008 report by the Public Health Agency of Canada, cancers, circulatory diseases, and injuries (this category includes both unintentional and intentional injuries) are the most common causes of premature mortality in Canada.[288] When combined with chronic respiratory disease, these 4 conditions together were found to cause more than 70% of all potential years of life lost in Canada. The Global Burden of Disease (GBD) study[289] has produced a country-specific report for Canada that includes "years of life lost" as a measure of premature mortality. This is similar to PYLL, although the GBD uses slightly different definitions than those adopted by Statistics Canada. The GBD identifies ischemic heart disease, lung cancer, and self-harm as the top 3 causes of years of life lost.

c. According to the GBD study,[289] the top contributors to years lived with disability in Canada (as of 2015) were low back pain, sense-organ diseases, and depressive disorders.

QUESTION 5

This rate describes the proportion of people with a specific disease that die from it and is therefore a case-fatality rate. For infectious diseases, the case-fatality rate is often a simple proportion. For other illnesses, it may be reported as the proportion dying during a specific time interval, as in this study.

QUESTION 6

Research usually starts with a question. Next, a study is designed to address that question. Analysis of the study data leads to an answer to the question. By contrast, surveillance routinely collects data to monitor health status, detect dangerous events in the population, and ensure appropriate action is taken. Research results are normally published in academic journals when they require communication to a scientific audience. The results of surveillance activities, however, require ongoing communication to audiences that implement public-health actions. Surveillance activities are based on (1) gathering information that is needed for public-health actions, rather than answering questions, (2) ongoing data collection, rather than discrete time-limited data collection, and (3) built-in methods of communicating findings to those who need to know.

QUESTION 7

Mortality data quantifies an important aspect of health status—the risk of death. However, it (1) treats deaths the same regardless of the age at death, and (2) ignores the fact that living with a disease is also important due to morbidity (e.g., suffering, diminished quality of life and functioning).

QUESTION 8

One component of the DALY is years of life lost—which is very similar to PYLL. The Global Burden of Disease study publishes estimates of years of life lost, essentially capturing all of the information comprising PYLL. In addition, the DALY has the major advantage of incorporating a measure of the morbidity associated with various diseases, which it quantifies in terms of years lived with disability.

QUESTION 9

If you interpret a ranking of contributions to disease burden (e.g., quantified using the DALY) as a way of setting health-system priorities, a concept is missed: modifiability. An argument can be made that health care resources should be invested in ways that lead to the most benefit, which is not necessarily the same as arguing that resource investments targeting a particular problem should be proportional to the burden of that health problem.

QUESTION 10

Canada has made efforts to develop a national capacity in health surveillance. The Public Health Agency of Canada, for example, operates the Chronic Diseases Surveillance System for conditions such as diabetes. Also, Statistics Canada and the Canadian Institute for Health Information collect and publish data relevant to health surveillance. However, in Canada, health care is a provincial responsibility, so much of the legislation and data collection occurs at a provincial rather than national level.

Chapter 5

QUESTION 1

The key feature of critical appraisal is that it adopts a critical stance towards research results. A critical appraiser does not read a study under the assumption that it was done correctly and that the results are valid. Instead, a critical appraiser looks for problems that may have introduced errors into the reported results (and also interpretations, conclusions, etc.). The popular media often do not approach health studies from a critical stance (although good reporters will seek opinions from several experts as they develop their stories). This sometimes leads to uncritical reporting of a "finding" (often an interpretation by an investigator) from a major study.

QUESTION 2

Random error is error that results from sampling variability. According to the law of large numbers, and assuming that there are no defects in a study's design, the extent of random error will predictably diminish with increasing sample sizes. The extent of random error can be quantified during the process of estimation by confidence intervals. The width of confidence intervals is the precision of the estimate.

QUESTION 3

The standard error of 0.42% (or 0.0042) indicates that an approximate 95% CI should be the point estimate (3%, or 0.03) plus or minus 2 times this quantity (roughly 0.8%). Therefore, an approximate 95% CI would be 2.2%–3.8%.

QUESTION 4

If the method of data collection (self-report over the phone) fails to detect some cases, the prevalence estimate will be too low. Increasing the sample size will not correct this problem, so this is not a form of random error. Rather, this is a form of systematic error (more specifically, a measurement bias). Consistent with the possibility of underreporting, a study conducted by Maclaren and Best[290] at the University of New Brunswick and Thompson Rivers University reported a higher prevalence. However, there are many other possible explanations for the divergent results.

QUESTION 5

Technically, it would be correct to say that, were this study conducted many times, the confidence intervals calculated from these repetitions would include the population value 95% of the time. However, this definition seems excessively technical, because studies are never conducted many times. A usual interpretive statement would be (assuming that the study methods are considered valid) that the study shows with 95% confidence that the population value is between 0.11 and 4.15 per 100 000.

QUESTION 6

This is a trick question. There is no good reason. Most people consider the 5% value to be arbitrary. Nevertheless, there seems to be some intuitive value to it, perhaps because 5% is equivalent to 1 in 20, and human beings have 20 fingers and toes.

QUESTION 7

Again, there is no good reason. If a type II error is for some reason less problematic than a type I error, perhaps it is reasonable to tolerate a higher risk of type II error. However, in epidemiology, a type II error might mean that a preventive opportunity is missed, which is serious.

QUESTION 8

Most epidemiologists would agree that reporting an exact P value is preferable. This provides more information since a P value of 0.001, for example, implies a much lower likelihood of a chance difference than a P value of 0.05.

QUESTION 9

A P value is a probability. It is the probability of the observed results, or results that are more extreme, occurring by chance under the assumption that a null hypothesis is true. This probability can never be 0 because it is not completely impossible that the observations could occur by chance even if the null hypothesis is true. Therefore, it is better to report a very small number than to say $P = 0$—for example, it would be reasonable to say $P < 0.0001$.

QUESTION 10

(1) Confidence intervals provide a range of plausible values for an estimated parameter, which P values do not. (2) Confidence intervals usually provide all of the information that a P value provides. If a 95% confidence interval does not include a null value, then that value would be significant at the 5% level of confidence. (3) Confidence intervals are more closely connected to the values in the underlying data. A confidence interval for a frequency is a range of frequencies. A P value is merely a probability.

Chapter 6

QUESTION 1

There are 21 subjects that have DVT according to the gold standard test. Of these, 8 are positive on the colour Doppler ultrasound test, which means the sensitivity is 8/21, or 38.1%. There are 298 that are negative for DVT, of whom 275 test negative, which means the specificity is 275/298, or 92.2%.

QUESTION 2

The odds of DVT are 21/298 or 0.07. These are the pretest odds: they represent the odds in the absence of any information about the test results. The pretest probability (or prevalence) of DVT can be calculated from these odds using the formula: proportion = odds ÷ (1 + odds). For this study, the result is 0.07 ÷ 1.07 = 0.066. Because the outcome is fairly uncommon, the prevalence proportion is quite similar to the prevalence odds.

QUESTION 3

The likelihood ratio positive can be calculated as: sensitivity ÷ (1 − specificity). In this study, the result is 0.38 ÷ (1 − 0.92) = 4.9.

QUESTION 4

The posttest odds are the pretest odds multiplied by the likelihood ratio positive, or 0.07 x 4.9, which is 0.35. Without knowing the test result, the best guess about the probability of DVT was the pretest odds of approximately 7%. The likelihood ratio positive indicates that a positive test increases this fivefold.

QUESTION 5

If the pretest odds are 1.0, then the likelihood ratio positive indicates that the posttest odds would be 4.94. Converting this to a proportion—so, proportion = odds ÷ (1 + odds)—results in a positive predictive value of 83%. Bayes' theorem, as always, produces the same result: (0.38 x 0.50) ÷ [(0.38 x 0.50) + (1 − 0.92) x (1 − 0.5)] = 0.83, or 83%.

QUESTION 6

Yes, this makes perfect sense. The result (a ratio of 2 odds) helps to quantify the association of test results and disease status. It has many favourable properties. For example, health scientists tend to be familiar with odds ratios. Also the log odds ratio tends to be approximately normally distributed, which is a useful property for some types of statistical analysis. The diagnostic odds ratio is a common metric for quantifying test performance.[169] In later chapters, we will encounter many different types of odds ratios. Question 6 from chapter 10 will ask you to calculate a diagnostic odds ratio from the data in Table 11.

QUESTION 7

Because the procedure used to treat the disease is risky, there are important repercussions of false-positive test results. People may end up receiving a dangerous treatment for no reason. The probability of a false-positive result is related to the specificity of the test. Since specificity is the probability that a person who does not have the disease will have a negative test, the complementary probability is 1 minus specificity, which is the probability that a person without the disease will have a positive test result. This is called the *false-positive rate*. To minimize the false-positive rate, it is essential that this diagnostic test be highly specific. For some screening tests, where the goal is not to miss a case (a false-negative result), the most important requirement is high sensitivity. The best tests have both high sensitivity and specificity.

QUESTION 8

Continuous variables should not be routinely categorized. The justification for categorizing them is that categories (such as diagnoses) often link well with clinical decisions. A diagnosis of hypertension, for example, implies that certain actions (such as monitoring and treatment) should be taken, which creates a connection to a research literature about the effectiveness and safety of such strategies. Another example of a continuous variable that is often transformed into nominal categories is body mass index (BMI). BMI is calculated by dividing a person's weight in kilograms by their height in metres squared. A BMI < 18.5 is categorized as underweight, 18.5–24.9 is normal weight, 25–29.9 is overweight, and 30+ is obese. The justification for this categorization is that these nominal categories are associated with risks of developing health problems. The same risks do not apply in children or pregnant women, so BMI is not calculated in these groups.

There are many other examples of categorizing continuous variables. For example, definitions of diabetes are often based on measures of blood glucose, a continuous variable. Some disease definitions are not based on a simple categorization of a single continuous variable, but rather on a pattern. For example, in diabetes, the abnormality may be defined as a pattern of blood glucose after a challenge test in which a person consumes a known quantity of glucose, or when they are known to be fasting.

Here's a related example: many mental-illness diagnoses require elevated symptom levels (usually measured as an ordinal rating obtained from a scale). Exceeding a threshold of symptom severity, however, is not enough to make a diagnosis— anxiety, for example, is normal in certain circumstances (e.g., before an exam). Therefore, mental-illness diagnoses require that elevated symptom levels be present for a prolonged period of time and in situations where their occurrence is problematic.

QUESTION 9

Since the chance of a positive "test" is 50% when the disease is present, the expected value of sensitivity is 50%. Since the chance of a negative test when the disease is absent is 50%, the specificity is also 50%.

QUESTION 10
Everybody with a positive test will have the disease, such that the positive predictive value, despite the uselessness of the test, will be 100%. What makes the test
useless is that the pretest probability was also 100%, so the test results deliver no
new information.

Chapter 7

QUESTION 1
a. The performance of the algorithm in this sample is good. However, the sample
   is small ($n = 20$ with parkinsonism and 20 controls). The actual sensitivity and
   specificity of the algorithm may differ from the 100% estimates due to random
   error. As a result, the future use of the algorithm could nevertheless contribute
   to misclassification bias in assessment of the prevalence of parkinsonism.
b. All cases of diabetes will be detected since the sensitivity is 100% (note, however, that the 100% sensitivity is itself an estimate). Seventy percent specificity
   means that false positives are expected to occur with this particular algorithm.
   This will inflate the estimated prevalence because the false positives will occur
   in the numerator of the formula for prevalence.

QUESTION 2
a. Imperfect measurement creates vulnerability to bias. Because the sensitivity
   for this particular condition was quite low, it is likely that the majority of cases
   would be missed, which would likely lead to bias. It should be noted that the
   interRAI rating system had excellent performance for several other conditions.
   Traumatic brain injury stood out in the Foebel et al study as a specific condition
   where the performance of interRAI was not very good.
b. Since interRAI was highly specific, few false positives are expected. Because its
   sensitivity for traumatic brain injury was low, those with traumatic brain injury
   will be underrepresented in the numerator of the prevalence formula, leading to
   a negative bias. The expected value of the estimate is too low.

QUESTION 3
a. This type of bias (where people hide an attribute due to an awareness that it
   is negatively perceived by others) is called *social desirability bias*. If the level of
   stigma reported by people is lower than the level of stigmatizing beliefs that
   they actually hold, this will introduce bias.
b. This would be a negative bias: the mean level of stigma that is estimated will be
   lower than the actual level in the real population. Notably, during the development of the scale, Kassam et al measured the effect of social desirability on the
   scores and argued that the scale was not highly vulnerable to this type of bias.

QUESTION 4
a. It is doubtful that even those mothers searching their memories for a cause for
   the malformation would produce false-positive recollections. The tendency
   to focus on such issues would, therefore, likely improve the sensitivity of their
   reporting of such exposures. If their sensitivity of recollection was 100% and if
   no false-positive reports occur (specificity = 100%), bias would not occur.

b. The best way to control misclassification bias is when the study is designed. By ensuring accurate measurement (e.g., built-in double-checks of the self-report, or cognitive interviewing techniques that provide cues to ensure highly accurate reporting) the possibility of misclassification bias is minimized.

QUESTION 5

This is a matter of opinion. In the past, there has been much criticism of the quality of information on medical charts. However, electronic medical records are evolving and may (or may not) contain better information than the old paper charts of the past. Marrie et al also reported kappa statistics, which quantified the level of agreement between the 2 data sources without assuming that the chart review was a gold standard. This assumption is built in to the definitions of sensitivity and specificity.

QUESTION 6

If people report that they have migraines when they actually have tension headaches, this creates false-positive test results and reflects an issue with the specificity of the measurement strategy. False-positive results inflate the numerator of the equation for prevalence, resulting in its overestimation.

QUESTION 7

In a prevalence study, a specificity of 99% implies that 1% of the population will be falsely classified as having the disease. Since the disease is very rare, a much larger number of false positives are expected, relative to true positives, which greatly inflates the prevalence estimate.

QUESTION 8

A case definition that requires only a single administrative code is likely to be highly sensitive, since everyone with MS is very likely to receive at least 1 such code. However, it may be nonspecific, because a patient may present with symptoms suggestive of MS and the G35 code may then be used to describe the focus of a visit even though the diagnosis is unconfirmed. Requiring 2 G35 codes 6 months apart is likely to make the diagnosis much more specific, since 6 months is usually long enough to confirm a diagnosis. Therefore, false positives are unlikely. However, people with an onset of MS within the past 6 months will be false negatives, leading to lower sensitivity.

QUESTION 9

The potential flaw in this approach is that the number of false negatives (due to imperfect sensitivity) and false positives (due to imperfect specificity) could balance, such that an inaccurate measure could nevertheless produce an unbiased prevalence estimate.

QUESTION 10

It has been shown that people tend to exaggerate their height and minimize their weight when these variables are measured using self-report.[291] This would produce false-negative results in a self-report survey and a systematic underestimation of prevalence.

Chapter 8

QUESTION 1

a. An unwillingness to disclose excessive use of substances could lower the sensitivity of the interview to detect these conditions. This could introduce bias, but it would not be selection bias. This would be a form of misclassification bias.

b. The fear of stigma may have caused people with mental illnesses to be less likely to participate in the survey than people without such difficulties. This would result in the numerator of the prevalence equation being diminished and in estimates that are negatively biased.

c. If there is no selection, then selection bias cannot occur. However, bias could still arise from problems affecting participation—for example, from problems with missing data. Investigators don't generally label bias due to missing data *selection bias*, although both types of bias occur through similar mechanisms if investigators handle missing data by excluding those participants from the calculations. *Bias due to missing data* is a better, descriptive label.

QUESTION 2

The question appears to state that the selection probabilities would be lower in people with dementia. Therefore, participation in the survey is related to the attribute whose frequency is being estimated. This is a typical situation in which selection bias could occur. However, if the target population is the household population, then the target of estimation is the prevalence of dementia in the household population (not the entire population, which would include household residents and others, such as residents of institutions and homeless people). For this reason, bias would not occur, at least not through the mechanism specified.

QUESTION 3

Such studies typically use the entire population in their denominator. This is the correct denominator, because universal health care in Canada essentially ensures that the entire population is registered with a provincial, or territorial, health care insurance plan. There are a few exceptions, such as members of the armed forces. The fact that some people with this condition may not have seen a physician during the study period (nor been admitted to hospital) would not be a cause of selection bias. This would be a form of misclassification bias: some of those people would have been misclassified as not having the illness, but they would still be included in the prevalence calculation (they would appear in the denominator).

QUESTION 4

a. Yes: if symptoms of the illness cause people with schizophrenia to be less likely to provide consent than others, selection bias would result.

b. The numerator of the prevalence equation would be too small, so that the prevalence of schizophrenia would be underestimated. The direction of bias is negative.

QUESTION 5

Yes: attrition affects participation in prospective studies. If an illness-related characteristic increases the risk of attrition, bias could occur in the estimated parameter—in this study, an incidence proportion. Bias due to attrition—because it is related to participation in a study and behaves similarly to other forms of selection bias—is often classified as a form of selection bias in epidemiology.

QUESTION 6

Socioeconomic status is a determinant, or at least a marker, of a reduced likelihood of participation in a study and is also associated with many health problems. If a study sample has reduced participation from people of lower socioeconomic status, it is likely to have reduced participation from those who have diseases, which would often lead to underestimation of prevalence. This problem can be avoided by designing studies in ways to ensure that every member of the target population has a known probability of selection, and a very high probability of full and successful participation in the study.

QUESTION 7

This would not cause selection bias since it does not influence who participates in a study. Instead, it would diminish the sensitivity of the measure, since patients or physicians unaware of a condition would misclassify cases of the disease as disease-free (false-negative misclassification). This would cause bias, but it would not be selection bias, it would be misclassification bias.

QUESTION 8

This situation will result in selection bias. People with glaucoma will be less likely to participate than people without glaucoma, which would lead to underestimation of prevalence. Increasing the sample size will not correct the problem. This bias arises due to a study-design defect that allows the probability of participation to depend on disease status. To eliminate this bias, the enrollment procedures would need to be changed (e.g., by using a verbal-consent procedure rather than a written form) so that the probability of participation no longer depends on disease status.

QUESTION 9

This is another example of a study-design defect that would lead to selection bias. If those with the syndrome are more likely to participate as a result of this defect, the prevalence will be overestimated. When estimating prevalence or a related (frequency-based) parameter, the solution is always the same—to ensure that the probability of participation is unrelated to disease status. These investigators should ensure that everyone, or almost everyone, in their sample is included in the study regardless of whether they are at home when the study personnel arrive. The study personnel may need to make multiple visits or make alternate arrangements to do their assessment. They must do whatever it takes to ensure a very high rate of participation in their sample.

QUESTION 10

Even though the study-design defect is related to measurement, this is not an error of classification. The respondents who refused to answer the question were not placed in the wrong cell of the 1×2 table, they were simply not included in the analysis. Therefore, this is an issue of participation rather than classification. When a participant is misclassified, they remain a participant in the study and appear in the 1×2 table from which prevalence is calculated. It may seem odd to label this type of bias as selection bias, since the selection of respondents is said to be perfect. But their participation is not perfect—indeed, since the probability of contributing to the estimate depends on the characteristic under assessment, selection bias will occur.

Chapter 9

QUESTION 1

a. This is indirect standardization. Note that values for the number of observed and expected cases have been reported.

b. The standardized mortality ratio (SMR) is 42/46.28 = 0.91.

c. This SMR does not suggest that increased mortality from this particular cause is associated with this exposure. An SMR less than 1 may reflect a healthy worker effect.

QUESTION 2

a. This a hugely elevated SMR. It indicates that these women are dying at a rate nearly 50 times that of the general population, after adjustment for age.

b. Intravenous drug use itself is dangerous. Many of these women would have also been homeless, and therefore vulnerable to violence, victimization, and many other risk factors for mortality (exposure, malnutrition, etc.). Socioeconomic deprivation is a major risk factor for mortality. HIV and sex-trade involvement were strongly associated with mortality in this analysis.

QUESTION 3

Indirect standardization can control for the effects of basic demographic variables such as age and sex (and also race, see question 4) because mortality rates for the general population are usually known for such variables. This allows an expected number of outcomes to be calculated for the exposed group. However, other confounders (e.g., smoking status) could account for an elevated SMR and are not addressed during the standardization procedure.

QUESTION 4

According to the authors: "Given that illicit drug users are often unaware of or misperceive the impacts of drug use on safe driving, it may be important for health-service or public-health interventions to address such biases and improve road safety." Long-term record linkage studies of this type may not provide the detailed information needed to formulate such interventions, but they do produce evidence relevant to the generation of such hypotheses.

QUESTION 5

Direct standardization is often used with mortality data, which is merely a specific type of incidence data. Direct and indirect standardization can both be used with other types of incident events. In this case, the value of the procedure is that the 3 ethnic groups can be compared without worrying that differences merely reflect the demographic characteristics adjusted for in the standardization (sex, and age based on 10-year age increments).

QUESTION 6

Standardization procedures make 2 different populations more comparable. If the goal is to plan services, then the actual number or proportion of the population with a health outcome is more appropriate than a standardized estimate.

QUESTION 7

Canadian studies usually use census data. Age and sex is collected in the census, which is conducted every 5 years in Canada. If the goal is to standardize for demographic features that are not contained in the basic census, the 2016 census included a "long form" component (this had been cancelled in the 2011 census) that includes detailed information. The WHO also offers a version of a standard population.[292]

QUESTION 8

An SMR of 2 should not cause concern because they are nursing home patients. This population is expected to have a higher mortality than the general population for reasons other than their age. The healthy worker effect has a similar basis, but going in the other direction. Workers are expected to be healthier than members of the general population, so an SMR of 1 is a cause for some concern.

QUESTION 9

The advantage of stratification is that the age-specific estimates remain accessible, providing a more detailed picture of the mortality pattern in the population. The disadvantage is that the stratum-specific estimates may be less precise (more subject to random error) than the overall standardized estimate.

QUESTION 10

This would defeat the purpose of doing the stratification. The point of the exercise is to make the estimates more comparable. Weighting them by their own (different) population values would not accomplish this.

Chapter 10

QUESTION 1

Advantages:

- Provides a snapshot of disease burden at a point in time, which is valuable information for those planning and administering health services. As cross-sectional studies often take the form of surveys they can adopt sampling procedures that are well suited to making population inference about prevalence.

- These studies can be completed on a shorter timeline and often with less expense than longitudinal studies of a comparable size and complexity.

- As examples such as the Canadian Community Health Survey attest, it is often possible to incorporate multiple exposures and multiple disease outcomes in a single cross-sectional survey.

- Since the data are collected at a single point in time there is not an issue with loss to follow-up in cross-sectional studies, as there may be in longitudinal studies.

Disadvantages:

- Only prevalence can be estimated from a cross-sectional survey, not incidence. Therefore, such studies cannot usually provide information about risk.

- The results of a cross-sectional study can be misleading if there are changes over time (e.g., seasonal changes) in prevalence.

- The design is not strong for determining causation because the temporal relationship between exposure and disease can generally not be elucidated by cross-sectional studies.

- These studies are inefficient for rare diseases and rare exposures since even large samples may include too few cases to allow precise estimation.

QUESTION 2

This statement is sometimes made, usually based on the (generally true) assertion that the temporal sequence of exposure and disease cannot be clarified from cross-sectional data. However, cross-sectional data provide clear temporality in some situations—for example, studies of the adult outcomes of birth or childhood-related exposures, genetic inheritance, and congenital malformations.

QUESTION 3

a. The prevalence calculation includes all those with the disease in the numerator, regardless of their exposure status: 420/3090, or 0.136.[167]

b. An approximate 95% CI can be calculated using the normal approximation of the binomial distribution. The standard error of the estimated proportion is:

$$\text{Standard Error} = \sqrt{\frac{p \times (1-p)}{n}}$$

For this study, the standard error is 0.006. The approximate confidence limits are then 0.136 +/− 1.96 x 0.006, leading to a 95% CI of 0.124–0.148. Of course, an exact confidence interval is always preferable and in this case the result (from statistical software) is 0.124–0.149. In this case, the approximate formula performed quite well.

QUESTION 4

The prevalence difference is the prevalence in the exposed (0.171) minus the prevalence in the nonexposed (0.069), which is 0.102, or 10.2%.

QUESTION 5

a. The odds in the exposed is 348/1692 = 0.21 and ln(0.21) = −1.58. Among the nonexposed, the odds are 72/978 = 0.074 and ln(0.074) = −2.61.

b. The first step is to calculate α. The indicator variable representing exposure has a value of 0 in the nonexposed group, which means −2.61 is α. The log odds in the exposed are −1.58. Since $\alpha + \beta$ must be −1.58 and α is −2.61 (see above), β must be 1.03. The linear equation is therefore: log odds of impulse control disorder = $-2.61 + 1.03X_e$.

c. The inverse log of β (which has a value of 1.027, rounded to 1.03 in the equation above) is 2.79. This is the odds ratio. In this kind of equation, β is a log odds ratio.

QUESTION 6

The diagnostic odds ratio reflects the association between having a condition and having a positive test. The calculation is the usual one. Using data from Table 11, the odds ratio is 8 x 275 / 23 x 13, which is 7.4.

QUESTION 7

a. In a cross-sectional study, information about exposure and disease is collected at a single point in time. However, studies may take several months to complete. For example, the Canadian Community Health Surveys collect cross-sectional data on a continuous year-round basis. It is correct to classify this study as a cross-sectional study.

b. A cross-sectional study that collects data during a specific season can produce estimates that do not reflect the health status of the population in other seasons. However, a cross-sectional study that collects data in different seasons can make valid comparisons among seasons. In this study, vitamin D insufficiency was found to be more common when blood was drawn in the spring than in the summer. This makes sense, since vitamin D is synthesized in skin exposed to sunlight. The suggestion that deficiency emerges during the winter may have important implications for future research and policy. Another example is a cross-sectional study looking at seasonality and depression in Canada.[293] This study found a higher prevalence of major depression in the winter months, which may have implications for planning of mental-health services. These 2 studies illustrate an important point about the listed advantages and disadvantages of study designs. Such lists can be useful as a general guide, but they should not be applied inflexibly to all studies.

QUESTION 8

One reason is that the temporality of the exposure and disease is usually unclear in cross-sectional studies. A cause must precede the effect, which can rarely be accurately confirmed by a cross-sectional study. A second reason is mortality. Prevalence is not only a reflection of risk in various groups, but also a reflection of survival and persistence of a disease. If an exposure increases the mortality associated with a disease, it will lower the prevalence. In a disease from which recovery is possible, an exposure that prolongs the disease will cause the prevalence to increase.

QUESTION 9

Generally speaking, it is fair to say that cross-sectional studies are descriptive in nature. However, many studies (both cross-sectional and otherwise) have both descriptive and analytic goals. As a result, when classifying study designs, it is usually best to focus on more tangible features than the descriptive-versus-analytic goals of a study. Many textbooks of epidemiology, however, continue to classify study designs according to whether they are predominantly descriptive or analytic.

QUESTION 10

Statistics Canada has conducted several longitudinal health studies (e.g., the National Population Health Survey, and the National Longitudinal Study of Children and Youth), but its emphasis is on cross-sectional studies. This emphasis is consistent with the critical role of Statistics Canada in health surveillance and hypothesis generation. National cross-sectional studies are very difficult for individual researchers to conduct. Statistics Canada, however—as a quasi-governmental agency—has the national infrastructure and expertise to make very high-quality cross-sectional estimates.

Chapter 11

QUESTION 1
Advantages:

- Very efficient for rare diseases.
- Can easily examine multiple exposures for a single disease.
- Compared to longitudinal studies they are inexpensive and can be relatively quick to complete.
- Able to cope with long induction and latency periods.

Disadvantages:

- Vulnerable to bias due to selection and misclassification.
- Cannot study multiple diseases.
- Inefficient for rare exposures.
- Cannot assess risk—only exposure-disease associations.

QUESTION 2
The incubation period is a period during which the infection has become established but has not yet progressed to where it is clinically evident. Therefore, this is best regarded as a latency period. In infectious diseases, the offending microbe is a necessary component cause, by definition, but is rarely sufficient. Since some exposed persons do not contract infectious diseases, there must be other component causes that these resilient individuals do not have.

QUESTION 3
a. The odds ratio is 0.82, as reported in the study.[170]
b. To calculate the percent reduction from a relative measure such as an odds ratio or risk ratio, subtract 1 from the odds ratio or risk ratio and multiply by 100. An odds ratio of 1.5 implies a percent increase of $(1.5 - 1.0) \times 100 = 50\%$ in the odds of disease. An odds ratio of 0.82 implies a $(0.82 - 1.0) \times 100 = -18\%$ reduction in the odds of rupture among those treated with angiotensin-converting enzyme (ACE) inhibitors.

QUESTION 4
The odds of rupture in those being treated with ACE inhibitors is only 0.82 that of those who are untreated. The results are interpreted in terms of odds, so there is no concern about the rare disease assumption. This assumption only reflects the extent to which odds and odds ratios can serve as an approximation of proportions and relative proportions.

QUESTION 5
This is not screening in the sense used in epidemiology and public health, where screening means secondary prevention or early intervention (during a detectable

preclinical or latent phase of the disease). A better term for the effort described in the question is *case finding*. Underdetection is not a de facto reason for screening, although it is occasionally regarded as such. A critique of "screening" for depression has been published by Thombs et al.[294]

QUESTION 6

If this statement were correct, there would be no basis for conducting case-control studies. Fortunately, it is not correct. The selection probabilities for cases are always higher than for controls in a case-control study. However, as long as selection probabilities do not differ in relation to exposure status in a way that depends on disease status, bias will not occur.

QUESTION 7

This is not true. Recall that bias indicates a systematic deviation of a study's estimate from the true underlying population value. The estimated odds ratio for a rare disease from a case-control study should be close to the underlying population odds ratio if the study meets the following standard: it uses incident data, it is free of study-design defects, and it has an adequate sample size. When a disease is not rare, however, the estimated odds ratio from a case-control study will not necessarily resemble the underlying risk ratio, since the rare disease assumption is violated. In a case-control study using prevalent cases of a common disease, and in the absence of study-design defects, the estimates will resemble the underlying prevalence odds ratio, but not the prevalence ratio.

QUESTION 8

In theory, primary prevention is best because it prevents the disease from occurring at all. However, the feasibility of primary prevention depends on the existence of modifiable risk factors.

QUESTION 9

There is no checklist to decide when screening is feasible, but a variety of factors play into this decision. A screening test must be very accurate and very safe if screening is to be feasible. Inaccurate tests either miss cases (lack of sensitivity) or detect false positives (lack of specificity). The latter is often particularly problematic as a positive screen requires further testing and may expose people to associated dangers. Since predictive value depends on the base rate of a disease, screening is usually more useful for fairly common diseases (when a disease is common, a larger proportion of positive screens will be true rather than false-positive results). There must also be a long enough latency phase to allow early detection. In addition, there must be beneficial, affordable, and safe ways of intervening during that latency phase. A common mistake is to assume that screening is always useful for diseases that are sometimes missed in clinical practice. But, for the reasons stated above, this is an inadequate justification for screening.

QUESTION 10

In a log-transformed model, the ß coefficient is the difference between 2 log odds, which, due to the properties of logarithms, is equivalent to the log of the ratio of those odds.

Chapter 12

QUESTION 1

a. Social desirability bias occurs when people attempt to present as normal by providing inaccurate answers. This would result in false-negative classification, or low sensitivity.

b. It seems unlikely that the sensitivity of these instruments would be affected by exposure, so the most likely type of bias would be nondifferential misclassification bias. However, since the investigators are concerned that impulsive behaviour may be caused by these drugs, it is conceivable that the exposure could change the measurement properties of the diagnostic instruments. For example, people might impulsively provide certain answers when taking these medications, potentially increasing the sensitivity or reducing the specificity among the exposed participants.

c. Nondifferential misclassification bias is predictably in the direction of the null value of the parameter being estimated. In the case of the odds ratio, the estimates would be biased towards the null value of 1.

QUESTION 2

a. Recall bias refers to increased recollection of past exposures among people with a disease. The term can mean other things, so more specific terminology is preferable—e.g., differential misclassification of exposure with greater sensitivity in the cases.

b. This type of bias in case-control studies tends to inflate the value of the odds ratio.

c. In a disease that causes cognitive problems (such as dementia), those with the disease may be less likely to recall past exposures than controls. Their defective recall could lead to bias in the other direction. This possibility illustrates the hazards of using nonspecific terminology such as *recall bias*.

QUESTION 3

Any type of misclassification can introduce bias. Administrative data are not collected for research purposes and may therefore be inaccurate. Such inaccuracy introduces bias into the estimation of epidemiologic parameters. The fact that inaccuracy of exposure classification would not depend on disease status in most situations does not mean that bias will not occur, only that the misclassification bias will be nondifferential.

QUESTION 4

a. The study used careful measurement strategies, so it is not vulnerable to misclassification bias. Theoretically, any degree of imperfection in measurement can introduce bias, but minor inaccuracy will normally be a minor threat to the validity of the study. No epidemiologic study is perfect.

b. Similarly, this form of bias is possible in theory, but only a tiny proportion of the population are likely to fall into this category. The impact of such bias will be negligible.

QUESTION 5

This is a situation where the type of misclassification bias is of critical importance. Because the bias is almost certainly nondifferential, the expected direction of bias is towards the null value and it is likely that the actual associations are stronger than reported.

QUESTION 6

The goal is always to produce a valid estimate, so in this sense they are both equally bad. When reporting a significant association between a risk factor and a disease, however, authors often argue that if misclassification bias may have occurred, it would have been nondifferential. The implication of such a claim is that any bias would be in the direction of the null value (e.g., towards 1.0 for an odds ratio or risk ratio, and towards 0 for a risk difference) and so could not invalidate the finding that an association exists. If the authors have shown an association and nondifferential misclassification is a possibility, this suggests that the actual association is probably even stronger than reported. In this scenario, the existence of an association is not challenged by the possible occurrence of nondifferential misclassification bias. A critical reader, however, would not ignore the fact that nondifferential misclassification introduces systematic error into an estimated association.

QUESTION 7

Differential misclassification occurs if the sensitivity or specificity of a measure of exposure differs between cases and controls. Procedures to prevent this include the use of objective measurement strategies that are not subject to errors in recall, and the blinding of interviewers to study hypotheses (which they may otherwise seek unconsciously to confirm) or to the case/control status of the person that they are interviewing. If self-reported recall of exposure is the only option, specialized cognitive interviewing techniques can help to ensure accuracy. For example, orienting or priming statements that are designed to increase the sensitivity of recall in controls can offset the lowered sensitivity that can lead to recall bias.

QUESTION 8

It is possible that a case definition would be slightly insensitive (failing to detect some cases) but also sufficiently nonspecific to offset this insensitivity with false positives, leading to a valid prevalence or incidence estimate. This inaccuracy of measurement would nevertheless cause nondifferential misclassification bias in an analytical study using this same case definition.

QUESTION 9

The usual problem is that cases spend more time reflecting on the possible causes of their disease. As a result, their recall of exposure is more sensitive compared to controls, who have no specific reason to reflect on their exposures. This lowered sensitivity in the controls leads to a lowered frequency of exposure in the controls, leading to overestimation of the odds ratio.

QUESTION 10

For exactly the same reason, increased sensitivity of recall for past exposure could lead to recall bias in a cross-sectional study.

Chapter 13

QUESTION 1

Advantages:

- They can clarify the temporal relationship between exposure and disease.
- They allow an assessment of risk as well as association.
- They can look at multiple outcomes of an exposure.
- Prospective cohort studies are protected from selection bias since, in order for selection bias to occur, participation must be affected both by exposure and disease. This is unlikely to occur in a prospective cohort study since the disease (or other outcome) has not occurred at the time of selection.

Disadvantages:

- They tend to be expensive, since subjects must be tracked prospectively over time.
- They can take a long time to produce results, especially in situations where induction periods are very long.
- They are usually not an effective way to study very rare outcomes.
- They are vulnerable to bias resulting from attrition.

QUESTION 2

It is too simple to say that one study design is better than another. The best study design must be chosen for a particular research question. A prospective cohort design may be impossible to apply for certain diseases (such as those with a very long induction period). A poorly conducted prospective cohort study may yield lower quality estimates than a higher quality case-control study.

QUESTION 3

a. 978/6 645 = 14.7%, which is the 10-year incidence proportion reported in the study.[197(p1476)]

b. To cause selection bias, attrition must be related to both exposure and disease. It seems plausible that people in poorer health, perhaps those having more fractures, would be more likely to drop out of the study. This would result in an underestimation of the incidence proportion, but would not necessarily cause bias in a measure of association. If multiple fractures tended to lead to drop out in the nonexposed subjects, but did not do this to the same extent in the exposed subjects, then the estimate could be biased in a positive direction: the incidence of fractures in the nonexposed group would be underestimated to a greater extent than in the exposed, diminishing the denominator of the risk ratio relatively more than the numerator. This would increase (inflate) the value of the estimated risk ratio. While this could occur in theory, it does not seem likely to occur. It seems perhaps more likely that depressed people (including many more of the exposed group) might be less able to cope with the pain of the fractures and more likely to drop out, which would create a negative bias in the risk ratio.

c. There is no reason to expect that the measurement of antidepressant use would be more or less accurate depending on subsequent fractures. Inaccurate classification of exposure could lead to bias, which would be nondifferential and in the direction of the null value. Bias of this type cannot explain the association observed, but leads to suspicion that it might be stronger than reported.

QUESTION 4

Any of these measures could be chosen. Since most people understand proportions better than odds, the odds ratio may not be the best choice. The risk ratio would be a good choice, but a long-term study may experience attrition from its sample, which is difficult to deal with using a risk ratio. A hazard ratio derives from survival analysis methods and can accommodate attrition by censoring observations at the time subjects leave the sample. This would therefore be the preferred measure.

QUESTION 5

A recurrent disease is very difficult to study cross-sectionally or retrospectively. It can be difficult for people to remember the onsets and remissions of their illness. The prospective cohort design allows this information to be collected prospectively, allowing much more accurate measurement.

QUESTION 6

This is a dynamic cohort. In a fixed cohort, all participants are recruited at a single point in time.

QUESTION 7

The odds ratio can be used, although it is not a requirement (as it is in a case-control study). Also, in a prospective cohort study, the odds ratio has the same issues as the risk ratio (not accounting for the departure of incident cases from the population at risk during follow-up) and only approximates the risk ratio if the incidence is low.

QUESTION 8

a. Yes. Retrospective cohort studies are often carried out in occupational settings. Since workers typically differ from the general population in terms of their age and sex, the SMR is often used as a measure of association in such studies. For example, see a study of Air Canada pilots by Band et al.[223]

b. In an occupational retrospective cohort study, the process of selecting an exposed cohort from an occupational setting leads to selection of a cohort that tends to be healthier than the general population. This better state of health is related to outcome as well as exposure. The error is systematic and is not corrected by increasing the sample size. It does not involve measurement error: it is related to selection. For these reasons, the healthy worker effect can be viewed as a type of selection bias.

QUESTION 9

Disease status can be confirmed at the start of a prospective cohort study at a time when the participants receive a detailed assessment. Indeed, assessment of incidence depends on known disease status at baseline, so investigators typically invest adequate resources in this. Also, biased application of measurement instruments in relation to outcome (differential misclassification) is impossible since the outcome has not occurred at this baseline time point. By contrast, during follow-up, exposure status is known, potentially resulting in closer surveillance of the exposed (leading to increased sensitivity of disease assessment in the exposed) and raising the spectre of differential misclassification bias.

QUESTION 10
This is a prospective cohort study. The analysis of data from a prospective cohort study must necessarily occur after completion of the study. This does not make it a retrospective study. The important point is this: the data were collected by following participants from a baseline time point into the future—in other words, forward in time.

Chapter 14

QUESTION 1
According to the traditional definition, a confounding variable:

- must be a risk factor for the outcome under investigation
- must be associated with the exposure
- must not occur on the causal pathway under investigation

According to a DAG-based definition of confounding, a confounding variable:

- ·must be a cause of the outcome under investigation
- must be a cause of the exposure

QUESTION 2
a. The β coefficient in the logistic regression model is a log odds ratio. Since the odds ratio is 2.72, the β coefficient is 1.001 (the log of 2.72).

b. The lack of change in the crude odds ratio with adjustment for these covariates indicates that these variables did not confound the association under investigation.

QUESTION 3
Since the adjusted odds ratio is essentially the same as the crude (unadjusted) odds ratio, the model shows that these variables did not act as confounding variables in the analysis.

QUESTION 4
a. This is not confounding. In confounding, the stratified estimates differ from the crude estimate, but resemble each another. Here, the stratum-specific estimates differ from each another, which indicates effect measure modification by age.

b. When there is effect measure modification, the stratum-specific estimates should be reported, as was done by these investigators.

QUESTION 5
a. Age is a strong determinant of mortality. If depression is more common in young people, age could be a strong confounder of the depression-mortality

association. Since depression is most common among young people, and younger people are much less likely to die, the possible effect of depression may be masked by the effect of age.

b. If variables such as smoking, which are independent determinants of mortality, are associated with depression, they may act as confounding variables. What appears to be an effect of depression in age- and sex-adjusted estimates may actually be due to the effect of variables such as smoking.

QUESTION 6

If wine drinking is protective and wine drinkers are more likely to use benzodiaze-pines, the protective effect of wine drinking will make the benzodiazepines appear less harmful. In the words of the authors: "The effect of not adjusting for these fac-tors was likely to be conservative."[175]

QUESTION 7

The authors' conclusion implies that interventions to reduce sodium intake may be valuable in people with hypertension who have high sodium diets, because this intervention may prevent cardiovascular events and deaths in this group. How-ever, very low sodium intake may be harmful in other groups, such as those with-out hypertension or those with hypertension but low sodium intake. The authors' conclusion reflects the importance of effect modification. If the effect of an inter-vention differs between groups, the intervention should target the group where it can convey benefits and not groups where it may convey harm. However, it is important to note that the authors' conclusion came after the publication of their study.[295,296]

QUESTION 8

This assertion makes a lot of sense. Whether a variable acts as a confounder depends on its association with exposure and disease, and confounding is detected during data analysis by determining whether an adjustment (e.g., in a regression model or in a stratified analysis) changes the estimated effect of an exposure. The statistical significance of the association between an extraneous variable and an outcome is not a good way to determine whether there is confounding.

QUESTION 9

The main goal of analytical epidemiology is to identify causal connections between modifiable risk factors and disease outcomes in order to allow prevention. In this case, public policies such as zoning regulations could be used to increase green-ness and thereby help to prevent prostate (and perhaps other) cancers. Increased physical activity and a lower odds of being overweight or obese are possible mechanisms—or links in a causal chain—by which greenness may lower the risk of prostate cancer. So, these are mediating variables that should not be treated as confounding variables.

QUESTION 10

This would cause confounding. Disease severity is associated with exposure if it affects treatment decisions, and disease severity is usually a determinant of out-come. This type of confounding is called confounding by severity. A related idea is that treatment decisions may be based on expected prognosis. For example, phy-sicians may prescribe particular treatments for patients who, in the estimation of the physicians, have a negative prognosis. This type of confounding is called *channelling bias*. This specialized terminology is not really necessary, as it is sufficient to specify that the threat to validity arises from confounding and to describe the underlying mechanism. The best solution to these difficult issues of confounding is randomization, which helps to ensure that the exposure (treatment) is unrelated to severity or prognosis.

Chapter 15

QUESTION 1
The best strategy is to measure all suspected or known risk factors for the outcome under study. Potential confounders must be associated with exposure as well as outcome, but there is rarely sufficient information to make a firm determination about whether a potential confounder is or is not associated with exposure. These determinations may engage information from diverse sources, such as basic science knowledge of the physiology of the disease, clinical observations, expert opinions, or plain common sense. They usually require a good literature review and consultation with experts.

QUESTION 2
A confounding variable must be associated with exposure and must be an independent determinant of disease. Female sex is associated with multiple sclerosis. However, in this study the exposed and nonexposed groups were matched on sex, so there will be no association between exposure and this potential confounding variable in the sample. Sex can therefore not act as a confounding variable.

QUESTION 3
This pattern is suggestive of effect measure modification and not confounding. After stratification for a confounding variable, the stratum-specific estimates should be different than the crude estimate and similar to each another. In this case, they appear to differ from each other.

QUESTION 4
Models can sometimes avoid the need for arbitrary stratification—for example, when a continuous variable such as age is a potential confounder. In doing so, they avoid the sparse-data problems that plague stratified analysis. They are better for examining multiple strata of a single potential confounding variable or for simultaneously examining the effects of multiple confounding variables.

QUESTION 5
Most epidemiologists believe that stratified analysis continues to play an important role. Stratified analysis involves making tables, so it may offer a better connection to the data than the more abstract output of regression modelling. In practice, many analysts carry out stratified analysis, but often include only model-based output in published studies.

QUESTION 6
It is never possible to ensure that every potentially relevant variable has been measured, since the etiology of disease is incompletely understood. In principle, any

variable that may modify an effect should be included. Since published information on effect modification is often scarce, it may be necessary to make these decisions based on what is known, or hypothesized, about the underlying biology. It is better to err on the side of inclusion in these decisions, since the modifying effects of an unmeasured variable cannot be assessed.

QUESTION 7

Study Finding	Interpretation	What should be reported?
No heterogeneity, stratified estimates resemble crude.	a	d
Heterogeneity	b	e
No heterogeneity, stratified estimates differ from crude.	c	f

Scenario *a* is a situation in which there is no effect modification or confounding. Scenario *b* represents effect modification. Scenario *c* represents confounding.

QUESTION 8

Scenario *d* is a situation in which the crude measure of effect may be reported. As there is no effect modification, stratified estimates do not need to be reported and, because there is no confounding, adjustment for confounding is not necessary. Scenario *e* requires that the stratum-specific effects be reported. Both the crude and adjusted estimates obscure the heterogeneity, thereby misrepresenting the findings. Scenario *f* represents the occurrence of confounding. An adjusted estimate must be reported. The stratified estimates are adjusted, but are likely to suffer from imprecision. Therefore an estimate with a model-based adjustment or a Mantel-Haenszel pooled estimate is preferable.

QUESTION 9

The odds ratio has the same interpretation as always: it is the ratio of odds of disease at a particular level of exposure to that of another level of exposure. In this case, it represents the change over 1 unit of age (in this case years). Often, the size of the estimate is tiny (e.g., an odds ratio of 1.01). In the case of age measured in years, this would suggest a 1% increase in the odds of disease per year—a sizable effect.

QUESTION 10

This way of thinking does not fit with the approach taken in epidemiological analysis. In epidemiology, the goal is usually to characterize an exposure-disease relationship, so modelling is primarily used as a tool to address the dual issues of confounding and effect modification. A decision to keep or remove a variable from a model therefore should not be based on its statistical significance, but rather on its effects (either in terms of effect modification or confounding) on an exposure-disease association. Nevertheless, you will encounter studies in which investigators have removed variables from a model because of a lack of statistical significance. This approach is not necessarily problematic, since the lack of significance may often indicate lack of association between the potential confounder and disease, in which case confounding would not occur.

Chapter 16

QUESTION 1

The key difference between a nested case-control study and a case-cohort study is that the case-control study selects a referent, or control, group that includes only respondents who do not have the disease. In contrast, a case-cohort study selects a subcohort representative of the entire cohort from which the cases later arose.

a. Case-cohort studies have an important advantage over nested case-control studies. In the nested case-control design, a new set of controls needs to be selected for each outcome examined. If a single control is to be selected for each case, controls should be selected from among those without the disease at the time when an incident case emerges. With the case-cohort design, multiple outcomes can be examined using the same subcohort as a referent group. This counteracts a limitation of the case-control design—its usual ability to examine only a single outcome.

b. The main advantage of case-cohort studies over prospective cohort studies is efficiency. Case-cohort studies can reduce costs by taking expensive measurements only in the cases and the subcohort, not the entire cohort.

QUESTION 2

a. This kind of study design is sometimes called an *interrupted time series*, since it looks for a change in the pattern of an outcome before and after some key event (in this case the introduction of sophisticated medical treatments). However, the study design is ecological. Ecological studies use aggregate units of analysis, which can be geographic areas, political units, or units of time. They are comparing a set of years before and after the introduction of the new treatments and are examining whether a difference in exposure within these years is associated with the rate of surgery (an aggregate measure).

b. Always be careful about making causal inference from ecological data, because of the possibility of ecological fallacy. Here, even though the rate of surgery declined in association with the introduction of the new medical therapies, the study does not actually confirm that the people who are avoiding surgery are getting the medical treatments instead.

QUESTION 3

In a retrospective cohort design, selection is usually based on an assessment of exposure. Typically, a comparison is made to the general population using an SMR, although some retrospective cohort studies have both exposed and nonexposed cohorts, which allow them to calculate parameters such as risk ratios or hazard ratios. These studies have a forward logical direction, from exposure to disease. In contrast, the case-cohort design has a backward logical direction, comparing a series of cases to a referent cohort in terms of their exposure frequency.

QUESTION 4

The main advantage of the case-crossover design is that—because this design makes comparisons within the same people, often over a short period—it can account (essentially through matching) for a large number of time-invariant personal characteristics that might otherwise act as confounding variables.

QUESTION 5

The key advantage of randomized controlled trials is the unique ability of randomization to address both measured and unmeasured confounding variables, by helping to ensure that any such variables will be approximately equally distributed between the comparison groups.

QUESTION 6

By matching its observations within individual people and basing comparisons on different time intervals, the case-crossover design is able to control confounding due to any personal characteristic that does not change over time. However, if changes occur over time in a personal characteristic that is an independent determinant of disease, the effects of this characteristic could become intermixed with the effect of exposure, and confounding could occur.

QUESTION 7

Many randomized controlled trials seek to evaluate the efficacy of treatments. Companies, such as drug companies, often sponsor these trials, and these companies have a vested interest in documenting the efficacy of their products. As such, it's a concern that stringent selection criteria might be motivated by a desire to magnify the effect of the treatment. This is an issue of generalizability, implying that the results of the trial may not apply to real-world populations. However, there is a scientific logic to the strategy of sacrificing some degree of generalizability for better validity, because validity and generalizability are hierarchical concepts. Generalizability is a meaningless concept for an invalid result, so it is essential that randomized controlled trials provide a valid assessment of efficacy before issues of generalizability can be fully considered.

QUESTION 8

A popular strategy is to conduct a randomized controlled trial in a real-world population, without the application of stringent selection and eligibility criteria. Such trials are called *pragmatic randomized controlled trials*.

QUESTION 9

In the study, the outcome is driving under the influence of cannabis, which is an individual-level outcome. Even though 2 exposures were area-based, the study is best regarded as a cross-sectional study. It is not uncommon for cross-sectional studies to include aggregate measures of exposure. These are not just rough approximations of individual exposure: they convey important information about the environment in which an individual lives. For example, commonly used indices for social and material deprivation are based on census information for a geographical area such as a census dissemination area.[242] This, in itself, does not make a study ecological.

QUESTION 10

Unlike most of the study designs used in epidemiologic research, ecological studies often use correlation coefficients. Ecological studies are usually looking for the sort of association that is best expressed as a correlation (e.g., whether mortality from cardiovascular disease tends to decrease as per capita consumption of fish increases). Ecological data cannot be used with more traditional parameters, such as risk ratios, odds ratios, and so on. The use of correlational methods is so common in ecological studies that, in the past, ecological studies were sometimes called *correlational studies.*

Chapter 17

QUESTION 1

a. The implication is that 9% of high blood pressure could be avoided if people kept their indoor living temperature above 18 degrees.

b. This interpretation depends on a series of assumptions, including that the cross-sectional estimate of association reflects a relative risk. Generally, prevalence ratios or prevalence odds ratios should not be accepted as a measure of relative risk. Risk cannot be estimated from cross-sectional data. Also, it must be assumed that the effect is causal, which is dubious in this case and cannot generally be determined from cross-sectional data at any rate.

QUESTION 2

Based on the formula used, the alcohol attributable fraction (AAF) is the attributable fraction (among the exposed). The formula presented is predicated on the idea that the odds ratio provides a good estimate of the relative risk.

QUESTION 3

It is not easy to explain. If all current smokers could be changed to never smokers, the incidence of myocardial infarction in the population could be reduced by 35.7%. In this case, the population attributable risk is a theoretical parameter, since current smokers can become former smokers, but they cannot become "never smokers."

QUESTION 4

a. Attributable risk among the exposed: 0.14

b. Attributable fraction among the exposed: 72.5%

c. Population attributable risk: 0.07

d. Population attributable risk percent: 56.0%

e. Confounding by indication may mean that the observed effect is not causal. The effects (if any) of the drugs are probably mixed with the effects of the illnesses that they treating. If this is the case, the effects should not be attributed to the drugs and the above parameters should not have been calculated.

QUESTION 5

The population attributable risk (PAR), expressed as a percentage, is the total population incidence (25/759) minus the incidence in the nonexposed (22/730), all divided by the total population incidence and multiplied by 100.

$$PAR\% = \frac{\left(\dfrac{25}{759} - \dfrac{22}{730} \right)}{\dfrac{25}{759}} \times 100 = 8.5\%$$

QUESTION 6

This statement refers to the general population rather than an exposed population. Therefore, this is a statement of population attributable risk.

QUESTION 7

The concept of causation in epidemiology is that removal of an exposure will cause the risk of disease to diminish. A valid estimate of attributable risk is in this sense a valid statement about causation.

QUESTION 8

The absolute difference is 10%, such that the number needed to treat is 1/0.1 or 10.

QUESTION 9

The absolute risk difference is 0.017, so that the number needed to treat is 58.8.

QUESTION 10

Both parameters are based on differences and provide complementary perspective parameters that are based on relative risk.

Chapter 18

QUESTION 1

Causal judgements are always somewhat subjective, so the weight placed on specific criteria varies by context. In general, a dose-response relationship is viewed as providing supportive evidence for causation, but due to the existence of threshold and saturation effects, the lack of a biological gradient does not usually provide evidence against causality.

QUESTION 2

Questions of causation cannot usually be settled by a single study and usually require accessing the broader literature. A case in point is the criterion of consistency, which requires examining the results of different studies.

QUESTION 3

They argued that all of the associations between diet and coronary heart disease investigated in this literature were biologically plausible, and therefore that this criterion was satisfied by default. They argued that analogy was too subjective to be useful. They also noted that most risk factors for coronary heart disease were inevitably nonspecific, so this criterion was not very meaningful to them.

QUESTION 4

a. Hill argues that important risk factors may not seem plausible when first reported in epidemiological studies. Epidemiological studies sometimes drive biological research and should therefore not be subordinated to it.

b. The counter argument is that temporality is the most important criterion, because it alone is a logical requirement for causation. In his discussion, Hill describes several situations in which extremely strong associations led to decisive conclusions—for example, the observation that mortality from cancer of the scrotum occurred 200 times more often in chimney sweeps. Such observations are indeed compelling, but they are not encountered very often in modern epidemiology.

QUESTION 5

This is a profound statement about the way in which causality is conceptualized in epidemiology. The word *links* refers to the concept of a causal chain. The opportunistic and pragmatic perspective adopted by epidemiologists is highlighted by optimism that disrupting key associations along causal chains are often sufficient to make a positive impact on population health.

QUESTION 6

The authors are drawing upon the concept of biological gradient for causal judgement. When an exposure causes a disease, it is often the case that higher levels of that exposure will be associated with a more marked increase in disease risk than lower levels of exposure. Here, the highest level of exposure shows a weaker association. As with all causal criteria, this criterion is imperfect. Exposures associated with saturation or threshold effects mean that important causal factors do not always produce a biological gradient.

QUESTION 7

1. Establish the existence of an outbreak.
2. Confirm the diagnosis.
3. Establish a case definition and count cases.
4. Relate outbreak to time, place, and person.
5. Determine who is at risk of becoming ill.
6. Formulate a tentative hypothesis.
7. Compare the hypothesis with the established facts.
8. Plan a detailed epidemiologic investigation.
9. Prepare a written report.
10. Implement control and prevention measures.

QUESTION 8

This would be a bad idea. The use of these sets of criteria as if they were algorithms would be risky. The intention of these criteria is merely to focus the reader's attention on a set of topics that should be considered in the process of formulating causal judgements.

QUESTION 9

a. There are 2 paths: ED and EAZBD.
b. ED is a causal path, but in EAZBD the arrows do not all point in the same direction. There is a collider variable, so this path is naturally blocked.
c. Since the noncausal path is blocked, an estimate of the exposure-disease relationship is valid without making any adjustments, under this causal model.

d. Adjusting for Z would open up the noncausal path and would cause collider bias. This is not a good idea because under this causal model the adjustment is unnecessary. However, adjustment for A or B (or both) would remove the collider bias by blocking the noncausal path.

QUESTION 10

The answer is the temporal relationship between exposure and disease. This can rarely be fully discerned from cross-sectional data.

Chapter 19

QUESTION 1

a. Ecological studies: the ecological fallacy.

b. Cross-sectional studies: their (usual) inability to clarify temporal effects.

c. Randomized controlled trials: external validity. These studies typically apply multiple inclusion and exclusion criteria, and often unfold in an idealized environment, which can draw their external validity into question.

d. Prospective cohort studies: selection bias, which can be introduced through attrition from the study cohort.

e. Case-control studies: misclassification and selection bias.

QUESTION 2

It is difficult to argue that there can be external validity of an estimate that is invalid. If an estimate is wrong, it has no value in the population in which it was estimated. It is not conceivable that such as estimate could be usefully exported to an external population. During the process of critical appraisal, this means that the issue of external validity (generalizability) doesn't need discussion if a determination has already been made that a study lacks internal validity. This is not the only situation in which the issue of validity takes precedence over other issues during critical appraisal. Confidence intervals are not very meaningful when the associated estimate is invalid, nor is it very meaningful to ask whether an invalid estimate of an association represents a causal effect.

QUESTION 3

The best answer to this question is "it depends." These 2 provinces are far apart geographically, and the demographic features and culture of their populations also have differences. However, there are also similarities. If the differences between the provinces are not relevant to the association under consideration, an estimate could be generalized. If differences between these populations could alter the disease-exposure association, it would be unwise to generalize such estimates. External validity always needs to be considered on a case-by-case basis.

QUESTION 4

a. This is a problem. In epidemiology, adjustment for effect modifiers as if they were confounding variables is considered inappropriate. When there is effect measure modification, there is a different strength of association depending on the presence of the effect-modifying variable. Any type of adjusted estimate that pools across those strata produces a meaningless average of the differing associations. In stratified analysis, the heterogeneity or homogeneity of stratum-specific effects are readily apparent, but there is often a lack of clarity on this issue in model-based analyses, which is worrisome when it occurs.

b. The idea that significant variables should be retained in models is widespread, but it is not entirely central to the process of reasoning in epidemiological analysis. In epidemiology, the clearest justification for making an adjustment is that the variable in question acts as a confounder. In other words, the intent is to estimate the effect of an exposure, and the effect of that exposure is mixed with the effect of another variable, making adjustment necessary. Confounding is detected during modelling by determining whether a measure of effect—such as an odds ratio, risk ratio, risk difference, or hazard ratio—changes when an adjustment is made for a potential confounder (assuming that it has already been determined that the variable is not an effect modifier). The detection of confounding is not based on determining whether that particular confounder is significantly associated with the outcome.

QUESTION 5

Supplementary materials could include:

- Flowcharts: these can delineate inclusions, exclusions, attrition, and missing data—all factors related to participation that can assist with assessment of selection bias.
- Detailed information about the performance of measurement instruments (such as results of internal validation studies).
- Detailed tables: print editions often can't publish detailed tables. These could include more detailed modelling output, which would allow the presentation of tests for interaction—often not reported in published studies.
- Detailed stratified analysis: published studies often only include regression models.
- Archived versions of original study protocols: they can be useful because they lay out the analysis plan for a study as it stood before the data were examined. This helps with the assessment of type I error since it clarifies which analyses were planned ahead of time and which arose during exploratory phases of the analysis. Results of the latter type are vulnerable to type I error and therefore require replication.
- Study data set: some investigators believe that the study data set itself should be published along with the study. This would allow investigators to replicate the analysis, or conduct the analysis differently, as a means of assessing the robustness of the study's conclusions.

QUESTION 6

The ecological fallacy refers to errors that can arise when a measure based on an aggregate group (e.g., a geographical area) is used as a proxy for an individual exposure. Conceivably, a social-deprivation index could be used as a proxy for deprivation experienced at the individual level, in which case the ecological fallacy would apply. However, a measure of this type may also have inherent value as a social measure and not a mere proxy for an individual exposure. For example, living in a deprived neighborhood may have negative health effects even for a person who is not deprived as an individual. To insist that aggregate measures are always vulnerable to the ecological fallacy would amount to a dismissal of the role of aggregate characteristics as determinants of health.

QUESTION 7

In epidemiology, such sweeping statements are usually too simplistic. While it is true that each study design has some characteristic vulnerabilities, these vulnerabilities are not absolute. For example, the most notorious vulnerability of cross-sectional studies is that they cannot clarify temporal relationships, and are therefore unable to support causal inference. However, there are some instances in which temporal clarity can be achieved in cross-sectional studies (e.g., in a study of the sequelae of birth traumas, or adult risks associated with a particular genotype). Similar considerations apply to questions of bias and random error. For example, a prospective study with poor measurement may be more vulnerable to misclassification bias than a study using another design but employing high-quality measurement strategies. Similarly, small sample sizes result in large risks of random error, regardless of the study design.

QUESTION 8

Prospective studies can take a long time to produce results. With unlimited funds, solutions could be found to many of the challenges of these studies, such as minimizing attrition and avoiding measurement error. In an urgent situation, however, such as an outbreak of an infectious disease, case-control and cross-sectional studies have the advantage of producing valuable knowledge much faster.

QUESTION 9

Most epidemiologists would agree that improved reporting is a positive development that will facilitate gains in knowledge provided by research. Thoughtful critical appraisal of published studies is of central importance to the science of epidemiology. Critical appraisal is compromised if studies report inadequate information. Reporting standards should help to avoid this situation. If a problem arises from the use of reporting standards, it would be an unintended consequence. For example, since many studies have unique and creative elements, it is unlikely that a checklist would be able capture all of the elements that should be reported in an individual study. All of the elements in these checklists should be reported, but doing so should not be interpreted as evidence that all important pieces of information have been reported. In other words, the limitations of checklists and guidelines must always be kept in mind. They should never be allowed to replace thoughtful analysis.

QUESTION 10

Because epidemiologic research occurs in the real world, no study is completely perfect. If perfection is demanded, each study would be discounted and the discipline could not advance. However, if flawed studies are accepted uncritically, then invalid results will lead to invalid (and potentially harmful) clinical and public-health actions. Studies should of course strive for perfection, seeking to minimize all relevant sources of error. The question is always whether the implications of study-design defects are sufficient to discount the information reported, or whether there is sufficient validity to guide actions capable of improving health.

Glossary

Adjusted estimate. An estimate of effect from which the confounding effects of an extraneous variable have been removed. Examples include stratified estimates, pooled estimates (e.g., the Mantel-Haenszel family of estimators), and estimates that have been adjusted using regression models.

Adjustment. A procedure to remove the effect of a confounding variable from an estimated parameter. Examples include direct and indirect standardization, as well as stratification or adjustments made using statistical models.

Alpha value. This is another name for the critical value used to determine when a statistical test is statistically significant.

Ambispective study. A study that includes both retrospective and prospective timing of data collection.

Analogy. A criterion employed in consideration of causation in epidemiology. It is rarely used because it is very subjective. It involves consideration of known causal pathways, and applying that information, by analogy, to a different health problem.

Analytical epidemiology. A branch of epidemiology that evaluates hypotheses, usually about disease etiology.

Annual prevalence. A type of period prevalence in which the prevalence period is 1 year. This is the proportion (or count) of a population that has the disease at any time during the preceding year.

Attack rate. An incidence proportion usually calculated during an outbreak or epidemic, in which the risk interval for the incidence proportion consists of the duration of the outbreak or epidemic.

Attributable burden. The amount of disease burden in a population that can be attributed to a risk factor. This is similar to attributable risk, except that a measure of burden, such as a disability-adjusted life-year (DALY), is used rather than a measure of risk.

Attributable risk. The estimated amount (expressed either as a difference in incidence or as a percentage) by which the occurrence of disease could be reduced by removing a risk factor from an exposed population or completely ameliorating its effects.

Attrition. This term usually applies to prospective studies, where it refers to loss of participants to a study (i.e., "drop outs").

Avoidable premature mortality. Deaths occurring before the age 75 due to causes of death that are either preventable or treatable. Avoidable premature mortality is a Canadian Institute of Health (CIHI) health indicators. Statistics Canada produces updated annual estimates of this parameter, expressed both as a mortality rate and potential years of life lost (PYLL).

Beneficence. An ethical principle that research should do good. Research should benefit people.

ß probability. The probability of making a type II error.

Bias. This term has many meanings in epidemiology. For example, judgement can be biased and testing procedures can also be biased. However, the most important meaning of this term in epidemiology relates to errors that studies make in their estimation of epidemiologic parameters. In this sense, bias is a systematic (as opposed to random) error in the estimation of a parameter that results from a defect in study design.

Biological gradient. A criterion that may be considered when weighing causal judgements. A biological gradient is a situation in which increasing levels of exposure lead to a stronger exposure-disease association. This is sometimes also called a dose-response relationship.

Biological plausibility. A criterion employed in consideration of causation in epidemiology. It refers to whether an association makes sense in view of biological data.

Blinding. Procedures to ensure that investigators and participants are unaware of treatment assignment (allocation) in a study or trial. If both investigators and participants are unaware of allocation, the study is double blind. If only the participants are unaware, the study is single blind.

Blocked path. In a directed acyclic graph, a path connecting exposure to disease that is blocked. It may be naturally blocked by a collider variable or due to conditioning (e.g., by adjustment in a regression model, stratification, or restriction) on a variable along the path.

Canadian Institute of Health Information (CIHI). An institute that "provides comparable and actionable data and information that are used to accelerate improvements in health care, health system performance and population health across Canada" (see cihi.ca).

CANSIM. A historical name for Statistics Canada's socioeconomic database. The name is an acronym for the Canadian Socioeconomic Information Management System. The CANSIM database is not limited to health. It comprises many categories of data. Statistics Canada no longer uses CANSIM, but you may find CANSIM tables, or references to CANSIM tables, among archived materials on the Statistics Canada web site.

CANUE. The Canadian Urban Environmental Health Research Consortium, which seeks to better understand the health impact of environments, especially urban environments. An important activity of CANUE is to produce data sets for environmental characteristics that can be shared or linked to other data sources.

Cardinal data. A term that is sometimes used to describe data consisting of quantities that can be counted (e.g., the number of people in a city).

Case-cohort study. A study, often considered a variant of the case-control design, in which the source population for the referent group includes a subset of all individuals in the population from which the cases derived, not just those without the disease.

Causal path. See *directed path.*

Census. The enumeration, or counting, of all persons in a town, city, or country.

Channelling bias. Bias that may occur in nonrandomized studies of treatment efficacy. Clinicians may preferentially prescribe specific treatments based on their perceptions of prognosis. This may result in treatment being channelled to patients who are more or less likely to have positive outcomes. This is a form of confounding since the effect of treatment is intermixed with that of various prognostic factors.

Cholera. An infectious disease caused by the bacterium *Vibrio cholerae.* Symptoms include severe diarrhea, which can lead to dehydration and death.

Clustering. A phenomenon that arises when samples are selected in multiple stages—for example, when households are selected within neighbourhoods. Clustering can produce an underestimation of the variability in the sample (i.e., confidence intervals that are too narrow) unless appropriate analysis methods are used to address it.

CNODES. The Canadian Network for Observational Drug Effect Studies

Coherence. This is a criterion employed in consideration of causation in epidemiology. It refers to whether an epidemiological observation is consistent with existing knowledge and theory.

Cohort effect. Variation in health outcomes that are associated with year of birth.

Collider variable. A variable caused by 2 or more other variables, such that, in a directed acyclic graph (DAG), the arrowheads appear to collide on the node representing the collider variable. This is a term used in the literature about causal diagrams.

Comma-delimited data file. A data file containing values for variables in columns. The values associated with different variables are separated by commas. This is sometimes called a comma-separated values (CSV) data file.

Comparative clinical trial. A trial whose referent group is a standard treatment rather than a placebo or sham treatment.

Complementary probabilities. Two outcomes are said to be complementary if 1 or the other must occur. For example, if the probability of dying in a particular context is 0.25, then the probability of not dying must be 1 minus this probability, or 0.75.

Component cause. An exposure that causes a disease through its participation in causal mechanisms that typically include combinations of causes. Such combinations, together, comprise a causal mechanism.

Concurrent validity. A type of criterion validity in which the criterion is measured at the same time as the test or classification procedure is performed. Sensitivity and specificity are examples of concurrent validity in which the criterion is a gold standard.

Conditioning. In descriptions of causal models such as directed acyclic graphs (DAGs), conditioning on a variable (represented as a node in the causal diagram) means adjusting for it in a regression model, stratification, or restriction.

Confidence interval (CI). An interval quantifying the degree of precision of an estimated epidemiologic parameter. A confidence interval provides a range of plausible parameters for a population parameter at a given level of confidence. Most commonly, a 95% level of confidence is used in the calculation.

Confidence limit. The number at the lower end of the range of a confidence interval (the lower limit) or at the upper end of the range (the upper limit).

Confounding. The intermixing (within a measure of association) of an effect of interest and the effect of an independent causal factor.

Confounding by indication. A special type of confounding that is a source of concern in the pharmacoepidemiology literature. Since drugs are prescribed for specific reasons (known as indications), the effects of the drug may be intermixed with the effects of the indication for its treatment.

Confusion matrix. An increasingly popular term that describes the contingency table of a classification procedure. It cross tabulates true status by classified status. With binary classification, this produces 4 cells containing true positives, false positives, true negatives, and false negatives.

Consistency. This is a criterion employed in consideration of causation in epidemiology. It refers to the consistency with which an association has been reported in different studies conducted in different populations.

Continuous data. Variables can be measured on a continuous scale if the variable can assume any value within an interval. This term applies to numerical data.

Convenience sample. Any approach to sampling that is not linked to probability through knowledge of selection probabilities in a defined target population. Such samples are decidedly inferior to probability samples.

Coroner. An official involved in confirmation and certification of causes of death. Coroners also conduct investigations into causes of death.

Correlation coefficient. The most common measure of association seen in ecological studies. There are several types, but they all seek to quantify the extent of linear relationship between 2 variables. They assume values between −1 (representing a perfect negative correlation) and +1 (representing a perfect positive correlation). A value of 0 means no correlation. Most approaches (e.g., Pearson product moment coefficient, Spearman rank correlation) are based on pairs of observations, but the intraclass correlation coefficient (ICC) is based on groups of observations.

Correlational study. See *ecological study*.

Counterfactual. A statement that is contrary to fact. For example, epidemiologists may be interested in the outcomes that would have occurred in an exposed group had they not been exposed, which is counterfactual since they were exposed.

COVID-19. A disease caused by the SARS-CoV-2 virus, declared a pandemic by the World Health Organization in March 2020.

Criterion validity. Assessment of validity of a measure based on how well it agrees with a criterion. Ideally, this criterion should be a gold standard, but such a standard is not always available.

Critical appraisal. Reading a study critically, with a view to identifying defects that could lead to inaccurate results.

Critical value. A cutpoint against which to judge whether an observed set of data is sufficiently unlikely to allow a null hypothesis to be rejected. This is sometimes called an *alpha value*, and is often set at 5%, or 0.05.

Cross-product term. A term formed by multiplying 2 variables together. Such terms are useful in regression modelling because they provide an assessment of statistical interaction between those variables. This contributes to the assessment of effect measure modification, which must precede assessment and control of confounding in epidemiological analyses.

Cross-sectional study. A study in which all data are collected at a single point in time.

Crude parameter. A parameter that is not stratified (or otherwise adjusted) for the occurrence of other factors such as confounding variables. The term *crude* can be used for proportions (e.g., crude prevalence) or for measures of association (e.g., crude odds ratio).

Cumulative incidence. The incidence proportion expressed in terms of an accumulation of cases in an at-risk population over time.

Death certificate. A form that provides official certification of death and records important information related to death.

Deaths due to treatable causes. Deaths that could have been averted by secondary or tertiary prevention. Premature deaths due to treatable causes are 1 of 2 components of the "avoidable premature mortality" indicator of the Canadian Institute for Health Information (CIHI).

Denominator. In a ratio (which is 1 number divided by another), the denominator is the number in the bottom of the fraction.

Dependent variable: A variable that depends on other factors. Since the term has its roots in laboratory science, whereas epidemiology is mostly an observational science, terms like *disease* or *disease outcome* or *health-related outcomes* are often used to describe the dependent variables in epidemiology.

Deprivation. A concept that reflects disadvantage of a person or group in accessing material or social resources.

Descriptive epidemiology. The study of the burden and distribution of diseases in populations. Describing these aspects of disease is essential for policy and planning purposes. Descriptive studies do not evaluate hypotheses about disease etiology, but sometimes generate such hypotheses.

Design effects. Complexities in the design of a study (usually this term is used when describing a survey that uses a complex sampling procedure) that must be accounted for in the way that the study data are analyzed.

Determinant. An exposure that determines the epidemiology of a disease, but not necessarily through a causal effect. Determinants can, for example, be exposures that alter mortality or prognosis, and therefore alter the connection between incidence and prevalence.

Deterministic record linkage. A procedure for linking 2 data sets using a single variable that uniquely identifies the same individual in the 2 data sets.

Diagnostic odds ratio. An odds ratio reflecting the association of disease and test status. This is a simple parameter reflecting diagnostic test accuracy.

Differential misclassification bias. Systematic error that occurs due to misclassification of exposure or disease in a way that differs depending on exposure status (in classification of disease) or disease status (in classification of exposure). An example of such bias is recall bias in case-control studies.

Direct standardization. A procedure for increasing the comparability of 2 potentially confounded parameters by weighting them both by the same standardizing population. The weights are the proportion of the standardizing population within each stratum defined by the potential confounding variable (most commonly age and sex). Directly standardized rates are not real entities and have no meaning in themselves: their purpose is to facilitate comparisons between different populations.

Directed acyclic graph (DAG). This is a type of diagram that uses a set of formal rules and specifies a causal model.

Directed path. A path on a causal graph, such as a directed acyclic graph (DAG), in which the arrows connecting a series of nodes all point in the same direction. The path always enters the arrow by the tail and leaves by the head. A directed path may also be called a causal path.

Disability-adjusted life-year (DALY). A composite measure of disease burden composed of years lived with disability due to a disease (weighted by the extent of disability or health loss associated with the disease) and years of life lost.

Discrete data. Data that consist of a countable number of possible values.

Dynamic cohort. A cohort in which study participants are added or removed at different times.

Ecological fallacy. A methodological concern for studies assessing associations at the ecological (aggregate) level. The fallacy is assuming that an association at the aggregate level must also exist at the individual level.

Ecological study. An observational study design that assesses an association at an aggregate level, such as average exposure rates or incidence rates measured at the level of regions, provinces, or countries.

Effect size. This term has different meanings in different disciplines. It is sometimes used to refer to a standardized measure of a treatment effect, but in epidemiology it usually refers to the strength of association of a health outcome with a risk factor.

Effectiveness. Unlike *efficacy*, which refers to the effect of a treatment under ideal conditions (as typically created in randomized controlled trials), *effectiveness* refers to the effect of a treatment in real-world conditions. Effectiveness is assessed by pragmatic clinical trials.

Efficacy. As distinguished from *effectiveness* (effect of a treatment in real-world conditions), *efficacy* refers to the effect of treatment under ideal conditions.

Endemic disease. A disease that is maintained in a population at a relatively stable level, or steady state. Changes in the prevalence of endemic diseases, since they occur slowly, tend to be viewed as long-term trends, rather than as epidemics.

Epidemic. The occurrence of cases of disease in excess of what would normally be expected. Deciding what is expected may involve consideration of the history of the afflicted community, the geographical area in which it occurs or, sometimes, the season.

Epidemiology. The study of the distribution and determinants of disease in human populations. There are many variants of this definition. Veterinary epidemiology is closely related to human epidemiology, so *human* is often omitted. Also, some definitions refer to the study of the distribution and determinants of disease frequency, to emphasize that epidemiological research focuses on populations rather than individual people.

EQUATOR network: A centralized network of reporting standards for studies—for example, the PRISMA and RECORD statements. These are typically reported in the form of a statement and a checklist to ensure and document compliance with the standard.

Equipoise. An ethical requirement for randomized controlled trials. It means there is neither enough evidence for or against a treatment to preclude its use as an intervention in research.

Extraneous variable. A variable whose effects fall outside of the exposure-disease association of primary interest.

Face validity. The concept of whether "on its face" a measure seems to be assessing what it is intended to measure.

False-negative rate (or proportion). The complement of sensitivity: the frequency with which people who have a disease are classified as not having it.

False-positive rate (or proportion). The complement of specificity: the frequency with which disease-free individuals are classified as having a disease.

Fatal discontinuity. An abrupt change in mortality rates due to a major event such as an epidemic, or a natural or man-made disaster.

Finite population correction factor. A statistical adjustment made to address issues that can arise when a study sample is a large proportion of a population.

Fixed cohort. A cohort in which all members begin their participation at a single point in time.

Fixed-effects meta-analysis. An approach to meta-analysis in which parameters are considered fixed (not subject to random variation) such that all of the estimates in a literature are estimating this same fixed parameter. See also *random effects meta-analysis.*

Frequency weight. A type of sampling weight in which the value of the weight depicts the number of people in the general population represented by a survey participant.

Funnel plot. A scatterplot frequently seen in reports of meta-analyses. Each point on the scatterplot represents 1 study. Precision (e.g., standard error, width of confidence intervals) is plotted against each study's estimate of effect (e.g., a risk difference, mean difference, odds ratio, etc.). An asymmetrical scatterplot suggests publication bias.

Gold standard. A test or classification procedure that does not make errors.

Hawthorne effect. Effect that occurs because study participants are aware of being observed. This effect tends to improve outcomes in study participants.

Hazard ratio. A measure of association based on time-to-event data in survival analysis.

Health-adjusted life expectancy (HALE). An alternative approach to estimating disease burden. HALE is calculated in a way that resembles the estimation of life expectancy, but it accounts for years lived in a state of less-than-full health.

Healthy worker effect. The tendency of working people to be healthier, on average, than nonworking people. This creates an expectation that a standardized mortality ratio (SMR) calculated from an occupational cohort should be less than 1.

Heterogeneity. This term describes a situation in which estimates differ from each other to a greater extent than can be accounted for by chance. In stratified analysis, heterogeneity often indicates effect modification. In meta-analysis, heterogeneity means that the results from different studies differ by some reason other than chance (e.g., due to features of their study designs).

Homogeneity. Estimates are homogeneous if they can be viewed as estimates of the same underlying effect—in other words, if they differ only by an amount that can be attributed to sampling variability. If homogeneity is observed across stratum-specific estimates, then there is a justification for pooling the estimates. If it is observed across studies in a meta-analysis, then there is also justification for pooling the estimates.

Imputation. A set of strategies for dealing with missing data by replacing the missing values with a substitute value. The preferred approach to imputation is called *multiple imputation.*

Incidence. The new occurrence of disease in those at risk of the disease. Incidence can be measured as a proportion, an odds, or an incidence rate. An incidence proportion is the proportion of an at-risk group that develops the disease in a defined risk interval. The incidence odds are the same thing, but quantified as an odds rather than a proportion. The incidence rate is an instantaneous rate of change in disease status within those at risk. Like all rates, the incidence rate has associated units, expressed in time^{-1} units, also called person-time units.

Incidence density sampling. This is a procedure for selecting cases for case-control studies. Each case is selected from a risk set that includes all members of a population at risk of disease at the specific time when an incident case develops the disease.

Incidence proportion. See *incidence.*

Incidence proportion ratio. A highly descriptive, but rarely used, term for a parameter consisting of a ratio of 2 incidence proportions. Also sometimes called a *cumulative incidence ratio, risk ratio,* or *relative risk.*

Incidence rate. See *incidence.*

Incubation period. The period of time between exposure to an infectious agent and the emergence of an infectious disease.

Independent variable. A variable that isn't changed by the value of other variables. This term is widely used in laboratory research, where the values of independent variables are fixed or determined by the investigator under tightly controlled conditions. Such conditions don't fit well with an observational science such as epidemiology, so epidemiology uses exposure instead.

Indirect evidence. A term used in the field of evidence synthesis as the opposite of direct evidence, which involves comparisons of exposed and nonexposed groups. Indirect evidence relies on exposure groups having common comparators. Network meta-analysis is an evidence-synthesis technique capable of estimating effects from indirect evidence.

Indirect standardization. An approach to standardization often encountered in the occupational health literature. The age and sex distribution of an occupational cohort, along with age- and sex-specific rates or frequencies from a standardizing population, is used to calculate an expected number of deaths (or cases), which is then compared to the observed number of deaths in a standardized mortality (or morbidity) ratio (SMR).

Individual matching. Matching multiple controls to each case in a study, which is different from pair matching. In pair matching, a study (usually a case-control study) seeks to match each case with a single control who has similar characteristics—in other words, pair matching involves pairs.

Individual person data meta-analysis. Most meta-analyses pool study results from a systematic review of literature. When data from the individual studies are available, an individual person data meta-analysis can be used to pool the results.

Induction period. The period of time between exposure to a risk factor and the establishment of a disease process. In the causal pie (or sufficient-component cause) model of etiology, the induction period is a period of time when exposure to other component causes is occurring. When a set of component causes forms a complete causal mechanism, disease onset occurs.

Infant mortality rate. The number of infant deaths (the death of a child under 1 year of age) divided by the number of live births in the same year.

Inference. The process of gaining information about a population by studying a sample drawn from that population.

Interaction. A situation in which the effects of 1 variable depend on the level of the another variable. Tests for interaction in statistical models are a way to detect effect measure modification.

International Classification of Disease. The international standard for classification of diseases and other health problems on death certificates and other administrative health records.

Interval data. A type of numerical data in which differences are meaningful.

Interventional study. A study in which investigators assign an exposure to study participants, for example, through a random process (randomization).

Inverse probability of attrition weights (IPAWs). Weights designed to reduce bias caused by attrition from a study. IPAWS are for use in weighted analysis.

I^2 (I-squared value). A statistic used in meta-analysis to quantify the amount of heterogeneity in a set of study estimates. It reflects the percent of variability in a set of study estimates that is due to heterogeneity rather than chance variation.

Justice. An ethical principle stating (in the context of epidemiological research) that groups that endure the risks and harms of research should stand to benefit from the research.

Kappa coefficient. A coefficient used to quantify agreement between 2 ratings (e.g., in the assessment of interrater or test-rest reliability) that are categorical.

Late fetal deaths. A baby born with no signs of life but of 28 or more weeks gestation. In Canada, this typically excludes such births when they are of unknown gestational age.

Law of large numbers. A law of probability indicating that when an experiment is repeated many times, the result gets closer and closer to an expected value.

Life expectancy. A construct consisting of a projection of the average age that a member of a hypothetical birth cohort (in the case of life expectancy at birth) can be expected to live. Life expectancy can be calculated at other ages, too (e.g., life expectancy at age 65).

Lifetime prevalence. A type of period prevalence in which the prevalence period is a person's life up to the point of sampling or measurement. Note that lifetime prevalence is **not** the proportion of people who will ever get the disease during their lifetime (which is a rarely seen parameter called *lifetime morbidity risk*).

Likelihood ratio. An alternative strategy for interpreting the results of a diagnostic test. This parameter allows posttest odds to be calculated from pretest odds using simple multiplication.

Listwise deletion. A procedure for dealing with missing data. Observations with missing data elements are deleted from the list of study participants. See also *pairwise deletion.*

Live birth. A product of conception that, subsequent to birth, shows any signs of life such as breathing or movement.

Living systematic review. A type of systematic review that is constantly updated, synthesizing new evidence as it become available.

Mantel-Haenszel estimators. A family of estimators that play a critical role in stratified analysis because they allow the pooling of stratum-specific estimates into a single, more precise, estimate of effect. This adjusts for confounding that arises from the variable on which the estimates were stratified.

Mantel-Haenszel test for homogeneity. A statistical test used in stratified analysis to determine whether 2 or more stratum-specific estimates differ from each other to a greater extent than could be explained by chance. The test provides a way of evaluating effect measure modification in stratified analysis.

Marginal sum. The sum of the values in the rows or columns in a contingency table.

Masking. See *blinding.*

Matching. Application of restriction rules to a referent group (e.g., controls in a case-control study or nonexposed participants in a prospective cohort study) to ensure that the distribution of a confounder, or confounders, is equal in the index (e.g., cases in a case-control study or exposed participants in a prospective cohort study) and referent groups, thereby controlling confounding. Study participants can be individually matched (as in pair matching), or frequency matched to ensure that groups being compared have the same frequency of exposure to potentially confounding variables.

Material deprivation. Disadvantage in access to material resources, including basic resources such as food and heating, and also important services such as transportation. The concept can be applied to individuals or to defined groups or areas. Food insecurity is an example of severe material deprivation.

Maternal death. Defined by the WHO as "the death of a woman while pregnant or within 42 days of termination of pregnancy, irrespective of the duration and site of the pregnancy, from any cause related to or aggravated by the pregnancy or its management but not from accidental or incidental causes."

Maternal mortality ratio. The ratio of maternal deaths to live births.

Mean. A measure of the central tendency of a variable. It is calculated as the sum of values of the variable divided by the number of observations.

Median. The midpoint in a range of values taken by a variable. Half the observed values are greater than the median and half are less.

Medical examiner's office. This term is used in some Canadian jurisdictions in lieu of the term *coroner's office*.

Mendelian randomization. A study design that uses genetic variants, such as single nucleotide polymorphisms or genetic risk scores that have a known function, to study exposure-disease associations. The goal is to make stronger causal inference than would normally be possible from observational studies.

Meta-analysis. A set of statistical techniques for combining a set of estimates into a single estimate. The goal is to increase precision.

Misclassification bias. Systematic error in the estimation of a parameter that is due to a study-design defect involving the classification of subjects into disease and exposure groups. In analytic studies, such bias can be differential or nondifferential.

Modelling. Statistical procedures used most often (in epidemiology) to produce estimates of the effect of an exposure that are unconfounded by the causal effects of other independent risk factors.

Modifiable determinant. A determinant of disease that can be changed, usually through public health action.

Morbidity. The diminishment from a healthy state caused by having a disease.

Mortality. Death. The rate of death in a population is the mortality rate. An unadjusted mortality rate is a crude mortality rate.

Mortality rate. The number of deaths divided by person-time at risk of death.

NACRS. The National Ambulatory Care Reporting System. This is a source of Canadian administrative data describing emergency room presentations, some outpatient clinic visits, and day surgeries.

Narrative synthesis. A review of evidence in a literature that uses narrative (words) rather than statistical approaches to synthesize available information.

Necessary cause. A component cause that is a member of all causal mechanisms for a disease.

Negative predictive value. The probability that a disease is not present given a negative diagnostic test or a negative result on another type of classification procedure.

Neonatal mortality rate. Neonatal deaths occur in the first month of life. The neonatal mortality rate is expressed as a proportion of neonatal deaths among live births.

Nested case-control study. A case-control study nested within a prospective cohort study.

Net survival. Another term for the relative survival proportion, usually calculated over a 5-year period.

Network meta-analysis. A set of methods used to understand the relative effects of multiple exposures (usually treatments) even when each exposure has not been directly compared to the others.

Nominal data. A type of nonnumerical data in which quantities can be named but not ordered.

Nondifferential misclassification bias. Systematic error from misclassification that does not differ across the categories on the other axis of the classic 2 × 2 contingency table. For example, misclassification of exposure that does not depend on disease status is nondifferential.

Nonmaleficence. An ethical principle that states that research should not do harm.

Nonmodifiable determinant. A determinant of disease that cannot be changed. Such variables are usually treated as extraneous variables in epidemiological studies because, although they do not generally identify opportunities for prevention, they can confound or modify associations between modifiable risk factors and disease outcomes.

Normal distribution. A symmetrical bell-shaped distribution that arises often in nature and in statistical theory.

Number needed to harm. The expected number of people who would need to receive an exposure for 1 extra person to be harmed by it.

Number needed to treat. The expected number of people who would need to receive a treatment for 1 extra person to be successfully treated.

Numerator. In a ratio (which is 1 number divided by another), the numerator is the number in the top of a fraction, and the denominator is the number in the bottom.

Numerical data. A type of data in which numbers are meaningful. This is distinguished from nominal or ordinal data.

Observational study. A study in which investigators do not assign exposure, as distinct from an interventional study (in which they do).

Observed survival proportion. This is the proportion of those with cancer who are alive after a specified period (usually 5 years). This parameter could be calculated for any condition, but the terminology is mostly used in the cancer literature.

Odds. A ratio in which the contents of the numerator are not counted in the denominator. For example, in a group of 10 people where 1 has a disease, you could say that the odds of disease are 1/9, which is equivalent to saying that the proportion with the disease is 1/10.

Odds ratio. A measure of association that is based on dividing the odds of disease in exposed study participants by the odds of disease in nonexposed study participants. Alternatively, the odds of exposure in diseased study participants could be divided by the odds of exposure in nondiseased study participants. This is the basic measure of association in case-control studies, but is widely used in other types of studies as well.

Omitted variable bias. The distortion of a study's estimates when there is failure to control for the effects of 1 or more confounding variables.

1-tailed test. A statistical test for deviation from the null hypothesis in a single, pre-specified direction.

Open science. A movement that encourages greater access to scientific data, results, and manuscripts. This movement has the ultimate goal of increasing the benefits of publicly funded research.

Ordinal data. A type of nonnumerical data in which quantities can be placed in a meaningful order.

Outbreak. The occurrence of cases of a (usually) infectious disease in excess of expectation.

Overadjustment. Adjustment for variables that mediate the effect of exposure on disease, usually by including them in a regression model. This will cause bias towards the null hypothesis.

P-hacking. The use of unscrupulous methods to produce "significant" *P* values—a misleading and unethical practice in research.

Pairwise comparison. A statistical comparison of 2 groups—for example, an exposed and unexposed group, or a group receiving active treatment and a group receiving placebo.

Pairwise deletion. An approach to the handling of missing data. Observations from individuals that are missing the specific data elements involved in a particular comparison are deleted, but data from comparisons that use other data elements are still used. The idea is to minimize the data loss that occurs with list-wise deletion.

Pampalon index. An index that for measuring social and material deprivation that can be calculated using Canadian census data for small geographical areas. It provides an area-base measure of deprivation.

Pandemic. An epidemic that crosses international boundaries.

Parameter. A characteristic that defines an epidemiological feature or relationship, such as prevalence or relative risk. A parameter is similar to a variable because it can take on different values, but it typically connects 1 or more variables. For example, an odds ratio connects information about exposure and disease variables into a single parameter.

Percent positive. See *positivity rate.*

Perinatal death. The death of a child under 1 week of age (0 to 6 days) or a stillbirth of 28 or more weeks gestation. The death of a child under 1 week of age is called an early neonatal death.

Perinatal mortality rate. The rate of occurrence of perinatal deaths (see above) during a year, usually expressed per 1000 births (where births include both live births and late fetal deaths) in that year.

Period prevalence. The prevalence (usually a proportion, but sometimes a count) of disease in a period of time. The numerator includes people with the disease at any time during the prevalence period. The most common type of period prevalence is annual prevalence.

Pharmacoepidemiology. The study of the use of drugs using epidemiologic methods and in real-world populations. These studies examine the beneficial and adverse effects of drugs in populations, and other topics such as frequency or appropriateness of drug use.

Phase 1 trials. Preliminary studies of a new treatment, most often a drug. These studies use small samples of health volunteers and often low dosages in order to gain preliminary evidence about safety.

Phase 2 trials. Testing of a new treatment on research participants with the condition targeted by the treatment. These studies are uncontrolled and seek to provide preliminary information on dosages, efficacy, and safety.

Phase 3 trials. Randomized controlled trials designed to provide decisive evidence about efficacy or effectiveness of a treatment.

Phase 4 trials. Studies (usually observational) that seek to quantify the performance of a treatment after its regulatory approval, when the treatment is being used in real-world practice. See also *pharmacoepidemiology*.

Physical distancing. Limiting close contact with others to control the outbreak of an infectious disease. Examples of measures include maintaining distance from others, avoiding crowds, limiting social interactions, and staying home when sick.

PICO. A framework to assist with stating a research question clearly. PICO stands for **p**atient/problem/population, **i**ntervention (or exposure), **c**omparison/control/comparator, and **o**utcome.

Placebo effect. Improvements that are due to experiences associated with receiving care rather than the specific actions of a treatment.

Point estimate. A single estimate of a parameter calculated directly from the available data.

Point prevalence. Prevalence of a disease at a point in time.

Population attributable risk. The extent to which the risk of disease could be diminished in an entire population by either removing a risk factor completely or completely ameliorating its effects.

Positive predictive value. The probability of disease given a positive diagnostic test or a positive result on another type of classification procedure.

Positivity rate. The percentage of diagnostic tests that are positive. Generally, this is interpreted as a rough indicator of the degree of prevalence. In the COVID-19 pandemic, increases in the positivity rate in various locations were interpreted as evidence of increasing community spread or, alternatively, undertesting.

Postal code conversion file (PCCF). A file that allows linkage between Canada Post Corporation's 6-character postal code and geographical areas for which census data are available. This is very useful for purposes of data integration.

Postcensal estimate. Estimates that use data from the most-current census to produce population estimates for the noncensus years that follow. The census is performed in Canada once every 5 years, but population estimates are needed for all years.

Postneonatal mortality rate. The proportion of infants who die 28 to 364 days after birth.

Potential outcome. A counterfactual scenario related to an exposure-disease outcome. The potential outcome is the outcome that would have occurred in an exposed cohort had they not been exposed, or the outcome that would have occurred in a nonexposed group had they been exposed.

Power calculation. A calculation that determines the power of an analysis to reject a null hypothesis, given parameters such as the sample size and an effect size.

Pragmatic clinical trial. A randomized trial that seeks to evaluate a treatment in a real-world population and under conditions realistic to clinical practice. Such trials can reap the benefits of randomization while minimizing the limitations in generalizability that often characterize randomized controlled trials. Pragmatic clinical trials evaluate effectiveness rather than efficacy.

Precision. The extent to which a study is free of vulnerability to random error. In epidemiology, precision is often quantified as the width of 95% CIs. Wide intervals indicate imprecision and narrow intervals indicate high precision.

Precision health. An emerging approach to health care that uses detailed information about individual people (e.g., their genes, their lifestyle characteristics) to personalize their health care. Epidemiologists are prominent in the field of precision health due to their understanding of the determinants of health and their expertise with statistical methods.

Preclinical phase. A phase in the development of a disease in which the disease process is established but the disease is not yet causing symptoms or signs that would make it clinically apparent. If the disease is detectable during this preclinical phase by using a screening test, then it may be possible to intervene earlier than would be possible in clinical practice through screening (secondary prevention).

Predictive validity. A type of criterion validity in which the criterion is a future event. The test or classification procedure predicts an event that it should predict if it is valid.

Preferred Reporting Items for Systematic Reviews and Meta-Analyses. See *PRISMA*.

Pregnancy-related death. A death within 42 days of termination of a pregnancy, regardless of the cause of death. This is a simplified alternative to defining a maternal death, for use in situations in which the cause of death is unknown or of uncertain accuracy.

Premature mortality. In Canada, deaths occurring before age 75.

Prevalence. There are 2 main types of prevalence. Point prevalence is the number or proportion of a population with a disease at a point in time. Period prevalence is the number or proportion of a population having a disease at any point during a defined interval of time—for example, annual prevalence is the number or proportion of a population having the disease at any point during a 1-year period.

Prevalence difference. A parameter quantifying the strength of association between an exposure and the prevalence of disease. It is calculated as the prevalence in exposed subjects minus the prevalence in nonexposed subjects.

Prevalence ratio. A parameter quantifying the strength of association between an exposure and the prevalence of disease. It is calculated as the prevalence in exposed subjects divided by the prevalence in nonexposed subjects.

Prevalences. The plural of prevalence. Use this term to avoid "prevalence rates," which is a misnomer since prevalence is a proportion, not a rate (see *rate*).

Preventable premature mortality. Deaths before age 75 that could have been avoided by primary preventive measures.

Preventive fraction. The proportion or percentage of disease that could be prevented in a population through exposure to a protective factor (such as a preventive intervention).

Primal prevention. See *primordial prevention*.

Primary prevention. Prevention of the incidence of disease. Primary prevention intervenes at the level of risk-factor (or component-cause) exposures and thereby reduces the occurrence of disease.

Primordial prevention. An approach to prevention that focuses on social and environmental conditions within which risk factors emerge. This approach to prevention involves changing these conditions by addressing the social determinants of health.

PRISMA. The most widely used reporting standard for systematic reviews. The acronym stands for **p**referred **r**eporting **i**tems for **s**ystematic **r**eviews and **m**eta-**a**nalyses.

Probabilistic record linkage. A procedure for linking 2 data sets by identifying individual records that have a high probability of being from the same person. This approach uses several variables, none of which on its own could act as unique individual identifier.

Probability sample. A form of random sample in which the probability of any member of the population being selected into a sample is known.

Propensity adjustments. Analyses (which may be based on matching, regression adjustment, or weighting) that use propensity scores to emulate a counterfactual referent group. This is compared to the exposed group to support causal judgements from observational data.

Propensity score. A predictive probability of exposure. Such scores are used in propensity adjustments to support causal inference from observational data.

Proportion. A proportion is a special type of ratio, in which the contents of the numerator are contained in the denominator. Descriptive epidemiology makes use of proportions a lot. For example, prevalence is usually expressed as a proportion and incidence can be expressed as a proportion.

Proportional mortality ratio. This ratio is calculated as the number of deaths due to a particular cause divided by the total number of deaths during an interval of time.

Protocol registration. A strategy to protect the integrity of an analysis, and increase readers' confidence in the results of a study, by publishing the study protocol, including an analysis plan, in advance of conducting the data analysis.

Proxy measure. A way of measuring an exposure that cannot itself be directly measured. A proxy measure uses a variable that is sufficiently correlated with the target of measurement that it can substitute for the target. This substitute variable is measured in place of the target.

Public Health Agency of Canada. Usually known as PHAC. A federal government agency with a mission to promote and protect the health of Canadians through leadership, partnership, innovation, and action in public health.

Publication bias. A type of bias that occurs in a literature when certain types of studies (e.g., those with more positive results) are more likely to be published, producing a distortion of the available evidence.

PulseNet Canada. An electronic network that links databases in public-health laboratories in Canada for purposes of surveillance of foodborne disease.

Qualitative Research. An approach to research that seeks to understand concepts, opinions, or experiences using specialized methods for collection and analysis of nonnumerical data.

Quality of life. According to the WHO, "an individual's perception of their position in life in the context of the culture and value system in which they live and in relation to their goals, expectations, standards and concerns."[91]

Quantitative research. Research methods that involve the collection and analysis of numerical data.

Quasi-experiment. An intervention study in which the exposure is not assigned randomly.

Random-effects meta-analysis. An approach to the pooling of study results that accounts for differences between the pooled studies (heterogeneity) by representing the pooled value as a distribution of possible values rather than a single fixed value (as in a fixed-effects model).

Random error. Error introduced into an estimate as a result of sampling variability. Increasing the sample size of a study reduces its vulnerability to random error.

Random sample. A sample in which the selection of subjects is not predictable: it follows no rules (is random). Note this term is distinct from *random allocation* (as in a randomized trial).

Randomization. A procedure used in some interventional studies by which a random (unpredictable) procedure is used to assign exposure to a subset of study participants.

Randomized controlled trial. An interventional variant of the prospective cohort design in which the exposure is assigned randomly to study participants. Such studies can use random assignment to active treatment versus placebo, or to active treatment versus a standard treatment (as in a comparative trial).

Rate. In mathematics, a ratio of 2 related quantities in different units. In epidemiology, this term is most properly used to quantify the amount of disease occurrence or the amount of mortality in a population at risk, where this is quantified as the number of new events per person-time unit of observation. The numerator is a count and the denominator is in person-time units. Unfortunately, many parameters that are not actually rates are often called rates in epidemiology, leading to terms such as "prevalence rate" and "attack rate."

Recall bias. A type of bias that arises from recall errors. Recall bias due to misclassification of exposure in case-control studies is a type of differential misclassification bias.

RECORD. A reporting standard for studies using routinely collected health data. In Canada, these are widely used to guide the reporting of studies based on administrative data sources. Part of the EQUATOR network.

Record linkage. The process of combining 2 data sources that contain the same individuals, so that data in each source can be connected to the same unique individuals.

Regression to the mean. If an observation is more extreme at its first observation (e.g., people being more often recruited into studies when they are more troubled by symptoms of an illness that has a variable course over time), it will tend to be closer to its average value over subsequent observations.

Relative survival proportion. The ratio of survival in a group with a particular cancer to that of a comparable group free of the cancer. While relative survival proportions could be calculated for many conditions, this parameter has the highest profile in cancer research. It is recommended over the observed survival proportion by the Canadian Cancer Society.

Replicate bootstrap weights. A set of (usually) 500 to 1000 sampling weights that have been developed using a bootstrap procedure. A large set of such weights can be used to offset design features of a survey, such as clustering and unequal selection probabilities.

Reportable disease. A disease that laboratories and health professionals are required, according to provincial legislation, to report to specified public-health authorities. The goal is to facilitate surveillance and expeditious action to prevent the spread of these diseases.

Residual confounding. A distortion in an estimate, due to confounding, that has persisted despite the use of a procedure to prevent or control confounding.

Respect for persons principle. An ethical principle stating that people's autonomy must be respected. Potential participants decide, without coercion, whether to participate in a research study based on a thorough understanding of what participation would involve.

Restriction. A procedure to control confounding. Participants are selected such that they are always or never exposed to a confounder, eliminating the possibility that any effects of that confounder would be intermixed in parameters intended to reflect the causal impact of an exposure.

Retrospective. Looking back in time, into the past.

Retrospective cohort study. A cohort study having a forward logical direction but a backward (looking into the past) temporal direction.

Risk factor. An exposure that causes a disease.

Risk indicator. An exposure that is associated with a higher risk of disease, but is not necessarily the cause of that elevated risk.

Risk set sampling. An approach to the selection of controls in case-control studies, often seen in nested case-control studies. In this approach, 1 or more controls is selected from the risk set (those at risk of disease) at the point in time when a case occurs.

Sample. A subset of a population. In epidemiology, this usually means a group of people sampled from a population.

Sample-size calculations. Calculations that determine the required sample size to achieve desired statistical power in the testing of a hypothesis or a desired level of precision in an estimate.

Sampling distribution. The distribution of values of an estimated parameter that is, or would be, observed when the parameter is calculated from a large number of samples drawn from a population.

Sampling frame. A list of population elements that serves as the basis for the selection of a sample.

Sampling weight. A weight used to offset unequal selection probabilities in survey research, allowing more valid estimates to be produced.

Sampling with replacement. An approach to sampling in which a sampled individual is returned to the population and remains eligible to be sampled again.

Sampling without replacement. An approach to sampling in which a sampled individual is not eligible to be sampled again.

Scatterplot. A type of graphic that can display information about 2 variables. Data are presented as points on a 2-dimensional surface with 1 variable determining the position of the point on the y-axis and the other variable determining the position of the point on the x-axis. An example of a scatterplot is a funnel plot, often used in meta-analysis.

Screening. In its strictest sense, screening means the detection of latent disease (in a detectable preclinical stage), facilitating better outcomes through earlier intervention. Increasingly, the term is being used to describe any attempt to routinely or selectively assess any type of nonobvious health condition.

Secondary attack rate. The proportion of a population at risk that develops a disease from exposure to a primary case—for example, the proportion of household residents who become infected after a household member develops an infectious disease.

Secondary prevention. This term is synonymous with the less formal term, *screening*. It describes efforts to achieve better outcomes by earlier detection (in the latency phase) and earlier treatment of diseases.

Selection bias. A form of systematic error that results from study-design defects involving participation, or nonparticipation, in a study.

Self-isolation. Isolating oneself after exposure to an active case of an infection or when one has symptoms that may indicate an infection. This is a means to slow the spread of infectious diseases.

Sensitivity. The expected proportion of positive tests (or positive results on another type of classification procedure) among people who actually have the condition being tested for.

Sentinel indicators. Health statistics that reflect factors relevant to the health of entire populations, even if, on the surface, the statistics are based on a single age range. The classic examples are perinatal and infant mortality rates.

Simple random sample. A sample in which each individual in the population has the same probability of selection.

Social deprivation. A concept of disadvantage that can apply to individuals, groups, or geographical areas. The deprivation involves disconnection from society, which can occur in many ways.

Social determinants of health. Social and environmental conditions that determine health outcomes.

Source population. The population from which a study sample is drawn. Ideally, a source population should be directly representative of the population to which inference is directed (see *target population*). Otherwise, issues of generalizability arise.

Specific mortality rate. A rate calculated after stratification for a characteristic. Common examples include age- or sex-specific mortality rates.

Specificity. The expected proportion of negative tests (or negative results on another type of classification procedure) among those who actually do not have the condition being tested for.

Standard error. The standard deviation of the sampling distribution of a parameter, such as prevalence or an incidence proportion. It represents the amount of variability in estimates of such a parameter.

Standardized incidence ratio. This is the same as a standardized mortality ratio (see below), except that it is a standardization of incidence rather than mortality. This is most often found in the cancer epidemiology literature, due to the ability of cancer registries to support estimation of incidence.

Standardized mortality (or morbidity) ratio. The ratio of observed to expected deaths (mortality) or cases of disease (morbidity) in a population.

Statistical test. A procedure for evaluating the role of chance. A statistical test conducted at the 5% level of confidence determines whether observed results, or results that are more extreme, would occur by chance more than 5% of the time given a null hypothesis of no effect.

Statistics Canada. Canada's national statistical agency. (See statcan.gc.ca.)

Stillbirth. A fetal death. In Canada, fetal deaths for which the product of conception has a birth weight of 500 grams or more, or the duration of pregnancy is 20 weeks or longer, are registered as stillbirths. Some stillbirths are also perinatal deaths. To be counted as a perinatal death, the gestation would need to be 28 or more weeks.

Stochastic error. This is another term for random error. Nonsystematic error in the estimation of study parameters. This form of error is reduced by increasing the sample size.

Stratification. A procedure to detect and control confounding. At its most basic level, it involves estimating measures of association within strata defined by a potential confounding variable.

Stratified sampling. This is a type of probability sampling, but it differs from a simple random sample. In stratified sampling, the population is divided into different strata and subjects are randomly selected from the strata using different selection probabilities.

Stratify. Dividing a sample or population into groups based on some characteristic. When the groups are defined by the presence or level of a confounding characteristic, stratification is used as a method of adjustment for the confounding.

Stratum. A layer. In epidemiology, a stratum is usually a range of values for a characteristic in a sample. The plural of *stratum* is *strata.*

Strength of association. This is a criterion employed in consideration of causation in epidemiology. Stronger associations are generally viewed as more suggestive of causal effects.

Study population. The population in a study. This term is confusing due to its use of the word *population* to describe a sample. Also, the term lacks consistent meaning in studies that use it.

Sufficient cause. In the causal pie model of etiology, a combination of component causes that produces a disease. Sometimes the term is used to refer to a single exposure that would be sufficient, in itself, to produce a disease.

Suppressor variable. A type of confounding variable. In the absence of appropriate adjustment for such a variable, the association appears smaller than it actually is. Since this is merely a type of confounding, the use of this terminology is not necessary.

Surveillance. Surveillance is a process of ongoing data collection, analysis, and communication of results (to those who need to know) for public health purposes.

Systematic review. A type of review article that uses systematic research methods to examine a literature. These systematic methods include systematic strategies for literature review, abstracting data from published papers, assessing publication bias, and others. When appropriate, systematic reviews may use meta-analytic techniques to produce pooled estimates.

Target population. A population to which inference is intended. This is the population that an epidemiologist is trying to learn about when conducting a research study.

Temporality. This is a criterion employed in consideration of causation in epidemiology. Since causes must precede effects, this criterion refers to the necessity of understanding the temporal relationship between exposure and disease before concluding that an association is causal.

Tertiary prevention. Efforts to diminish the negative impact of established diseases.

Theory. In epidemiology, a system of ideas that helps to explain the distribution and determinants of disease. Biological and psychological theories can also guide epidemiologic research.

Tri-Council Policy Statement: Ethical Conduct for Research Involving Humans. A joint statement of research ethics by Canada's 3 major research-funding councils. The statement covers ethical issues applicable to all types of research.

2-tailed test. An approach to statistical testing that does not assume deviations from the null hypothesis can go only in 1 direction.

Type I error. A statistical error that results in rejection of a null hypothesis that is true.

Type II error. A statistical error that results in failure to reject a null hypothesis that is false.

Umbrella review. A method for synthesizing the results of multiple systematic reviews. This is an increasingly popular type of study.

Under-5 mortality rate. The probability of dying by age 5. This parameter is expressed as a proportion of live births.

Unnecessary adjustment. Including variables that are neither confounders nor mediators in a regression model. With the models most often used in epidemiology, this does not cause bias but leads to a loss of precision.

Utilitarian principle. An ethical principle stating that the potential for research to harm may be allowable if offset by a suitable potential to do good. This is the idea that the potential harms of research can be weighed against the potential benefits.

Validity. This word has many different meanings in epidemiology. In every case, it refers to whether a result is accurate or correct. Where a diagnostic test is concerned, validity refers to the truthfulness of measurement. In critical appraisal, validity refers to the accuracy of an epidemiologic estimate.

Variable. A feature or factor that can assume different values.

References

1. Darwich R, Ghazawi FM, Le M, et al. Epidemiology of invasive ocular surface squamous neoplasia in Canada during 1992-2010. *Br J Ophthalmol.* 2020;104(10):1368–1372.

2. Darwich R, Ghazawi FM, Rahme E, et al. Epidemiology of ophthalmic lymphoma in Canada during 1992-2010. *Br J Ophthalmol.* 2020;104(8):1176–1180.

3. Pappaioanou M, Spencer H. "One Health" initiative and ASPH. *Public Health Rep.* 2008;123(3):261. Medline:19006965

4. Chakraborty R, Parvez S. COVID-19: an overview of the current pharmacological interventions, vaccines, and clinical trials. *Biochem Pharmacol.* 2020;180:114184. https://doi.org/10.1016/j.bcp.2020.114184.

5. Johnson S. *The ghost map.* New York: The Penguin Group; 2006.

6. London School of Hygiene and Tropical Medicine. John Snow Bicentenary. London (UK): London School of Hygiene and Tropical Medicine; 2013.

7. Koch, R. Investigations into the etiology of traumatic infective diseases [Internet]. London (UK): New Sydenham Society; 1858 [cited 2014 September 19]. Available from: http://nrs.harvard.edu/urn-3:HMS.COUNT:1149035.

8. Howard-Jones N. Robert Koch and the cholera vibrio: a centenary. *Br Med J (Clin Res Ed).* 1984;288(6414):379–381. http://dx.doi.org/10.1136/bmj.288.6414.379. Medline:6419937

9. GBD 2015 child mortality collaborators. Global, regional, national, and selected subnational levels of stillbirths, neonatal, infant, and under-5 mortality, 1980-2015: a systematic analysis for the Global Burden of Disease Study 2015. *Lancet.* 2016;388(10053):1725–1774.

10. Riley DL, Krepostman S, Stewart DE, et al. A mixed methods study of continuity of care from cardiac rehabilitation to primary care physicians. *Can J Cardiol.* 2009;25(6):e187–e192. http://dx.doi.org/10.1016/S0828-282X(09)70096-0. Medline:19536388

11. Hong KL, Babiolakis C, Zile B, et al. Canada-wide mixed methods analysis evaluating the reasons for inappropriate emergency department presentation in patients with a history of atrial fibrillation: the multicentre AF-ED trial. *BMJ open.* 2020;10(4):e033482.

12. Huang C, Wang Y, Li X, et al. Clinical features of patients infected with 2019 novel coronavirus in Wuhan, China. *Lancet.* 2020;395(10223):497–506.

13. Wang C, Horby PW, Hayden FG, et al. A novel coronavirus outbreak of global health concern. *Lancet.* 2020;395(10223):470-473.

14. Bernstein CN, Wajda A, Svenson LW, et al. The epidemiology of inflammatory bowel disease in Canada: a population-based study. *Am J Gastroenterol.* 2006;101(7):1559–1568. http://dx.doi.org/10.1111/j.1572-0241.2006.00603.x. Medline:16863561

15. Maxwell CJ, Dalby DM, Slater M, et al. The prevalence and management of current daily pain among older home care clients. *Pain.* 2008;138(1):208–216. http://dx.doi.org/10.1016/j.pain.2008.04.007. Medline:18513871

16. Tyas SL, Manfreda J, Strain LA, et al. Risk factors for Alzheimer's disease: a population-based, longitudinal study in Manitoba, Canada. *Int J Epidemiol.* 2001;30(3):590–597. http://dx.doi.org/10.1093/ije/30.3.590. Medline:11416089

17. Vigen, T. Spurious Correlations [Internet]. [Cambridge (MA)]: Tyler Vigen; [cited 2014 June 24]. Available from: http://www.tylervigen.com.

18. Doll R, Hill AB. Smoking and carcinoma of the lung; preliminary report. *Br Med J.* 1950;2(4682):739–48. http://dx.doi.org/10.1136/bmj.2.4682.739. Medline:14772469

19. Statistics Canada. Smoking, 2019 [Internet]. Ottawa (ON): Government of Canada; 2020 October 22 [cited 2020 December 6]. Available from: https://www150.statcan.gc.ca/n1/pub/82-625-x/2020001/article/00003-eng.htm.

20. Statistics Canada. Table 13-10-0112-01 Cancer incidence, by selected sites of cancer and sex, three-year average, census metropolitan areas [Internet]. Ottawa (ON): Government of Canada; [updated 2020 November 30; cited 2020 November 30]. doi: https://doi.org/10.25318/1310011201-eng.

21. Statistics Canada. Asthma, by sex, provinces and territories [Internet]. Ottawa (ON): Government of Canada; [updated 2020 December 6; cited 2020 December 6]. Available from: http://www.statcan.gc.ca/tables-tableaux/sum-som/l01/cst01/health50a-eng.htm.

22. Statistics Canada. Table 17-10-0005-01 Population estimates on July 1st, by age and sex [Internet]. Ottawa (ON): Government of Canada; [updated 2020 December 6; cited 2020 December 6]. doi: https://doi.org/10.25318/1710000501-eng.

23. Patten SB, Williams JV, Haynes L, et al. The incidence of delirium in psychiatric inpatient units. Can J Psychiatry. 1997;42(8):858–863. Medline:9356775

24. Tenenhouse A, Joseph L, Kreiger N, et al, and the CaMos Research Group. Canadian Multicentre Osteoporosis Study. Estimation of the prevalence of low bone density in Canadian women and men using a population-specific DXA reference standard: the Canadian Multicentre Osteoporosis Study (CaMos). Osteoporos Int. 2000;11(10):897–904. http://dx.doi.org/10.1007/s001980070050. Medline:11199195

25. Ebly EM, Parhad IM, Hogan DB, et al. Prevalence and types of dementia in the very old: results from the Canadian Study of Health and Aging. Neurology. 1994;44(9):1593–1600. http://dx.doi.org/10.1212/WNL.44.9.1593. Medline:7936280

26. Gravel R, Béland Y. The Canadian Community Health Survey: mental health and well-being. Can J Psychiatry. 2005;50(10):573–579. Medline:16276847

27. Patten SB, Williams JVA, Lavorato D, et al. Descriptive epidemiology of major depression in Canada in 2012. Can J Psychiatry. 2014;60(1):23–30.

28. Takeshima T, Wan Q, Zhang Y, et al. Prevalence, burden, and clinical management of migraine in China, Japan, and South Korea: a comprehensive review of the literature. J Headache Pain. 2019;20(1):111.

29. American Psychiatric Association. Diagnostic and statistical manual of mental disorders. 5th ed. Washington (DC): American Psychiatric Publishing; 2013.

30. Patten SB, Wang JL, Williams JV, et al. Descriptive epidemiology of major depression in Canada. Can J Psychiatry. 2006;51(2):84–90. Medline:16989107

31. Kessler RC, Andrews G, Mroczek D, et al. The World Health Organization Composite International Diagnostic Interview short-form (CIDI-SF). Int J Methods Psychiatr Res. 1998;7(4):171–185. http://dx.doi.org/10.1002/mpr.47.

32. Fiest KM, Dykeman J, Patten SB, et al. Depression in epilepsy: a systematic review and meta-analysis. Neurology. 2013;80(6):590–599. http://dx.doi.org/10.1212/WNL.0b013e31827b1ae0. Medline:23175727

33. Stubbs JL, Thornton AE, Sevick JM, et al. Traumatic brain injury in homeless and marginally housed individuals: a systematic review and meta-analysis. Lancet Public Health. 2020;5(1):e19-e32.

34. Streiner DL, Patten SB, Anthony JC, et al. Has 'lifetime prevalence' reached the end of its life? An examination of the concept. Int J Methods Psychiatr Res. 2009;18(4):221–8. http://dx.doi.org/10.1002/mpr.296. Medline:20052690

35. Pringsheim T, Wiltshire K, Day L, et al. The incidence and prevalence of Huntington's disease: a systematic review and meta-analysis. Mov Disord. 2012;27(9):1083–1091. http://dx.doi.org/10.1002/mds.25075. Medline:22692795

36. Bonaparte JP, Grant IA, Benstead TJ, et al. ALS incidence in Nova Scotia over a 20-year-period: a prospective study. Can J Neurol Sci. 2007;34(1):69–73. Medline:17352350

37. Wallington T, Berger L, Henry B, et al, and the SARS Investigation Team. Update: severe acute respiratory syndrome--Toronto, 2003. Can Commun Dis Rep. 2003;29(13):113–117. Medline:12861660

38. Jing QL, Liu MJ, Zhang ZB, et al. Household secondary attack rate of COVID-19 and associated determinants in Guangzhou, China: a retrospective cohort study. Lancet Infect Dis. 2020;20(10):1141–1150.

39. Wilkinson K, Chen X, Shaw S. Secondary attack rate of COVID-19 in household contacts in the Winnipeg Health Region, Canada. *Can J Pub Health*. 2020 [published online ahead of print: 2020 November 17]:1–5. doi: 10.17269/s41997-020-00451-x.

40. Gotay CC, Katzmarzyk PT, Janssen I, et al. Updating the Canadian obesity maps: an epidemic in progress. *Can J Public Health*. 2013;104(1):e64–e68. Medline:23618109

41. Belzak L, Halverson J. The opioid crisis in Canada: a national perspective. *Health Promot Chronic Dis Prev Can*. 2018;38(6):224–233.

42. GBD 2015 HIV collaborators. Estimates of global, regional, and national incidence, prevalence and mortality of HIV, 1980-2015: the Global Burden of Disease Study 2015. *Lancet HIV*. 2016;3(8): e361–e368.

43. Murray CJL, Lopez AC. *Global burden of disease and injury*. Boston: Harvard School of Public Health; 1996.

44. Murray CJ, Ezzati M, Flaxman AD, et al. GBD 2010: design, definitions, and metrics. *Lancet*. 2012;380(9859):2063–2066. http://dx.doi.org/10.1016/S0140-6736(12)61899-6. Medline:23245602

45. Barendregt JJ, Van Oortmarssen GJ, Vos T, et al. A generic model for the assessment of disease epidemiology: the computational basis of DisMod II. *Popul Health Metr*. 2003;1(1):4. http://dx.doi.org/10.1186/1478-7954-1-4. Medline:12773212

46. United Nations. *Handbook of vital statistical methods*. Series F, No 7, Studies in methods. New York: United Nations; 1955.

47. Wellcome Library. Introduction to mortality statistics in England and Wales: 17th-20th century [Internet]. London (UK): Wellcome Library; [cited 2014 July 9]. Available from: https://search.wellcomelibrary.org/iii/encore/record/C__Rb1748256?lang=eng.

48. Statistics Canada. Deaths and mortality rate, by selected grouped causes, sex and geography-Canada [Internet]. Ottawa (ON): Government of Canada; 2015 November 27 [cited 2017 July 24]. Available from: http://www.statcan.gc.ca/pub/84f0209x/2009000/tablesectlist-listetableauxsect-eng.htm.

49. Government of Ontario. *Handbook on medical certification of death: prepared for registered nurses (extended class)*. Thunder Bay (ON): Office of the Registrar, Ontario Ministry of Consumer and Business Services; 2010.

50. World Health Organization. The 11th Revision of the International Classification of Diseases (ICD-11) is due by 2018! [Internet]. Geneva (SU): World Health Organization: 2017 [cited 2017 July 24]. Available from: http://www.who.int/classifications/icd/revision/en/.

51. World Health Organization. The international classification of functioning, disability and health (ICF) [Internet]. Geneva (SU): World Health Organization; 2001 [updated 2017 January 27; cited 2017 February 15]. Available from: http://www.who.int/classifications/icf/en/.

52. Statistics Canada. Table 13-10-0394-01 Leading causes of death, total population, by age group [Internet]. Ottawa (ON): Government of Canada; [updated 2020 December 6; cited 2020 December 6]. doi: https://doi.org/10.25318/1310039401-eng.

53. Ashmore JP, Krewski D, Zielinski JM, et al. First analysis of mortality and occupational radiation exposure based on the National Dose Registry of Canada. *Am J Epidemiol*. 1998;148(6):564–574. http://dx.doi.org/10.1093/oxfordjournals.aje.a009682. Medline:9753011

54. Hwang SW. Mortality among men using homeless shelters in Toronto, Ontario. *JAMA*. 2000;283(16):2152–2157. http://dx.doi.org/10.1001/jama.283.16.2152. Medline:10791509

55. Aronson H, Tough SC. Horse-related fatalities in the Province of Alberta, 1975-1990. *Am J Forensic Med Pathol*. 1993;14(1):28–30. https://www.ncbi.nlm.nih.gov/labs/articles/8493964/. Medline:8493964

56. Boyd J, Haegeli P, Abu-Laban RB, et al. Patterns of death among avalanche fatalities: a 21-year review. *CMAJ*. 2009;180(5):507–512. Medline:19213801

57. Sinyor M, Reis C, Schaffer A. An observational study of suicide death in homeless and precariously housed people in Toronto. *Can J Psychiatry*. 2017;62(7):501–505. Medline:28525964

58. Service Nova Scotia and Municipal Relations. A handbook for physicians and medical examiners: medical certification of death and stillbirth [Internet]. Halifax (NS): Service Nova Scotia and Municipal Relations; 2002 [cited 2017 July 24]. Available from: https://www.novascotia.ca/snsmr/pdf/ans-vstat-physicians-handbook.pdf.

59. Choi BC. Perspectives on epidemiologic surveillance in the 21st century. *Chronic Dis Can.* 1998;19(4):145–151. Medline:10029510

60. Public Health Agency of Canada. Public health notices [Internet]. Ottawa: Public Health Agency of Canada; [updated 2017 July 14; cited 2017 July 24]. Available from: http://www.phac-aspc.gc.ca/phn-asp/index-eng.php.

61. Public Health Agency of Canada. Notifiable Disease Surveillance System [Internet]. Ottawa (ON): Government of Canada; 2014 March 31 [cited 2014 July 11]. Available from: http://dsol-smed.phac-aspc.gc.ca/dsol-smed/ndis/index-eng.php.

62. Bethell J, Bondy SJ, Lou WY, et al. Emergency department presentations for self-harm among Ontario youth. *Can J Public Health.* 2013;104(2):e124–e130. Medline:23618204

63. Statistics Canada. Postal code conversion file (PCCF), reference guide [Internet]. Ottawa: Government of Canada; [updated 2016 February 12; cited 2017 February 22]. Available from: http://www.statcan.gc.ca/pub/92-154-g/92-154-g2016001-eng.htm.

64. Public Health Agency of Canada. Public Health Agency of Canada Chronic Disease Infobase [Internet]. Ottawa (ON): Government of Canada; [updated 2017 January 14; cited 2017 July 24]. Available from: http://infobase.phac-aspc.gc.ca/.

65. Statistics Canada. Table 13-10-0710-01 Mortality rates by age group. (formerly CANSIM 102-0504) [Internet]. Ottawa (ON): Government of Canada; [updated 2020 November 26; cited 2020 Novmber 29]. Available from: https://doi.org/10.25318/1310071001-eng.

66. Statistics Canada. Table 13-10-0714-01 Perinatal mortality (late fetal deaths and early neonatal deaths) [Internet]. Ottawa (ON): Government of Canada; [updated 2020 December 6; cited 2020 December 6]. doi: https://doi.org/10.25318/1310071401-eng.

67. Statistics Canada. Table 13-10-0368-10 Infant mortality, by birth weight [Internet]. Ottawa (ON): Government of Canada; [updated 2020 December 9; cited 2020 December 9]. Available from: https://www150.statcan.gc.ca/t1/tbl1/en/tv.action?pid=1310036801.

68. Chen L, Xiao L, Auger N, et al. Disparities and trends in birth outcomes, perinatal and infant mortality in Aboriginal vs. non-Aboriginal populations: a population-based study in Quebec, Canada 1996–2010. *PLoS One.* 2015;10(9):e0138562. Medline:26397838

69. United Nations. Sustainable development goals [Internet]. Geneva (SU); United Nations; 2016 [cited 2017 February 15]. Available from: http://www.un.org/sustainabledevelopment/sustainable-development-goals/.

70. UN Inter-agency Group for Child Mortality Estimation. Child mortality estimates [Internet]. [place unknown]: UN Inter-agency Group for Child Mortality Estimation; [updated 2017 September 9; cited 2017 February 15]. Available from: http://www.childmortality.org/.

71. Statistics Canada. Health fact sheet: preterm live births in Canada, 2000 to 2013 [Internet]. Ottawa (ON): Government of Canada; 2016 October 26 [cited 2017 February 22]. Available from: http://www.statcan.gc.ca/pub/82-625-x/2016001/article/14675-eng.htm.

72. World Health Organization. Maternal mortality fact sheet [Internet]. Geneva (SU): WHO; 2017 [cited 2020 December 9]. Available from: https://www.who.int/news-room/fact-sheets/detail/maternal-mortality.

73. Statistics Canada. Table 13-10-0756-01 Number of maternal deaths and maternal mortality rates for selected causes [Internet]. Ottawa (ON): Government of Canada; [updated 2020 December 6; cited 2020 December 6]. doi: https://doi.org/10.25318/1310075601-eng.

74. Maskalyk J, Hoey J. SARS update. *CMAJ.* 2003;168(10):1294–5. Medline:12743077

75. Canadian Medical Association. SARS: the struggle for containment. *CMAJ.* 2003;168(10):1229, 1231. Medline:12743047

76. Abdollahi E, Champredon D, Langley JM, et al. Temporal estimates of case-fatality rate for COVID-19 outbreaks in Canada and the United States. *CMAJ.* 2020;192(25):E666–E670.

77. Canadian Cancer Society's Advisory Committee in Cancer Statistics. Canadian cancer statistics 2014. Special topic: skin cancers. Toronto (ON): Canadian Cancer Society; 2014.

78. Canadian Cancer Statistics Advisory Committee. Canadian cancer statistics 2019 [Internet]. Toronto (ON): Canadian Cancer Society; 2020 [cited 2020 December 7]. Available from: https://www.canada.ca/en/public-health/services/reports-publications/health-promotion-chronic-disease-prevention-canada-research-policy-practice/vol-39-no-8-9-2019/notice-canadian-cancer-statistics-2019.html.

79. Statistics Canada. Table 13-10-0742-01 Mortality and potential years of life lost, by selected causes of death and sex, three-year average, Canada, provinces, territories, health regions and peer groups occasional (number) [Internet]. Ottawa (ON): Government of Canada; [updated 2020 December 7; cited 2020 December 7]. doi: https://doi.org/10.25318/1310074201-eng.

80. Canadian Institute for Health Information. Indicator library: list of conditions for potentially avoidable mortality and mortality from preventable and treatable causes indicators. Ottawa (ON): Canadian Institute for Health Information; May 2018.

81. Statistics Canada. Table: 13-10-0744-01 Premature and potentially avoidable mortality, Canada, provinces and territories [Internet]. Ottawa (ON): Government of Canada; [updated 2020 November 14; cited 2020 November 14]. Available from: https://www150.statcan.gc.ca/t1/tbl1/en/tv.action?pid=1310074401.

82. Martel L, Provost M, Lebel A, et al. Methods for constructing life tables for Canada, provinces and territories [Internet]. Report 84-538-X. Ottawa: Government of Canada (Statistics Canada); 2017 July 12 [cited 2017 August 28]. Available from: http://www.statcan.gc.ca/pub/84-538-x/84-538-x2017001-eng.htm.

83. Statistics Canada. Table 13-10-0114-01 Life expectancy and other elements of the life table, Canada, all provinces except Prince Edward Island [Internet]. Ottawa (ON): Government of Canada; [updated 2020 November 30; cited 2020 November 30]. doi: https://doi.org/10.25318/1310011401-eng.

84. World Health Organization. Life expectancy data by WHO region [Internet]. Geneva (SU): World Health Organization; 2016 [cited 2017 February 15]. Available from: http://apps.who.int/gho/data/view.main.SDG2016LEXREGv?lang=en.

85. Statistics Canada. Life expectancy [Internet]. Ottawa: Government of Canada; [updated 2016 September 28; cited 2017 April 29]. Available from: http://www.statcan.gc.ca/eng/help/bb/info/life.

86. Ratnasingham S, Cairney J, Manson H, et al. The burden of mental illness and addiction in Ontario. Can J Psychiatry. 2013;58(9):529–537. Medline:24099501

87. Public Health Agency of Canada. Health-Adjusted Life Expectancy (HALE) in Canada 2012 [Internet]. Ottawa (ON): Government of Canada; [updated 2012 September 25; cited 2014 July 13]. Available from: https://www.canada.ca/en/public-health/services/publications/science-research-data/health-adjusted-life-expectancy-canada-2012-report-public-health-agency-canada.html.

88. Institute for Health Metrics and Evaluation. Mortality visualization: frequently asked questions [Internet]. Seattle: University of Washington; 2017 [cited 2017 March 29]. Available from: https://vizhub.healthdata.org/mortality/faq.

89. Statistics Canada. Prevalence of migraine in the Canadian household population [Internet]. Ottawa (ON): Government of Canada; 2014 June 18 [cited 2014 July 9]. Available from: http://www.statcan.gc.ca/daily-quotidien/140618/dq140618c-eng.pdf.

90. Ellison LF, Wilkins K. Canadian trends in cancer prevalence. Health Rep. 2012;23(1):7–16. Medline:22590801

91. World Health Organization. Measuring quality of life. Geneva (SU): World Health Organization; 1997.

92. Oemar M, Janssen B. EQ-5D-5L user guide: basic information on how to use the EQ-5D-5L instrument. Rotterdam (NL): EuroQol Group; 2013.

93. Feng Y, Bernier J, McIntosh C, et al. Validation of disability categories derived from Health Utilities Index Mark 3 scores. Health Rep. 2009;20(2):43–50. Medline:19728585

94. Horsman J, Furlong W, Feeny D, et al. The Health Utilities Index (HUI): concepts, measurement properties and applications. *Health Qual Life Outcomes.* 2003;1(1):54. http://dx.doi.org/10.1186/1477-7525-1-54. Medline:14613568

95. Marra F, Cloutier K, Oteng B, et al. Effectiveness and cost effectiveness of human papillomavirus vaccine: a systematic review. *Pharmacoeconomics.* 2009;27(2):127–147. http://dx.doi.org/10.2165/00019053-200927020-00004. Medline:19254046

96. Vos T, Flaxman AD, Naghavi M, et al. Years lived with disability (YLDs) for 1160 sequelae of 289 diseases and injuries 1990-2010: a systematic analysis for the Global Burden of Disease Study 2010. *Lancet.* 2012;380(9859):2163–2196. http://dx.doi.org/10.1016/S0140-6736(12)61729-2. Medline:23245607

97. GBD 2019 Diseases and Injuries Collaborators. Global burden of 369 diseases and injuries in 204 countries and territories, 1990–2019: a systematic analysis for the Global Burden of Disease Study 2019. *Lancet.* 2020;396(10258):1204–1222.

98. Lang JJ, Alam S, Cahill LE, et al. Global Burden of Disease Study trends for Canada from 1990 to 2016. *CMAJ.* 2018;190(44):E1296–E1304.

99. Alam S, Lang JJ, Drucker AM, et al. Assessment of the burden of diseases and injuries attributable to risk factors in Canada from 1990 to 2016: an analysis of the Global Burden of Disease Study. *CMAJ.* 2019;7(1):E140–E148.

100. Sadovnick AD, Eisen K, Ebers GC, et al. Cause of death in patients attending multiple sclerosis clinics. *Neurology.* 1991;41(8):1193–1196. http://dx.doi.org/10.1212/WNL.41.8.1193. Medline:1866003

101. Johansen HL, Wielgosz AT, Nguyen K, et al. Incidence, comorbidity, case fatality and readmission of hospitalized stroke patients in Canada. *Can J Cardiol.* 2006;22(1):65–71. http://dx.doi.org/10.1016/S0828-282X(06)70242-2. Medline:16450021

102. Neumann PJ, Cohen JT, Weinstein MC. Updating cost-effectiveness—the curious resilience of the $50,000-per-QALY threshold. *N Engl J Med.* 2014;371(9):796–797. Medline:25162885

103. Shields M. Youth smoking. *Health Rep.* 2005;16(3):53–57. Medline:15971516

104. Cochrane Canada [Internet]. London (UK): Cochrane Collaboration; 2017 [cited 2017 April 20]. Available from: http://canada.cochrane.org/.

105. Liberati A, Altman DG, Tetzlaff J, et al. The PRISMA statement for reporting systematic reviews and meta-analyses of studies that evaluate health care interventions: explanation and elaboration. *PLoS Med.* 2009;6(7):e1000100. Medline:19621070

106. Moher D, Liberati A, Tetzlaff J, et al, and the PRISMA Group. Preferred reporting items for systematic reviews and meta-analyses: the PRISMA statement. *PLoS Med.* 2009;6(7): e1000097. doi:10.1371/journal.pmed1000097.

107. Elliott JH, Synnot A, Turner T, et al. Living systematic review: 1. Introduction-the why, what, when, and how. *J Clin Epidemiol.* 2017;91:23–30.

108. Schunemann HJ, Khabsa J, Solo K, et al. Ventilation techniques and risk for transmission of coronavirus disease, including COVID-19: a living systematic review of multiple streams of evidence. *Ann Intern Med.* 2020;173(3):204–216.

109. Siemieniuk RA, Bartoszko JJ, Ge L, et al. Drug treatments for covid-19: living systematic review and network meta-analysis. *BMJ.* 2020;370:m2980.

110. Thombs BD, Bonardi O, Rice DB, et al. Curating evidence on mental health during COVID-19: a living systematic review. *J Psychosom Res.* 2020;133:110113.

111. United Nations Educational, Scientific and Cultural Organization. Open science [Internet]. Paris: UNESCO; [cited 2020-09-26]. Available from: https://en.unesco.org/science-sustainable-future/open-science.

112. Government of Canada. Open government and COVID-19 [Internet]. Ottawa (ON): Government of Canada; updated 2020 September 30 [cited 2020 October 25]. Available from: https://open.canada.ca/en/coronavirus.

113. Center for Open Science. Open science framework [Internet]. Charlottesville (VA); [cited 2020 October 25]. Available from: https://osf.io/.

114. Aromataris E, Fernandez R, Godfrey CM, et al. Summarizing systematic reviews: methodological development, conduct and reporting of an umbrella review approach. *Int J Evid Based Healthc*. 2015;13(3):132–140.

115. Veronese N, Demurtas J, Celotto S, et al. Is chocolate consumption associated with health outcomes? An umbrella review of systematic reviews and meta-analyses. *Clin Nutr*. 2019;38(3):1101–1108.

116. Richardson WS, Wilson MC, Nishikawa J, et al. The well-built clinical question: a key to evidence-based decisions. *ACP J Club*. 1995;123(3):A12–A13.

117. Johnston BC, Alonso-Coello P, Friedrich JO, et al. Do clinicians understand the size of treatment effects? A randomized survey across 8 countries. *CMAJ*. 2016;188(1):25–32. Medline:26504102

118. Thege BK, Colman I, El-guebaly N, Hodgins DC, Patten SB, Schopflocher D, Wolfe J, Wild TC. Substance-related and behavioural addiction problems: two surveys of Canadian adults. *Addict Res Theory*. 23(1), 34-42. http://hdl.handle.net/1880/50545.

119. Kessler RC, Andrews G, Colpe LJ, et al. Short screening scales to monitor population prevalences and trends in non-specific psychological distress. *Psychol Med*. 2002;32(6):959–976. http://dx.doi.org/10.1017/S0033291702006074. Medline:12214795

120. Oremus M, Oremus C, Hall GB, et al, and the ECT & Cognition Systematic Review Team. Inter-rater and test-retest reliability of quality assessments by novice student raters using the Jadad and Newcastle-Ottawa Scales. *BMJ Open*. 2012;2(4):e001368. http://dx.doi.org/10.1136/bmjopen-2012-001368. Medline:22855629

121. Kassam A, Papish A, Modgill G, et al. The development and psychometric properties of a new scale to measure mental illness related stigma by health care providers: the Opening Minds Scale for Health Care Providers (OMS-HC). *BMC Psychiatry*. 2012;12(1):62. http://dx.doi.org/10.1186/1471-244X-12-62. Medline:22694771

122. Selected abstracts presented at the annual conference of the Canadian Society of Clinical Chemists (CSCC), Ottawa, June 3–6, 2018. *Clinical Biochemistry*. 2018;61;50–71.

123. Joseph L, Gyorkos TW, Coupal L. Bayesian estimation of disease prevalence and the parameters of diagnostic tests in the absence of a gold standard. *Am J Epidemiol*. 1995;141(3):263–272. Medline:7840100

124. Davidson BL, Elliott CG, Lensing AW, and the the RD Heparin Arthroplasty Group. Low accuracy of color Doppler ultrasound in the detection of proximal leg vein thrombosis in asymptomatic high-risk patients. *Ann Intern Med*. 1992;117(9):735–738. http://dx.doi.org/10.7326/0003-4819-117-9-735. Medline:1416575

125. Oremus M, Postuma R, Griffith L, et al, and the CLSA Algorithms Validation Group. Validating chronic disease ascertainment algorithms for use in the Canadian Longitudinal Study on Aging. *Can J Aging*. 2013;32(3):232–239. http://dx.doi.org/10.1017/S0714980813000275. Medline:23924995

126. Foebel AD, Hirdes JP, Heckman GA, et al, and the ideas PNC research team. Diagnostic data for neurological conditions in interRAI assessments in home care, nursing home and mental health care settings: a validity study. *BMC Health Serv Res*. 2013;13(1):457. http://dx.doi.org/10.1186/1472-6963-13-457. Medline:24176093

127. Marrie RA, Yu BN, Leung S, et al, and the CIHR Team in the Epidemiology and Impact of Comomrbidity on Multiple Sclerosis. The utility of administrative data for surveillance of comorbidity in multiple sclerosis: a validation study. *Neuroepidemiology*. 2013;40(2):85–92. http://dx.doi.org/10.1159/000343188. Medline:23095571

128. Modgill G, Jette N, Wang JL, et al. A population-based longitudinal community study of major depression and migraine. *Headache*. 2012;52(3):422–432. Medline:22084834

129. Higgins JPT, Green S (editors). Cochrane handbook for systematic reviews of interventions [Internet]. Version 5.1.0. London (UK): Cochrane Collaboration; 2011 [cited 2017 April 19]. Available from: http://handbook.cochrane.org/chapter_8/table_8_4_a_a_common_classification_scheme_for_bias.htm.

130. Statistics Canada. Canadian Community Health Survey - Annual Component [Internet]. Ottawa (ON): Government of Canada; 2013 September 30 [cited 2017 June 24]. Available from: http://www23.statcan.gc.ca/imdb/p2SV.pl?Function=getSurvey&SDDS=3226&lang=en&db=imdb&adm=8&dis=2.

131. Wells JE, Oakley Browne MA, Scott KM, et al, and the New Zealand Mental Health Survey Research Team. Te Rau Hinengaro: the New Zealand Mental Health Survey: overview of methods and findings. *Aust N Z J Psychiatry.* 2006;40(10):835–844. http://dx.doi.org/10.1111/j.1440-1614.2006.01902.x. Medline:16959009

132. Watson EK, Firman DW, Heywood A, et al. Conducting regional health surveys using a computer-assisted telephone interviewing method. *Aust J Public Health.* 1995;19(5):508–511. http://dx.doi.org/10.1111/j.1753-6405.1995.tb00419.x. Medline:8713202

133. Potthoff RF. Telephone sampling in epidemiologic research: to reap the benefits, avoid the pitfalls. *Am J Epidemiol.* 1994;139(10):967–978. Medline:8178785

134. Patten SB, Schopflocher D. Longitudinal epidemiology of major depression as assessed by the Brief Patient Health Questionnaire (PHQ-9). *Compr Psychiatry.* 2009;50(1):26–33. http://dx.doi.org/10.1016/j.comppsych.2008.05.012. Medline:19059510

135. Kish L. *Survey sampling.* New York: John Wiley & Sons Inc; 1995:1–34.

136. Jette N, Johnston M, Pringsheim T, et al. The case for neurological registry best practice guidelines in Canada. *Can J Neurol Sci.* 2013;40(4 Suppl 2):S1–S3. Medline:23787261

137. Bladen CL, Rafferty K, Straub V, et al. The TREAT-NMD Duchenne muscular dystrophy registries: conception, design, and utilization by industry and academia. *Hum Mutat.* 2013;34(11):1449–1457. http://dx.doi.org/10.1002/humu.22390. Medline:23913485

138. Furlan JC, Fehlings MG. The National Trauma Registry as a Canadian spine trauma database: a validation study using an institutional clinical database. *Neuroepidemiology.* 2011;37(2):96–101. http://dx.doi.org/10.1159/000330835. Medline:21921642

139. McLellan BA. A Canadian national trauma registry: the time is now. *J Trauma.* 1997;42(5):763–768. http://dx.doi.org/10.1097/00005373-199705000-00001. Medline:9191652

140. Shevell M, Dagenais L, Oskoui M. The epidemiology of cerebral palsy: new perspectives from a Canadian registry. *Semin Pediatr Neurol.* 2013;20(2):60–64. http://dx.doi.org/10.1016/j.spen.2013.06.008. Medline:23948680

141. Ivan M, Schopflocher DP, Svenson LW, et al. Estimating the infection rate of West Nile Virus in Alberta [Internet]. Edmonton (AB): 2005 [cited 2017 July 26]. 51 p. Available from: https://open.alberta.ca/dataset/097e5df0-6a52-47ec-8801-528e33386716/resource/e06bc3f2-8c0b-4168-a75b-51f55ddf2463/download/WNv-Infection-Rate-Study-05.pdf.

142. CRDCN: Canadian Research Data Centre Network [Internet]. Hamilton (ON): c2000 [cited 2017 July 26]. Available from: https://crdcn.org/.

143. Statistics Canada. Microdata access portal application process [Internet]. Ottawa (ON): Government of Canada; [updated 2020 June 24; cited 2020 December 7]. Available from: https://www.statcan.gc.ca/eng/microdata/data-centres/access.

144. Canadian Institutes of Health Research; Natural Sciences and Engineering Research Council of Canada; Social Sciences and Humanities Research Council of Canada. TCPS 2—2nd edition of Tri-Council Policy Statement: Ethical Conduct for Research Involving Humans [Internet]. Ottawa (ON): Government of Canada; 2010 [cited 2014 August 31]. Available from: http://www.pre.ethics.gc.ca/eng/policy-politique/initiatives/tcps2-eptc2/Default/.

145. Velasquez JC. MK-ULTRAViolence: or, how McGill pioneered psychological torture. *McGill Daily.* 2012;102(2):8–9.

146. Mosby I. Administering colonial science: nutrition research and human biomedical experimentation in aboriginal communities and residential schools, 1942–1952. *Soc Hist.* 2013;46(91):27.

147. Panel on Research Ethics. TCPS 2: CORE—Tutorial [Internet]. Ottawa: Government of Canada; [cited 2017 May 2]. Available from: https://tcps2core.ca/welcome.

148. Statistics Canada. Canadian Community Health Survey - Mental Health and Wellbeing [Internet]. Ottawa (ON): Government of Canada; 2013 December 18 [updated 2020 January 1; cited 2020 December 9] Available from: https://www23.statcan.gc.ca/imdb/p2SV.pl?Function=getSurvey&SDDS=3226.

149. Barnabe C, Joseph L, Bélisle P, et al. Prevalence of autoimmune inflammatory myopathy in the First Nations population of Alberta, Canada. *Arthritis Care Res (Hoboken).* 2012;64(11):1715–1719. http://dx.doi.org/10.1002/acr.21743. Medline:22623451

150. Supina AL, Patten SB. Self-reported diagnoses of schizophrenia and psychotic disorders may be valuable for monitoring and surveillance. *Can J Psychiatry*. 2006;51(4):256–259. Medline:16629350

151. Statistics Canada. Table 17-10-0005-01 Population estimates on July 1st, by age and sex (formerly CANSIM 051-0001) [Internet]. Ottawa (ON): Government of Canada; [updated 2020 September 29; cited 2020 November 30]. Available from: https://doi. org/10.25318/1710000501-eng.

152. Statistics Canada. Table 17-10-0005-01 Population estimates on July 1st, by age and sex (formerly CANSIM 051-0001) [Internet]. Ottawa (ON): Government of Canada; [updated 2020 November 29; cited 2020 November 29]. Available from: https://doi. org/10.25318/1710000501-eng.

153. Statistics Canada. Population estimates on July 1st, by age and sex [Internet]. Ottawa (ON): Government of Canada; [updated 2020 September 29; cited 2020 November 30]. Available from: https://open.canada.ca/data/en/dataset/ecdee020-5919-4996-8d3d-c3df75f50ca0.

154. Statistics Canada. Table 13-10-0800-01 Deaths and mortality rate (age standardization using 2011 population), by selected grouped causes [Internet]. Ottawa (ON): Government of Canada; [updated 2020 November 29; cited 2020 November 29]. doi: https://doi. org/10.25318/1310080001-eng.

155. Government of Nunavut, Department of Executive and Intergovernmental Affairs. Nunavut population estimates by sex and single years of age, 1997 to 2020 [Internet]. Iqaluit (NU): [cited 2020 November 29]. Available from: https://www.gov.nu.ca/executive-and-intergovernmental-affairs/information/population-data.

156. Statistics Canada. Data liberation initiative [Internet]. Ottawa (ON): Government of Canada; [updated 2017 May 5; cited 2017 August 5]. Available from: http://www.statcan. gc.ca/eng/dli/dli.

157. Statistics Canada. Data liberation initiative. Participating institutions and their contacts [Internet]. Ottawa (ON): Government of Canada; [updated 2017 August 1; cited 2017 August 5]. Available from: http://www.statcan.gc.ca/eng/dli/contact.

158. Yergens DW, Dutton DJ, Patten SB. An overview of the statistical methods reported by studies using the Canadian community health survey. *BMC Med Res Methodol*. 2014;14(1):15. http://dx.doi.org/10.1186/1471-2288-14-15. Medline:24460595

159. Zablotska LB, Lane RS, Frost SE, et al. Leukemia, lymphoma and multiple myeloma mortality (1950-1999) and incidence (1969-1999) in the Eldorado uranium workers cohort. *Environ Res*. 2014;130:43–50. http://dx.doi.org/10.1016/j.envres.2014.01.002. Medline:24583244

160. Spittal PM, Hogg RS, Li K, et al. Drastic elevations in mortality among female injection drug users in a Canadian setting. *AIDS Care*. 2006;18(2):101–108. http://dx.doi. org/10.1080/09540120500159292. Medline:16338767

161. Karamanis G, Skalkidou A, Tsakonas G, et al. Cancer incidence and mortality patterns in women with anorexia nervosa. *Int J Cancer*. 2014;134(7):1751–1757. http://dx.doi. org/10.1002/ijc.28495. Medline:24114497

162. Callaghan RC, Gatley JM, Veldhuizen S, et al. Alcohol- or drug-use disorders and motor vehicle accident mortality: a retrospective cohort study. *Accid Anal Prev*. 2013;53:149–155. http://dx.doi.org/10.1016/j.aap.2013.01.008. Medline:23434842

163. Nijjar AP, Wang H, Quan H, et al. Ethnic and sex differences in the incidence of hospitalized acute myocardial infarction: British Columbia, Canada 1995-2002. *BMC Cardiovasc Disord*. 2010;10(1):38. http://dx.doi.org/10.1186/1471-2261-10-38. Medline:20723259

164. Afifi TO, MacMillan HL, Boyle M, et al. Child abuse and mental disorders in Canada. *CMAJ*. 2014;186(9):E324–E332. http://dx.doi.org/10.1503/cmaj.131792. Medline:24756625

165. Minaker LM, Bonham A, Elton-Marshall T, et al. Under the influence: examination of prevalence and correlates of alcohol and marijuana consumption in relation to youth driving and passenger behaviours in Canada. A cross-sectional study. *CMAJ Open*. 2017;5(2):E386-E394.

166. Health Canada. Summary of results for the Canadian Student Tobacco, Alcohol and Drugs Survey 2018-19 [Internet]. Ottawa (ON): Government of Canada; [updated 2019 December 23; cited 2020 November 10]. Available from: https://www.canada.ca/en/health-canada/services/canadian-student-tobacco-alcohol-drugs-survey/2018-2019-summary.html.

167. Weintraub D, Koester J, Potenza MN, et al. Impulse control disorders in Parkinson disease: a cross-sectional study of 3090 patients. Arch Neurol. 2010;67(5):589–595. http://dx.doi.org/10.1001/archneurol.2010.65. Medline:20457959

168. Riverin B, Dewailly E, Cote S, et al. Prevalence of vitamin D insufficiency and associated factors among Canadian Cree: a cross-sectional study. Can J Public Health. 2013;104(4):e291–e297. Medline:24044468

169. Glas AS, Lijmer JG, Prins MH, et al. The diagnostic odds ratio: a single indicator of test performance. J Clin Epidemiol. 2003;56(11):1129–1135. Medline:14615004

170. Hackam DG, Thiruchelvam D, Redelmeier DA. Angiotensin-converting enzyme inhibitors and aortic rupture: a population-based case-control study. Lancet. 2006;368(9536):659–665. http://dx.doi.org/10.1016/S0140-6736(06)69250-7. Medline:16920471

171. Pahwa P, Karunanayake CP, Dosman JA, et al. Multiple myeloma and exposure to pesticides: a Canadian case-control study. J Agromedicine. 2012;17(1):40–50. Medline:22191502

172. Pan SY, de Groh M, Morrison H. A case-control study of risk factors for salivary gland cancer in Canada [Internet]. J Cancer Epidemiol. 2017; Article ID 4909214. Available from: https://www.hindawi.com/journals/jce/2017/4909214/.

173. Friedenreich CM, Speidel TP, Neilson HK, et al. Case-control study of lifetime alcohol consumption and endometrial cancer risk. Cancer Causes Control. 2013;24(11):1995–2003. http://dx.doi.org/10.1007/s10552-013-0275-0. Medline:23929278

174. Rothwell DM, Bondy SJ, Williams JI. Chiropractic manipulation and stroke: a population-based case-control study. Stroke. 2001;32(5):1054–1060. http://dx.doi.org/10.1161/01.STR.32.5.1054. Medline:11340209

175. de Gage SB, Moride Y, Ducruet T, et al. Benzodiazepine use and risk of Alzheimer's disease: case-control study. BMJ. 2014;349:g5205.

176. Berkson J. Limitations of the application of fourfold table analysis to hospital data. Biometrics. 1946;2(3):47–53. Medline:21001024

177. Rothman KJ, Greenland S, Poole C, et al. Causation and causal inference. In: Rothman KJ, Greenland S, Lash TL, editors. Modern epidemiology. Philadelphia: Lippincott Williams & Wilkins; 2008. pp. 5–31.

178. Health Canada. Strong Foundation, Renewed Focus - An Overview of Canada's Federal Tobacco Control Strategy 2012-17 [Internet]. Ottawa (ON): Government of Canada; [updated 2014 January 23; cited 2014 August 4]. Available from: http://www.hc-sc.gc.ca/hc-ps/pubs/tobac-tabac/fs-sf/index-eng.php.

179. Walboomers JM, Jacobs MV, Manos MM, et al. Human papillomavirus is a necessary cause of invasive cervical cancer worldwide. J Pathol. 1999;189(1):12–19. https://www.ncbi.nlm.nih.gov/pubmed/10451482. Medline:10451482

180. Canadian Public Health Association. What are the social determinants of health? [Internet]. Ottawa (ON): Canadian Public Health Association; [cited 2020 November 4]. Available from: https://www.cpha.ca/what-are-social-determinants-health#f2.

181. Raphael D, Bryant T, Mikkonen J, et al. Social determinants of health: the Canadian facts. Oshawa (ON): Ontario Tech University Faculty of Health Sciences; and Toronto (ON): York University School of Health Policy and Management; 2020.

182. Kleinbaum DG, Morgenstern H, Kupper LL. Selection bias in epidemiologic studies. Am J Epidemiol. 1981;113(4):452–463. Medline:6971055

183. Li Q, Guan X, Wu P, et al. Early transmission dynamics in Wuhan, China, of novel coronavirus-infected pneumonia. N Engl J Med. 2020;382(13):1199–1207.

184. Friedenreich CM, Biel RK, Lau DC, et al. Case-control study of the metabolic syndrome and metabolic risk factors for endometrial cancer. Cancer Epidemiol Biomarkers Prev. 2011;20(11):2384–2395. http://dx.doi.org/10.1158/1055-9965.EPI-11-0715. Medline:21921255

185. Villeneuve PJ, Jerrett M, Brenner D, et al. A case-control study of long-term exposure to ambient volatile organic compounds and lung cancer in Toronto, Ontario, Canada. *Am J Epidemiol*. 2014;179(4):443–451. http://dx.doi.org/10.1093/aje/kwt289. Medline:24287467

186. Crighton EJ, Ragetlie R, Luo J, et al. A spatial analysis of COPD prevalence, incidence, mortality and health service use in Ontario. *Health Rep*. 2015;26(3):10-18. Medline:25785665

187. Komenda P, Yu N, Leung S, et al. Determination of the optimal case definition for the diagnosis of end-stage renal disease from administrative claims data in Manitoba, Canada. *CMAJ Open*. 2015;3(3):E264-E269.

188. Canadian Longitudinal Study on Aging/ Étude longitudinale canadienne sur le vieillissement. Canadian Longitudinal Study on Aging/ Étude longitudinale canadienne sur le vieillissement [Internet]. Hamilton (ON): Canadian Longitudinal Study on Aging/ Étude longitudinale canadienne sur le vieillissement; 2009 [cited 2014 August 5]. Available from: https://www.clsa-elcv.ca/.

189. Canadian Partnership Against Cancer/Partenariat canadien contre le cancer. Canadian Partnership for Tomorrow Project [Internet]. Toronto (ON): Canadian Partnership Against Cancer; [cited 2014 August 5]. Available from: http://www.partnershipagainstcancer.ca/about-this-site/.

190. Sanmartin C, Decady Y, Trudeau R, et al. Linking the Canadian Community Health Survey and the Canadian Mortality Database: an enhanced data source for the study of mortality. *Health Rep*. 2016;27(12):10–18.

191. Patten SB, Williams JV, Bulloch AG. Major depressive episodes and mortality in the Canadian household population. *J Affect Disord*. 2019;242:165–171.

192. Nurses' Health Study. The Nurses' Health Study [Internet]. Boston (MA): [publisher unknown]; [cited 2014 August 5]. Available from: http://www.channing.harvard.edu/nhs/.

193. Centers for Disease Control and Prevention. National Health and Nutrition Examination Survey [Internet]. Atlanta (GA): CDC; [updated 2014 July 30; cited 2014 August 5]. Available from: http://www.cdc.gov/nchs/nhanes.htm.

194. Sackett DL. Bias in analytic research. *J Chronic Dis*. 1979;32(1-2):51–63. http://dx.doi.org/10.1016/0021-9681(79)90012-2. Medline:447779

195. Weuve J, Tchetgen Tchetgen EJ, Glymour MM, et al. Accounting for bias due to selective attrition: the example of smoking and cognitive decline. *Epidemiology*. 2012;23(1):119–128. Medline:21989136

196. Sterne JA, White IR, Carlin JB, et al. Multiple imputation for missing data in epidemiological and clinical research: potential and pitfalls. *BMJ*. 2009;338:b2393.

197. Moura C, Bernatsky S, Abrahamowicz M, et al. Antidepressant use and 10-year incident fracture risk: the population-based Canadian Multicentre Osteoporosis Study (CaMoS). *Osteoporos Int*. 2014;25(5):1473–1481. http://dx.doi.org/10.1007/s00198-014-2649-x. Medline:24566587

198. Gray SL, Dublin S, Yu O, et al. Benzodiazepine use and risk of incident dementia or cognitive decline: prospective population based study. *BMJ*. 2016;352:i90. Medline:26837813

199. Patten SB, Williams JV, Lavorato D, et al. Mortality associated with major depression in a Canadian community cohort. *Can J Psychiatry*. 2011;56(11):658–666. Medline:22114920

200. Harroud A, Richards JB. Mendelian randomization in multiple sclerosis: A causal role for vitamin D and obesity? *Mult Scler*. 2018;24(1):80–85.

201. Swanson SA, Tiemeier H, Ikram MA, et al. Nature as a trialist?: Deconstructing the analogy between Mendelian randomization and randomized trials. *Epidemiology*. 2017;28(5):653–659.

202. Rothwell PM. External validity of randomised controlled trials: "to whom do the results of this trial apply?". *Lancet*. 2005;365(9453):82–93. http://dx.doi.org/10.1016/S0140-6736(04)17670-8. Medline:15639683

203. Albanes D. Beta-carotene and lung cancer: a case study. *Am J Clin Nutr*. 1999;69(6):1345S–1350S.

204. Schisterman EF, Cole SR, Platt RW. Overadjustment bias and unnecessary adjustment in epidemiologic studies. *Epidemiology*. 2009;20(4):488–495.

205. Mente A, O'Donnell M, Rangarajan S, et al. Associations of urinary sodium excretion with cardiovascular events in individuals with and without hypertension: a pooled analysis of data from four studies. *Lancet*. 2016;388(10043):465–475. Medline:27216139

206. Simera I, Moher D, Hoey J, et al. The EQUATOR Network and reporting guidelines: helping to achieve high standards in reporting health research studies. *Maturitas*. 2009;63(1):4–6. Medline:19372017

207. Demoury C, Thierry B, Richard H, et al. Residential greenness and risk of prostate cancer: a case-control study in Montreal, Canada. *Environ Int*. 2017;Jan(98):129–136. Medline:27823799

208. Vinceti M, Bonvicini F, Rothman KJ, et al. The relation between amyotrophic lateral sclerosis and inorganic selenium in drinking water: a population-based case-control study. *Environ Health*. 2010;9(1):77. http://dx.doi.org/10.1186/1476-069X-9-77. Medline:21134276

209. Stark CR, Mantel N. Effects of maternal age and birth order on the risk of mongolism and leukemia. *J Natl Cancer Inst*. 1966;37(5):687–698. Medline:4224604

210. Julious SA, Mullee MA. Confounding and Simpson's paradox. *BMJ*. 1994;309(6967):1480–1481. http://dx.doi.org/10.1136/bmj.309.6967.1480. Medline:7804052

211. MacKinnon DP, Krull JL, Lockwood CM. Equivalence of the mediation, confounding and suppression effect. *Prev Sci*. 2000;1(4):173–181. Medline:11523746

212. Greenland S, Pearl J, Robins JM. Causal diagrams for epidemiologic research. *Epidemiol*. 1999;10(1):37–48. Medline:9888278

213. Cole SR, Platt RW, Schisterman EF, et al. Illustrating bias due to conditioning on a collider. *Int J Epidemiol*. 2010;39(2):417–420. Medline:19926667

214. Tjepkema M, Wilkins R, Long A. Socio-economic inequalities in cause-specific mortality: a 16-year follow-up study. *Can J Public Health*. 2013;104(7):e472–e478. Medline:24495823

215. Cheng I, Caberto CP, Lum-Jones A, et al. Type 2 diabetes risk variants and colorectal cancer risk: the Multiethnic Cohort and PAGE studies. *Gut*. 2011;60(12):1703–1711. http://dx.doi.org/10.1136/gut.2011.237727. Medline:21602532

216. Frachon I, Etienne Y, Jobic Y, et al. Benfluorex and unexplained valvular heart disease: a case-control study. *PLoS One*. 2010;5(4):e10128. http://dx.doi.org/10.1371/journal.pone.0010128. Medline:20405030

217. Jadidi E, Mohammadi M, Moradi T. High risk of cardiovascular diseases after diagnosis of multiple sclerosis. *Mult Scler*. 2013;19(10):1336–1340. http://dx.doi.org/10.1177/1352458513475833. Medline:23364857

218. Vandenbroucke JP, Pearce N. Case-control studies: basic concepts. *Int J Epidemiol*. 2012;41(5):1480–1489.

219. Verhave JC, Tagalakis V, Suissa S, et al. The risk of thromboembolic events in kidney transplant patients. *Kidney Int*. 2014;85(6):1454–1460. http://dx.doi.org/10.1038/ki.2013.536. Medline:24429408

220. Di Bartolomeo S, Valent F, Sbrojavacca R, et al. A case-crossover study of alcohol consumption, meals and the risk of road traffic crashes. *BMC Public Health*. 2009;9(1):316. http://dx.doi.org/10.1186/1471-2458-9-316. Medline:19723319

221. Redelmeier DA, Tibshirani RJ, Evans L. Traffic-law enforcement and risk of death from motor-vehicle crashes: case-crossover study. *Lancet*. 2003;361(9376):2177–2182. http://dx.doi.org/10.1016/S0140-6736(03)13770-1. Medline:12842370

222. Suissa S, Henry D, Caetano P, et al. CNODES: the Canadian Network for Observational Drug Effect Studies. *Open Med*. 2012;6(4):e134–e140.

223. Band PR, Le ND, Fang R, et al. Cohort study of Air Canada pilots: mortality, cancer incidence, and leukemia risk. *Am J Epidemiol*. 1996;143(2):137–143. http://dx.doi.org/10.1093/oxfordjournals.aje.a008722. Medline:8546114

224. Dimich-Ward H, Lorenzi M, Teschke K, et al. Mortality and cancer incidence in a cohort of registered nurses from British Columbia, Canada. *Am J Ind Med*. 2007;50(12):892–900. http://dx.doi.org/10.1002/ajim.20505. Medline:17853402

225. Villeneuve PJ, Morrison HI. Coronary heart disease mortality among Newfoundland fluorspar miners. *Scand J Work Environ Health*. 1997;23(3):221–226. http://dx.doi.org/10.5271/sjweh.202. Medline:9243733

226. Villeneuve PJ, Lane RS, Morrison HI. Coronary heart disease mortality and radon exposure in the Newfoundland fluorspar miners' cohort, 1950-2001. *Radiat Environ Biophys*. 2007;46(3):291–296. http://dx.doi.org/10.1007/s00411-007-0108-1. Medline:17453229

227. Lipscombe LL, Austin PC, Alessi-Severini S, et al. Atypical antipsychotics and hyperglycemic emergencies: multicentre, retrospective cohort study of administrative data. *Schizophr Res*. 2014;154(1-3):54-60.

228. Schulz KF. Subverting randomization in controlled trials. *JAMA*. 1995;274(18):1456–1458. Medline:7474192

229. Wechsler ME, Kelley JM, Boyd IO, et al. Active albuterol or placebo, sham acupuncture, or no intervention in asthma. *N Engl J Med*. 2011;365(2):119–126. Medline:21751905

230. Schulz KF, Altman DG, Moher D, and the CONSORT Group. CONSORT 2010 statement: updated guidelines for reporting parallel group randomised trials. *PLoS Med*. 2010;7(3):e1000251. http://dx.doi.org/10.1371/journal.pmed.1000251. Medline:20352064

231. Darsaut TE, Findlay JM, Magro E, et al. Surgical clipping or endovascular coiling for unruptured intracranial aneurysms: a pragmatic randomised trial. *J Neurol Neurosurg Psychiatry*. 2017;88(8):663–668. Medline:28634280

232. Lam RW, Levitt AJ, Levitan RD, et al. The Can-SAD study: a randomized controlled trial of the effectiveness of light therapy and fluoxetine in patients with winter seasonal affective disorder. *Am J Psychiatry*. 2006;163(5):805–812. http://dx.doi.org/10.1176/appi.ajp.163.5.805. Medline:16648320

233. Rossouw JE, Anderson GL, Prentice RL, et al, and the Writing Group for the Women's Health Initiative Investigators. Risks and benefits of estrogen plus progestin in healthy postmenopausal women: principal results From the Women's Health Initiative randomized controlled trial. *JAMA*. 2002;288(3):321–333. http://dx.doi.org/10.1001/jama.288.3.321. Medline:12117397

234. van Lonkhuijzen L, Kirsh VA, Kreiger N, et al. Endometrial cancer and meat consumption: a case-cohort study. *Eur J Cancer Prev*. 2011;20(4):334–339. http://dx.doi.org/10.1097/CEJ.0b013e328344747c. Medline:21422932

235. Rohan TE, Soskolne CL, Carroll KK, et al. The Canadian Study of Diet, Lifestyle, and Health: design and characteristics of a new cohort study of cancer risk. *Cancer Detect Prev*. 2007;31(1):12–17.

236. Arthur RS, Kirsh VA, Rohan TE. Dietary B-vitamin intake and risk of breast, endometrial, ovarian and colorectal cancer among Canadians. *Nutr Cancer*. 2019;71(7):1067–1077.

237. WHO Mortality Database [database]. Geneva (SU): World Health Organization; [updated 2104]. Available from: http://www.who.int/healthinfo/mortality_data/en/.

238. Cheng JJ, Schuster-Wallace CJ, Watt S, et al. An ecological quantification of the relationships between water, sanitation and infant, child, and maternal mortality. *Environ Health*. 2012;11(1):4. http://dx.doi.org/10.1186/1476-069X-11-4. Medline:22280473

239. Durbin A, Lin E, Taylor L, et al. First-generation immigrants and hospital admission rates for psychosis and affective disorders: an ecological study in Ontario. *Can J Psychiatry*. 2011;56(7):418–426. Medline:21835105

240. Stieb DM, Evans GJ, To TM, et al. An ecological analysis of long-term exposure to PM2.5 and incidence of COVID-19 in Canadian health regions. *Environ Res*. 2020;191:110052.

241. Canadian Urban Environmental Health Research Consortium [homepage on the Internet]. Available from: https//:canue.ca.

242. Pampalon R, Hamel D, Gamache P, et al. A deprivation index for health planning in Canada. *Chronic Dis Can*. 2009;29(4):178–191.

243. Auger N, Zang G, Daniel M. Community-level income inequality and mortality in Québec, Canada. *Public Health*. 2009;123(6):438–443. http://dx.doi.org/10.1016/j.puhe.2009.04.012. Medline:19482322

244. Reich KM, Chang HJ, Rezaie A, et al. The incidence rate of colectomy for medically refractory ulcerative colitis has declined in parallel with increasing anti-TNF use: a time-

trend study. *Aliment Pharmacol Ther.* 2014;40(6):629–638. http://dx.doi.org/10.1111/apt.12873. Medline:25039715

245. Hanley JA. A heuristic approach to the formulas for population attributable fraction. *J Epidemiol Community Health.* 2001; 55(7):508–514. Medline:11413183

246. Freedman MS, Montalban X, Miller AE, et al. Comparing outcomes from clinical studies of oral disease-modifying therapies (dimethyl fumarate, fingolimod, and teriflunomide) in relapsing MS: assessing absolute differences using a number needed to treat analysis. *Mult Scler Relat Disord.* 2016;Nov(10):204–212. Medline:27919491

247. Slobogean BL, Jackman H, Tennant S, et al. Iatrogenic ulnar nerve injury after the surgical treatment of displaced supracondylar fractures of the humerus: number needed to harm, a systematic review. *J Pediatr Orthop.* 2010;30(5):430–436. Medline:20574258

248. Shiue I, Shiue M. Indoor temperature below 18°C accounts for 9% population attributable risk for high blood pressure in Scotland. *Int J Cardiol.* 2014;171(1):e1–e2. http://dx.doi.org/10.1016/j.ijcard.2013.11.040. Medline:24315341

249. Kuendig H, Hasselberg M, Laflamme L, et al. Acute alcohol consumption and injury: risk associations and attributable fractions for different injury mechanisms. *J Stud Alcohol Drugs.* 2008;69(2):218–226. Medline:18299762

250. Yusuf S, Hawken S, Ounpuu S, et al, and the INTERHEART Study Investigators. Effect of potentially modifiable risk factors associated with myocardial infarction in 52 countries (the INTERHEART study): case-control study. *Lancet.* 2004;364(9438):937–952. http://dx.doi.org/10.1016/S0140-6736(04)17018-9. Medline:15364185

251. Patten SB, Williams JV, Love EJ. Depressive symptoms attributable to medication exposure in a medical inpatient population. *Can J Psychiatry.* 1996;41(10):651–654. Medline:8978945

252. Arseneault L, Cannon M, Witton J, et al. Causal association between cannabis and psychosis: examination of the evidence. *Br J Psychiatry.* 2004;184(2):110–117. http://dx.doi.org/10.1192/bjp.184.2.110. Medline:14754822

253. Hill AB. The environment and disease: association or causation? *Proc R Soc Med.* 1965;58:295–300. Medline:14283879

254. Surgeon General's Advisory Committee on Smoking and Health. Smoking and health: report of the advisory committee to the surgeon general of the public health service. Washington (DC): US Public Health Service, Office of the Surgeon General; 1964.

255. Wilson JM, Jungner G, and the World Health Organization. Principles and practice of screening for disease. Geneva (SU): World Health Organization; 1968. https://apps.who.int/iris/handle/10665/37650.

256. Smith RA. Can we improve on Wilson and Jungner's principles of screening for disease? *CMAJ.* 2018;190(14):E414–E415.

257. Dobrow MJ, Hagens V, Chafe R, et al. Consolidated principles for screening based on a systematic review and consensus process. *CMAJ.* 2018;190(14):E422–E429.

258. Bosch FX, Lorincz A, Muñoz N, et al. The causal relation between human papillomavirus and cervical cancer. *J Clin Pathol.* 2002;55(4):244–265. http://dx.doi.org/10.1136/jcp.55.4.244. Medline:11919208

259. Gottlieb MS, Schroff R, Schanker HM, et al. Pneumocystis carinii pneumonia and mucosal candidiasis in previously healthy homosexual men: evidence of a new acquired cellular immunodeficiency. *N Engl J Med.* 1981;305(24):1425–1431.

260. Textor J, van der Zander B, Gilthorpe MK, et al. Robust causal inference using directed acyclic graphs: the R package 'dagitty'. *Int J Epidemiol.* 2016;45(6):1887–1894.

261. Manitoba Health, Communicable Disease Control Unit. Communicable disease management protocol manual: epidemiological investigation of outbreaks [Internet]. Winnipeg (MN): Government of Manitoba; [cited 2017 May 2]. Available from: http://www.gov.mb.ca/health/publichealth/cdc/protocol/investigation.pdf.

262. Harvey RR, Heiman Marshall KE, Burnworth L, et al. International outbreak of multiple Salmonella serotype infections linked to sprouted chia seed powder—USA and Canada, 2013–2014. *Epidemiol Infect.* 2017;145(8):1535–1544. Medline:28318456

263. VanderWeele TJ, Robins JM. The identification of synergism in the sufficient-component-cause framework. *Epidemiology.* 2007;18(3):329–339. http://dx.doi.org/10.1097/01. ede.0000260218.66432.88. Medline:17435441

264. Au B, Smith KJ, Gariépy G, Schmitz N. C-reactive protein, depressive symptoms, and risk of diabetes: results from the English Longitudinal Study of Ageing (ELSA). *J Pschosom Res.* 2014;77(3):180–186.

265. Mente A, de Koning L, Shannon HS, et al. A systematic review of the evidence supporting a causal link between dietary factors and coronary heart disease. *Arch Intern Med.* 2009;169(7):659–669. http://dx.doi.org/10.1001/archinternmed.2009.38. Medline:19364995

266. Hodgson C. What is the distribution of deaths due to cerebrovascular disease in Ontario? *CMAJ.* 1998;159(6 Suppl):s25–s31.

267. Richards JB, Papaioannou A, Adachi JD, et al, and the Canadian Multicentre Osteoporosis Study Research Group. Effect of selective serotonin reuptake inhibitors on the risk of fracture. *Arch Intern Med.* 2007;167(2):188–194. http://dx.doi.org/10.1001/archinte.167.2.188. Medline:17242321

268. Agrawal S, Ebrahim S. Association between legume intake and self-reported diabetes among adult men and women in India. *BMC Public Health.* 2013;13(1):706. http://dx.doi.org/10.1186/1471-2458-13-706. Medline:23915141

269. Cedergren MI, Källén BA. Maternal obesity and infant heart defects. *Obes Res.* 2003;11(9):1065–1071. http://dx.doi.org/10.1038/oby.2003.146. Medline:12972676

270. Petitti DB, Harlan SL, Chowell-Puente G, et al. Occupation and environmental heat-associated deaths in Maricopa county, Arizona: a case-control study. *PLoS One.* 2013;8(5):e62596. http://dx.doi.org/10.1371/journal.pone.0062596. Medline:23734174

271. Heneghan C. Clinical epidemiology for the uninitiated [Internet]. Oxford (UK): Centre for Evidence-Base Medicine; 2016 January [cited 2016 November 11]. Available from: https://www.cebm.net/wp-content/uploads/2016/01/Clinical-Epidemiology-for-the-unitiated.pdf.

272. Centre for Evidence-based Medicine. Oxford Centre for Evidence-based Medicine—levels of evidence [Internet]. Oxford: [updated 2009 March; cited 2017 May 2]. Available from: http://www.cebm.net/oxford-centre-evidence-based-medicine-levels-evidence-march-2009/.

273. O'Keefe JH, Lavie CJ. Run for your life ... at a comfortable speed and not too far. *Heart.* 2013;99(8):516–519. http://dx.doi.org/10.1136/heartjnl-2012-302886. Medline:23197444

274. O'Keefe JH, Schnohr P, Lavie CJ. The dose of running that best confers longevity. *Heart.* 2013;99(8):588–590. http://dx.doi.org/10.1136/heartjnl-2013-303683. Medline:23512971

275. Weber T. Response to 'Run for your life ... at a comfortable speed and not too far'. *Heart.* 2013;99(8):588. http://dx.doi.org/10.1136/heartjnl-2012-303556. Medline:23512970

276. Keyes KM, Utz RL, Robinson W, et al. What is a cohort effect? Comparison of three statistical methods for modeling cohort effects in obesity prevalence in the United States, 1971–2006. *Soc Sci Med.* 2010;70(7):1100–1108. Medline:20122771

277. Critical Appraisal Skills Programme [homepage on the Internet]. Available from: https://casp-uk.net.

278. Guyatt GH, Rennie D. Users' guides to the medical literature. *JAMA.* 1993;270(17):2096–2097.

279. Downs SH, Black N. The feasibility of creating a checklist for the assessment of the methodological quality both of randomised and non-randomised studies of health care interventions. *J Epidemiol Community Health.* 1998;52(6):377–384.

280. Wells GA, Shea B, O'Connell D, et al. The Newcastle-Ottawa Scale (NOS) for assessing the quality of nonrandomized studies in meta-analysis [Internet]. Ottawa (ON): Ottawa Hospital Research Institute; 2019 [cited 2020 November 2]. Available from: http://www.ohri.ca/programs/clinical_epidemiology/oxford.asp.

281. Sterne JAC, Savovic J, Page MJ, et al. RoB 2: a revised tool for assessing risk of bias in randomised trials. *BMJ.* 2019;366:l4898.

282. Evidence Partners and the Clarity Group. Methodological resources [Internet]. Ottawa (ON): Evidence Partners; [cited 2020 November 21]. Available from: https://www.evidencepartners.com/resources/methodological-resources/.

283. Joanna Briggs Institute. Critical appraisal tools [Internet]. Adelaide (AU): Joanna Briggs Institute; [cited 2020 November 22]. Available from: https://joannabriggs.org/critical-appraisal-tools.

284. Von Elm E, Altman DG, Egger M, et al. The Strengthening the Reporting of Observational Studies in Epidemiology (STROBE) statement: guidelines for reporting observational studies. *Ann Intern Med*. 2007;147(8):573–577. Medline:17938396

285. Equator Network. REporting of studies Conducted using Observational Routinely-collected Data (RECORD) [Internet]. Oxford (UK): Equator Network; [updated 2017 14 July; cited 2017 July 31]. Available from: http://www.equator-network.org/reporting-guidelines/record/.

286. Equator Network [homepage on the Internet]. Oxford (UK): Equator Network; [cited July 31, 2017]. Available from: http://www.equator-network.org/.

287. Statistics Canada. Table 13-10-0394-01 Leading causes of death, total population, by age group [Internet]. Ottawa (ON): Government of Canada; [updated 2020 November 30; cited 2020 November 30]. doi: https://doi.org/10.25318/1310039401-eng.

288. Public Health Agency of Canada. The Chief Public Health Officer's report on the state of public health in Canada 2008 [Internet]. Chapter 3: causes of death. Ottawa (ON): Government of Canada; 2008 [cited 2017 September 1]. Available from: https://www.canada.ca/en/public-health/corporate/publications/chief-public-health-officer-reports-state-public-health-canada/report-on-state-public-health-canada-2008/chapter-3d.html#2.

289. Institute for Health Metrics and Evaluation. GBD profile: Canada [Internet]. Seattle (WA): Institute for Health Metrics and Evaluation, University of Washington; 2015 [Accessed 2017-04-19]. Available from: http://www.healthdata.org/canada.

290. MacLaren VV, Best LA. Multiple addictive behaviors in young adults: student norms for the Shorter PROMIS Questionnaire. *Addict Behav*. 2010;35(3):252–255. http://dx.doi.org/10.1016/j.addbeh.2009.09.023. Medline:19879058

291. Shields M, Connor Gorber S, Janssen I, et al. Bias in self-reported estimates of obesity in Canadian health surveys: an update on correction equations for adults. *Health Rep*. 2011;2(3):35–45.

292. Ahmad OB, Boschi-Pinto C, Lopez AD, et al. Age standardization of rates: a new WHO standard [Internet]. GPE Discussion Paper Series No. 31. Geneva (SU): WHO; 2001 [cited 2017 August 5]. Available from: http://www.who.int/healthinfo/paper31.pdf.

293. Patten SB, Williams JVA, Lavorato DH, et al. Seasonal variation in major depressive episode prevalence in Canada. *Epidemiology Psychiatr Sci*. 2017;26(2):169–176. Medline:26751782

294. Thombs BD, Coyne JC, Cuijpers P, et al. Rethinking recommendations for screening for depression in primary care. *CMAJ*. 2012;184(4):413–418. http://dx.doi.org/10.1503/cmaj.111035. Medline:21930744

295. Katz J. Sodium and cardiovascular disease. *Lancet*. 2016;388(10056):2112–2113. Medline:27968748

296. Cappuccio FP. Sodium and cardiovascular disease. *Lancet*. 2016;388(10056):2112. Medline:27968749

Index